IMMUNE SYSTEM DISORDERS SOURCEBOOK

Health Reference Series

Volume Eighteen

IMMUNE SYSTEM DISORDERS SOURCEBOOK

Basic Information about Lupus, Multiple Sclerosis, Guillain-Barré Syndrome, Chronic Granulomatous Disease, and More, along with Statistical and Demographic Data and Reports on Current Research Initiatives

Edited by
Allan R. Cook

Omnigraphics, Inc.

Penobscot Building / Detroit, MI 48226

BIBLIOGRAPHIC NOTE

This volume contains individual publications issued by the National Institutes of Health (NIH), its sister agencies, and sub-agencies. Numbered publications in this category are: NIH 90-2990, 90-3015, 91-2414, 92-2261, 92-2902, 93-529, 93-2114, 93-3219, 93-3413, 94-3422, 94-3774, NIH Pub No. 1990:241-292/00003, *NIH Consensus Statement,* volume 8, number 5, May 21-23, 1990, DHHS 89-1080. The unnumbered publication is: *Chronic Granulomatous Disease: A Guide for CGD Patients and Their Families.* Also included are reprints from the following issues of the *FDA Consumer:* April 1992, July/August 1992, November 1992, and October 1995. In addition, the volume includes one copyrighted article from John C. Keesy, M.D. with the Myasthenia Gravis Foundation, ©1994; 15 articles excerpted from the Immune Deficiency Foundation's *Patient and Family Handbook for the Primary Immune Deficiency Diseases,* ©1987, 1993; 2 articles compiled from 12 pamphlets from the *Lupus Foundation of America: What is Lupus, Lupus and Infections and Immunizations, Pregnancy and Lupus, Lupus in Men, Laboratory Tests Used in the Diagnosis of Lupus, Living Well with Lupus, Joint and Muscle Pain in Lupus,* ©1995, *Anti-Malarials in the Treatment of Lupus, Steroids in the Treatment of Lupus, Lupus and Vasculitis,* ©1994, *Nonsteroidal Anti-inflammatory Drugs (NSAIDS), Imuran, Cytoxan and Related Drugs* ©1993; and one from *Scientific American,* December 1995. These documents are used by permission.

Edited by Allan R. Cook

Peter D. Dresser, Managing Editor, Health Reference Series
Karen Bellenir, Series Editor, Health Reference Series

Omnigraphics, Inc.

Matthew P. Barbour, Production Manager
Laurie Lanzen Harris, Vice President, Editorial
Peter E. Ruffner, Vice President, Administration
James A. Sellgren, Vice President, Operations and Finance
Jane J. Steele, Vice President, Research

Frederick G. Ruffner, Jr., Publisher

Copyright © 1997, Omnigraphics, Inc.

Library of Congress Cataloging-in-Publication Data

Immune system disorders sourcebook : basic information for the layperson about lupus, multiple sclerosis, Guillain-Barré syndrome, chronic granulomatous disease, and more, along with statistical and demographic data an reports on current research initiatives / edited by Allan R. Cook.
   p. cm. — (Health reference series ; 18)
   Includes bibliographical references and index.
   ISBN 0-7808-0209-8 (lib. bdg. : alk. paper)
   1. Immunologic diseases—Popular works.   I. Cook, Allan R.
II. Series.
RC582.I4626   1996   96-33469
616.07'9—dc20   CIP

∞

This book is printed on acid-free paper meeting the ANSI Z39.48 Standard. The infinity symbol that appears above indicates that the paper in this book meets that standard.

Printed in the United States of America

Table of Contents

Part III: Autoimmune Diseases and Disorders

Part IV: Neuroimmunology: Immunity and the Nervous System

Part V: Treatments and Therapies

Part VI: Manipulating the Immune System

Part VII: Socioeconomic Implications

Part VIII: Glossary of Common Medical Terms

Preface

About This Book

We live in a dangerous world, filled with potentially harmful bacteria, viruses, fungi, parasites, and both natural and man-made chemicals. Luckily, our bodies also have an ever-watchful guardian network of immune system organs and millions of specialized cells, a system easily as complex as the brain and nervous system. Identifying individual cells as either self (belonging to our bodies) or non-self (foreign), the immune system efficiently targets and destroys dangerous invaders that manage to penetrate the skin barrier. But sometimes the immune system gets it wrong; it identifies self as non-self and begins to attack the cells of its own body, or it fails to react allowing dangerous microbes to establish infections inside the body. The result is seldom fatal, more often debilitating, painful, and long-term. The National Institute of Allergy and Infectious Disease estimates that one in ten Americans is affected by some form of immunologic disorder. However, the old, the young, and minorities are the most common victims.

This book contains basic information for the layperson on the operation of the immune system, the most common ways in which it fails, details on specific forms of immunologic diseases, treatments and coping strategies, some tips on handling the question of health insurance, and an analysis of the economic implications of immune disorders. Patients, friends, family members, and the interested general

ix

public will find this volume a good place to begin to understand the complexities of immune-system reactions. However, some topics are handled in more detail in other volumes of this series: the *Diabetes Sourcebook, AIDS Sourcebook, Arthritis Sourcebook, Allergies Sourcebook,* and the *Skin Disorders Sourcebook.*

How To Use This Book

This book is divided into parts and chapters. Parts focus on broad areas of interest and chapters on specific topics within those areas.

Part I: *The Immune System* examines the mechanism of human immunity, describing the specific components and functions of the immune network. It also considers the question of inheritance and the ways in which the potential for immune disorders can be passed from parent to child. Finally, it explains the "special case" of the developing fetus within the mother's womb, and the immunologic benefits of breast feeding for both mother and baby.

Part II: *Immunodeficiency Diseases and Disorders* describes the special class of immune disorders which result in a reduced immune function. In these disorders, the immune system fails to identify an invading body as non-self, allowing it unimpeded entry. The result can be either an attack on a specific organ or site of the body or a more general invasion. This section identifies the major forms of immunodeficiency diseases, their diagnoses, treatment, and future expectations for the patient.

Part III: *Autoimmune Diseases and Disorders* describes the class of immune disorders in which the immune system incorrectly identifies self as non-self and mounts an attack on the patient's own body. The condition may affect the entire body or specific organs. This section identifies the major forms of auto-immune disorders, their diagnoses, treatment, and future expectations for the patient. One chapter examines organ-specific disorders in detail.

Part IV: *Neuroimmunology: Immunity and the Nervous System* describes the link between the nervous system and the immune system and the potential this link holds for new, more effective treatments for immune disorders. It identifies specific disorders which may now be described and investigated by the newly-developing field of psychoneuroimmunology and some of the novel therapies now being tested.

Part V: *Treatments and Therapies* describes the traditional methods and common drugs used in treating immune disorders as well as some of the newer methods.

Part VI: *Manipulating the Immune System* focuses on the ways in which researchers and physicians are using their knowledge of the immune system to treat other diseases, disorders, and disabilities. Particularly, it notes the advances in immune suppression drugs in organ transplantation and immune stimulation in the treatment of infectious diseases.

Part VII: *Socioeconomic Implications* examines the costs of immune disorders, both economic and human. It also describes the intricate nature of health insurance coverage and the particular concerns of immune disorder patients. The section ends with a glossary of medical insurance terms designed to help demystify the language of health insurance professionals.

Part VIII: *Glossary of Common Medical Terms* provides a listing and short explanation of some common medical terms used throughout this volume.

Index: gives page references and cross-references for key words and phrases used in the various articles.

Acknowledgements

The editor gratefully acknowledges the assistance of the many people who helped produce this volume and the private organizations which agreed to grant permission to reprint their articles: *Scientific American*, the Lupus Foundation of America, the Myasthenia Gravis Foundation, and the Immune Deficiency Foundation. Special thanks to Margaret Mary Missar for her patient uncovering of the documents that make up this volume, Karen Bellenir for her technical assistance and advice, and Bruce the Scanman and special assistant Mike for their electronic prestidigitation.

Note from the Editor

This book is part of Omnigraphics' *Health Reference Series*. The series provides basic information about a broad range of medical concerns. It is not intended to serve as a tool for diagnosing illness, in prescribing treatments, or as a substitute for the physician/patient relationship. All persons concerned about medical symptoms or the possibility of disease are encouraged to seek professional care from an appropriate health care provider.

Part One

The Immune System

Chapter 1

Understanding the Immune System

The Body's Automatic Defense System

The immune system is a complex network of specialized cells and organs that has evolved to defend the body against attacks by "foreign" invaders. When functioning properly it fights off infections by agents such as bacteria, viruses, fungi, and parasites. When it malfunctions, however, it can unleash a torrent of diseases, from allergy to arthritis to cancer to AIDS.

The immune system evolved because we live in a sea of microbes. Like man, these organisms are programmed to perpetuate themselves. The human body provides an ideal habitat for many of them and they try to break in; because the presence of these organisms is often harmful, the body's immune system will attempt to bar their entry or, failing that, to seek out and destroy them.

The immune system, which equals in complexity the intricacies of the brain and nervous system, displays several remarkable characteristics. It can distinguish between "self" and "nonself." It is able to remember previous experiences and react accordingly. Once you have had chicken pox, your immune system will prevent you from getting it again. The immune system displays both enormous diversity and extraordinary specificity. Not only is it able to recognize many millions of distinctive nonself molecules, it can produce molecules and cells to match up with and counteract each one of them. And it has at its command a sophisticated array of weapons.

NIH Pub No. 93-529

3

The success of this system in defending the body relies on an incredibly elaborate and dynamic regulatory-communications network. Millions and millions of cells, organized into sets and subsets, pass information back and forth like clouds of bees swarming around a hive. The result is a sensitive system of checks and balances that produces an immune response that is prompt, appropriate, effective, and self-limiting.

Self and Nonself

At the heart of the immune system is the ability to distinguish between self and nonself. Virtually every body cell carries distinctive molecules that identify it as self.

The body's immune defenses do not normally attack tissues that carry a self marker. Rather, immune cells and other body cells coexist peaceably in a state known as self-tolerance. But when immune defenders encounter cells or organisms carrying molecules that say "foreign," the immune troops move quickly to eliminate the intruders.

Any substance capable of triggering an immune response is called an antigen. An antigen can be a virus, a bacterium, a fungus, or a parasite, or even a portion or product of one of these organisms. Tissues or cells from another individual, except an identical twin whose cells carry identical self-markers, also act as antigens; because the immune system recognizes transplanted tissues as foreign, it rejects them. The body will even reject nourishing proteins unless they are first broken down by the digestive system into their primary, non-antigenic building blocks.

An antigen announces its foreignness by means of intricate and characteristic shapes called epitopes, which protrude from its surface. Most antigens, even the simplest microbes, carry several different kinds of epitopes on their surface; some may carry several hundred. However, some epitopes will be more effective than others at stimulating an immune response.

In abnormal situations, the immune system can wrongly identify self as nonself and execute a misdirected immune attack. The result can be a so-called autoimmune disease such as rheumatoid arthritis or systemic lupus erythematosus.

In some people, an apparently harmless substance such as ragweed pollen or cat hair can provoke the immune system to set off the inappropriate and harmful response known as allergy; in these cases the antigens are known as allergens.

Genes and the Markers of Self

Molecules that mark a cell as self are encoded by a group of genes that is contained in a section of a specific chromosome known as the major histocompatibility complex (MHC). The prefix "histo" means tissue; the MHC was discovered in the course of tissue transplantation experiments. Because MHC genes and the molecules they encode vary widely in the details of their structure from one individual to another (a diversity known as polymorphism), transplants are very likely to be identified as foreign by the immune system and rejected.

Scientists eventually discovered a more natural role for the MHC: it is essential to the immune defenses. MHC markers determine which antigens an individual can respond to, and how strongly. Moreover, MHC markers allow immune cells such as B cells, T cells, and macrophages to recognize and communicate with one another.

One group of proteins encoded by the genes of the MHC are the markers of self that appear on almost all body cells. Known as class I MHC antigens, these molecules alert killer T cells to the presence of body cells that have been changed for the worse—infected with a virus or transformed by cancer—and that need to be eliminated.

A second group of MHC proteins, class II antigens, are found on B cells, macrophages, and other cells responsible for presenting foreign antigen to helper T cells. Class II products combine with particles of foreign antigen in a way that showcases the antigen and captures the attention of the helper T cell.

This focusing of T cell antigen recognition through class I and class II molecules is known as MHC (or histocompatibility) restriction.

The Anatomy of the Immune System

The organs of the immune system are stationed throughout the body. They are generally referred to as *lymphoid organs* because they are concerned with the growth, development, and deployment of lymphocytes, the white cells that are the key operatives of the immune system. Lymphoid organs include the *bone marrow* and the *thymus*, as well as *lymph nodes, spleen, tonsils* and *adenoids*, the *appendix*, and clumps of lymphoid tissue in the small intestine known as *Peyer's patches*. The blood and lymphatic vessels that carry lymphocytes to and from the other structures can also be considered lymphoid organs.

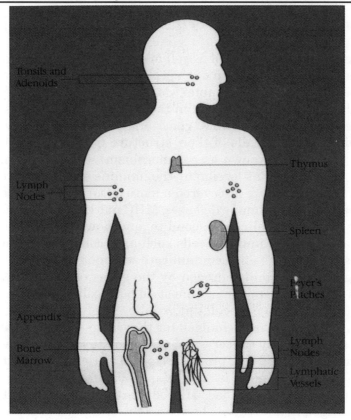

Figure 1.1. Organs of the immune system.

Cells destined to become immune cells, like all other blood cells, are produced in the bone marrow, the soft tissue in the hollow shafts of long bones. The descendants of some so-called stem cells become lymphocytes, while others develop into a second major group of immune cells typified by the large, cell-and particle-devouring white cells known as phagocytes.

The two major classes of lymphocytes are B cells and T cells. B cells complete their maturation in the bone marrow. T cells, on the other hand, migrate to the thymus, a multilobed organ that lies high behind the breastbone. There they multiply and mature into cells capable of producing an immune response—that is, they become immunocompetent. In a process referred to as T cell "education," T cells in the thymus learn to distinguish self cells from nonself cells; T cells that would react against self antigens are eliminated.

Upon exiting the bone marrow and thymus, some lymphocytes congregate in immune organs or lymph nodes. Others—both B and T cells—travel widely and continuously throughout the body. They use the blood circulation as well as a bodywide network of *lymphatic vessels* similar to blood vessels.

Laced along the lymphatic routes—with clusters in the neck armpits, abdomen, and groin—are small, bean-shaped lymph nodes. Each lymph node contains specialized compartments that house platoons of B lymphocytes, T lymphocytes, and other cells capable of enmeshing antigen and presenting it to T cells. Thus, the lymph node brings together the several components needed to spark an immune response.

The *spleen*, too, provides a meeting ground for immune defenses. A fist-sized organ at the upper left of the abdomen, the spleen contains two main types of tissue—the red pulp, where worn-out blood cells are disposed of, and the white pulp, which contains lymphoid tissue. Like the lymph nodes, the spleen's lymphoid tissue is subdivided into compartments that specialize in different kinds of immune cells. Microorganisms carried by the blood into the red pulp become trapped by the immune cells known as macrophages. (Although people can live without a spleen, persons whose spleens have been damaged by trauma or by disease such as sickle cell anemia are highly susceptible to infection; surgical removal of the spleen is especially dangerous for young children and the immunosuppressed.)

Nonencapsulated clusters of lymphoid tissue are found in many parts of the body. They are common around the mucous membranes lining the respiratory and digestive tracts—areas that serve as gateways to the body. They include the tonsils and adenoids, the appendix, and Peyer's patches.

The lymphatic vessels carry *lymph*, a clear fluid that bathes the body's tissues. Lymph, along with the many cells and particles it carries—notably lymphocytes, macrophages, and foreign antigens, drains out of tissues and seeps across the thin walls of tiny lymphatic vessels. The vessels transport the mix to lymph nodes, where antigens can be filtered out and presented to immune cells.

Additional lymphocytes reach the lymph nodes (and other immune tissues) through the bloodstream. Each node is supplied by an artery and a vein; lymphocytes enter the node by traversing the walls of very small specialized veins.

All lymphocytes exit lymph nodes in lymph via outgoing lymphatic vessels. Much as small creeks and streams empty into larger rivers, the lymphatics feed into larger and larger channels. At the base of the neck large lymphatic vessels merge into the *thoracic duct*, which empties its contents into the bloodstream.

Once in the bloodstream, the lymphocytes and other assorted immune cells are transported to tissues throughout the body. They patrol everywhere for foreign antigens, then gradually drift back into the lymphatic vessels, to begin the cycle all over again.

The Cells and Secretions of the Immune System

The immune system stockpiles a tremendous arsenal of cells. Some staff the general defenses, while others are trained on highly specific targets. To work effectively, however, most immune cells require the active cooperation of their fellows. Sometimes they communicate through direct physical contact, sometimes by releasing versatile chemical messengers.

In order to have room for enough cells to match millions of possible foreign invaders, the immune system stores just a few of each specificity. When an antigen appears, those few specifically matched cells are stimulated to multiply into a full-scale army. Later, to prevent this army from overexpanding wildly, like a cancer, powerful suppressor mechanisms come into play.

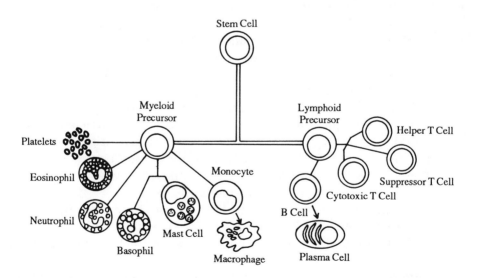

Figure 1.2. Cells of the immune system.

Lymphocytes

Lymphocytes are small white blood cells that bear the major responsibility for carrying out the activities of the immune system; they number about one trillion. The two major classes of lymphocytes are B cells, which grow to maturity independent of the thymus, and T cells, which are processed in the thymus. Both B cells and T cells recognize specific antigen targets.

B cells work chiefly by secreting soluble substances called antibodies into the body's fluids, or humors. (This is known as humoral immunity.) Antibodies typically interact with circulating antigens such as bacteria and toxic molecules, but are unable to penetrate living cells. T cells, in contrast, interact directly with their targets, attacking body cells that have been commandeered by viruses or warped by malignancy. (This is cellular immunity.)

Although small lymphocytes look identical, even under the microscope, they can be told apart by means of distinctive molecules they carry on their cell surface. Not only do such markers distinguish between B cells and T cells, they distinguish among various subsets of cells that behave differently. Every mature T cell, for instance, carries a marker known as T3 (or CD3); in addition, most helper T cells carry a T4 (CD4) marker, a molecule that recognizes class II MHC antigens. A molecule known as T8 (CD8), which recognizes class I MHC antigens, is found on many suppressor/cytotoxic T cells. In addition, different T cells have different kinds of antigen receptors—either alpha/beta or gamma/delta.

B Cells and Antibodies. Each B cell is programmed to make one specific antibody. For example, one B cell will make an antibody that blocks a virus that causes the common cold, while another produces antibody that zeros in on a bacterium that causes pneumonia.

When a B cell encounters its triggering antigen (along with collaborating T cells and accessory cells), it gives rise to many large *plasma cells*. Every plasma cell is essentially a factory for producing antibody. Each of the plasma cells descended from a given B cell (which are all members of the same family, or clone) manufactures millions of identical antibody molecules and pours them into the bloodstream.

A given *antibody* matches an antigen much as a key matches a lock. The fit varies: sometimes it is very precise, while at other times it is little better than that of a skeleton key. To some degree, however, the antibody interlocks with the antigen and thereby marks it for destruction.

9

Antibodies belong to a family of large molecules known as immunoglobulins. Immunoglobulins are proteins, made up of chains of polypeptides, strings of the basic units known as amino acids. Each antibody has two identical heavy polypeptide chains and two identical light chains, shaped to form a Y. The sections that make up the tips of the Y's arms vary greatly from one antibody to another, creating a pocket uniquely shaped to enfold a specific antigen. This is called the variable (V) region. The stem of the Y serves to link the antibody to other participants in the immune defenses. This area is identical in all antibodies of the same class, and is called the constant (C) region.

Scientists have identified nine chemically distinct classes of human immunoglobulins (Ig)—four kinds of IgG and two kinds of IgA, plus IgM, IgE, and IgD. Each type plays a different role in the immune defense strategy. IgG, the major immunoglobulin in the blood, is also able to enter tissue spaces; it works efficiently to coat microorganisms, speeding their uptake by other cells in the immune system. IgM, which usually combines in star-shaped clusters, tends to remain in the bloodstream, where it is very effective in killing bacteria. IgA concentrates in body fluids—tears, saliva, the secretions of the respiratory and gastrointestinal tracts—guarding the entrances to the body. IgE, which under normal circumstances occurs only in trace amounts, probably evolved as a defense against parasites, but it is more familiar as the villain in allergic reactions (see Allergy). IgD is almost exclusively found inserted into the membranes of B cells, where it somehow regulates the cell's activation.

Antibodies can work in several ways, depending on the nature of the antigen. Antibodies that interlock with toxins produced by certain bacteria can disable them directly (and are known as antitoxins). Other antibodies, by coating (or opsonizing) bacteria, make the microbes highly palatable to scavenger cells equipped to engulf and destroy them. More often, an antigen-antibody combination unleashes a group of lethal serum enzymes known as complement (see Complement). Yet other antibodies block viruses from entering into cells (a quality that is exploited in making vaccines). And, in a phenomenon known as antibody-dependent cell-mediated cytotoxicity (ADCC), cells coated with antibody become vulnerable to attack by several types of white blood cells.

T Cells and Lymphokines. T cells contribute to the immune defenses in two major ways. Regulatory T cells are vital to orchestrating the elaborate system. (B cells, for instance, cannot make antibody

10

against most substances without T cell help.) Cytotoxic T cells, on the other hand, directly attack body cells that are infected or malignant.

Chief among the regulatory T cells are "helper/inducer" cells. Typically identifiable by the T4 cell marker, helper T cells are essential for activating B cells and other T cells as well as natural killer cells and macrophages. Another subset of T cells acts to turn off or "suppress" these cells.

Cytotoxic T cells, which usually carry the T8 marker, are killer cells. In addition to ridding the body of cells that have been infected by viruses or transformed by cancer, they are responsible for the rejection of tissue and organ grafts. (Although suppressor/cytotoxic T cells are often called T8 cells, in reality the two are not always synonymous. The T8 molecule, like the T4 molecule, determines which MHC molecule, class I or class II, the T cell will recognize, but not how the T cell will behave.)

T cells work primarily by secreting substances known as cytokines or, more specifically, *lymphokines*. Lymphokines (which are also secreted by B cells) and their relatives, the *monokines* produced by monocytes and macrophages, are diverse and potent chemical messengers. Binding to specific receptors on target cells, lymphokines call into play many other cells and substances, including the elements of the inflammatory response. They encourage cell growth, promote cell activation, direct cellular traffic, destroy target cells, and incite macrophages. A single cytokine may have many functions; conversely, several different cytokines may be able to produce the same effect.

One of the first cytokines to be discovered was interferon. Produced by T cells and macrophages (as well as by cells outside the immune system), interferons are a family of proteins with antiviral properties. Interferon from immune cells, known as immune interferon or gamma interferon, activates macrophages. Two other cytokines, closely related to one another, are lymphotoxin (from lymphocytes) and tumor necrosis factor (from macrophages). Both kill tumor cells; tumor necrosis factor (TNF) also inhibits parasites and viruses.

Many cytokines are initially given descriptive names but, as their basic structure is identified, they are renamed as "interleukins"—messengers between leukocytes, or white cells. Interleukin-1, or IL-1, is a product of macrophages (and many other cells) that helps to activate B cells and T cells. IL-2, originally known as T cell growth factor, or TCGF, is produced by antigen-activated T cells and promotes the rapid growth or differentiation of mature T cells and B cells. IL-3 is a T-cell derived member of the family of protein mediators known as colony-stimulating factors (CSF); one of its many functions is to nurture the development of immature precursor cells into a variety of mature blood cells. IL-4, IL-5, and IL-6 help B cells grow and differentiate; IL-4 also affects T cells, macrophages, mast cells, and granulocytes.

A number of cytokines, obtained in quantity through recombinant DNA technology (see Genetic Engineering), are now being used—alone, in combination, linked to toxins—in clinical trials for patients with cancers, blood disorders, and immunodeficiency diseases (including AIDS), as well as people receiving bone marrow transplants. Their versatility, however, makes it difficult to predict the full range of their effects.

Natural Killer Cells. *Natural Killer (NK) cells* are yet another type of lethal lymphocyte. Like cytotoxic T cells, they contain granules filled with potent chemicals. They are called "natural" killers because they, unlike cytotoxic T cells, do not need to recognize a specific antigen before swinging into action. They target tumor cells and protect against a wide variety of infectious microbes. In several immunodeficiency diseases, including AIDS, natural killer cell function is abnormal. Natural killer cells may also contribute to immunoregulation by secreting high levels of influential lymphokines.

Both cytotoxic T cells and natural killer cells kill on contact. The killer binds to its target, aims its weapons, and then delivers a lethal burst of chemicals that produces holes in the target cell's membrane. Fluids seep in and leak out, and the cell bursts.

Phagocytes, Granulocytes, and Their Relatives

Phagocytes (literally, "cell eaters") are large white cells that can engulf and digest marauding microorganisms and other antigenic particles. Some phagocytes also have the ability to present antigen to lymphocytes.

Important phagocytes are *monocytes* and *macrophages*. Monocytes circulate in the blood, then migrate into tissues where they develop into macrophages ("big eaters"). Macrophages are seeded throughout body tissues in a variety of guises. Specialized macrophages include alveolar macrophages in the lungs, mesangial phagocytes in the kidneys, microglial cells in the brain, and Kupffer cells in the liver.

Macrophages are versatile cells that play many roles. As scavengers, they rid the body of worn-out cells and other debris. Foremost among the cells that "present" antigen to T cells, having first digested and processed it, macrophages play a crucial role in initiating the immune response. As secretory cells, monocytes and macrophages are vital to the regulation of immune responses and the development of inflammation: they churn out an amazing array of powerful chemical substances (monokines), including enzymes, complement proteins, and regulatory factors such as interleukin-1. At the same time, they carry receptors for lymphokines that allow them to be "activated" into single-minded pursuit of microbes and tumor cells.

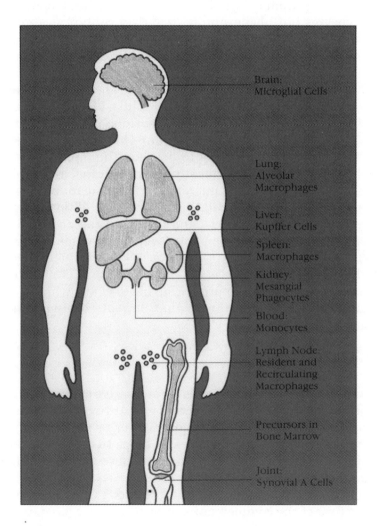

Brain:
Microglial Cells

Lung:
Alveolar
Macrophages

Liver:
Kupffer Cells

Spleen:
Macrophages

Kidney:
Mesangial
Phagocytes

Blood:
Monocytes

Lymph Node:
Resident and
Recirculating
Macrophages

Precursors in
Bone Marrow

Joint:
Synovial A Cells

Figure 1.3. Phagocytes in the body.

Macrophages are not the only cells to present antigen to lymphocytes. Other antigen-presenting cells include B cells, as noted above, and dendritic cells, irregularly shaped white blood cells found in the spleen and other lymphoid organs. Dendritic cells typically have long threadlike tentacles that enmesh lymphocytes and antigens. Langerhans cells are dendritic cells that travel about in the skin, picking up antigen and transporting it to nearby lymph nodes. Many other types of body cells, properly stimulated, can also be recruited to present antigens to lymphocytes.

Another critical phagocyte is the *neutrophil*. Neutrophils are not only phagocytes but also granulocytes: they contain granules filled with potent chemicals. These chemicals, in addition to destroying microorganisms, play a key role in acute inflammatory reactions.

Also known as polymorphonuclear leukocytes or polymorphs (because their nuclei come in "many shapes"), granulocytes include *eosinophils* and *basophils* as well as neutrophils. (The cells are named for the way they stain in the laboratory: eosinophils, for instance, have an affinity for acidic dyes such as eosin.) The phagocytic neutrophil uses its prepackaged chemicals to degrade the microbes it ingests eosinophils and basophils typically "degranulate," releasing their chemicals to work on cells or microbes in their surroundings.

The *mast cell* is a non-circulating counterpart of the basophil. Located in the lungs, skin, tongue, and linings of the nose and intestinal tract, the mast cell is responsible for the symptoms of allergy (see Allergy).

Another related structure is the *blood platelet*. Platelets, too, contain granules. In addition to promoting blood clotting and wound repair, platelets release substances that activate components of the immune system.

Complement

The complement system is made up of a series of about 25 proteins that work to "complement" the activity of antibodies in destroying bacteria, either by facilitating phagocytosis or by puncturing the bacterial cell membrane. Complement also helps to rid the body of antigen-antibody complexes. In carrying out these tasks, it induces an inflammatory response.

Complement proteins circulate in the blood in an inactive form. When the first of the complement substances is triggered, usually by antibody interlocked with an antigen, it sets in motion a ripple effect.

As each component is activated in turn, it acts upon the next in a precise sequence of carefully regulated steps known as the "complement cascade."

In the so-called "classical" pathway of complement activation, a series of proteins gives rise to a complex enzyme capable of cleaving a key protein, C3. In the "alternative" pathway, which can be triggered by suitable targets in the absence of antibody, C3 interacts with a different set of factors and enzymes. But both pathways end in the creation of a unit known as the membrane attack complex. Inserted in the wall of the target cell, the membrane attack complex constitutes a channel that allows fluids and molecules to flow in and out. The target cell rapidly swells and bursts. Meantime, various fragments flung off during the course of the cascade can produce other consequences. One byproduct causes mast cells and basophils to release their contents, producing the redness, warmth, and swelling of the inflammatory response. Another stimulates and attracts neutrophils. Yet another, C3b, opsonizes or coats target cells so as to make them more palatable to phagocytes, which carry a special receptor for C3b.

The C3b fragment also appears to play a major role in the body's control of immune complexes. By opsonizing antigen-antibody complexes, C3b helps prevent the formation of large and insoluble (and thus potentially damaging) immune aggregates. Moreover, receptors for C3b are also present on red blood cells, which appear to use the receptors to pick up complement-coated immune complexes and deliver them to the Kupffer cells in the liver.

Mounting an Immune Response

Infections remain the most common cause of human disease. Produced by bacteria, viruses, parasites, and fungi, infections may range from relatively mild respiratory illnesses such as the common cold, to debilitating conditions like chronic hepatitis, to life-threatening diseases such as AIDS and meningitis.

To fend off the threatening horde, the body has devised astonishingly intricate defenses. Microbes attempting to enter the body must first find a chink in the body's external protection. The skin and the mucous membranes that line the body's portals not only pose a physical barrier, they are also rich in scavenger cells and IgA antibodies.

Next, invaders must elude a series of *nonspecific* defenses: those cells and substances equipped to tackle infectious agents without regard for their antigenic peculiarities. Many potential infections are cut short when microbes are intercepted by patrolling scavenger cells or disabled by complement or other enzymes or chemicals. Virus-infected cells, for instance, secrete interferon, a chemical that rouses natural killer cells.

Microbes that breach the nonspecific barriers are confronted by specific weapons tailored to fit each one. These may be cellular responses directed both by cells, primarily T lymphocytes and their secretions (lymphokines), and against cells that have been infected. Or they may be humoral responses, the work of antibodies secreted by B lymphocytes into the body's fluids or humors.

Most antigens are recognized by a limited number of specific immune cells (and their offspring). A few antigens, however, are capable of rousing large classes of T cells, setting off an immune response so massive that it is harmful. Dubbed "superantigens," these substances include bacterial toxins such as those responsible for the toxic shock syndrome.

Although immunologists traditionally distinguished between cellular and humoral immunity, it has become increasingly clear that the two arms of the immune response are closely intertwined. Almost all antigens evoke both a humoral response and a cellular response—and most B cell responses require T cell help. In practice, however, one arm is usually more effective than the other, and regulatory mechanisms end up skewing the response toward either the cellular or the humoral side.

The *cell-mediated* response is initiated by a macrophage or other antigen-presenting cell. The *antigen-presenting cell* takes in the antigen, digests it, and then displays antigen fragments on its own surface. Bound to the antigen fragment is an MHC molecule. It takes both of these structures, together, to capture the T cell's attention.

A T cell whose receptor fits this antigen-MHC complex binds to it. The binding stimulates the antigen-presenting cell to secrete interleukins required for T cell activation and performance.

Before activated T cells can set to work, however, they need a second go-ahead signal. In a maneuver known as *co-stimulation*, the antigen-presenting cell displays a special molecule that engages specific receptor molecules on the T cell, including one known as CD28. Without co-stimulation, activated T cells fall into a state of unresponsiveness known as *anergy*. Anergy arrests T cell growth by blocking its ability to produce or respond to signals to proliferate.

Once up and going, some subsets of T cells synthesize and secrete lymphokines. Interleukin-2, for instance, spurs the growth of more

T cells. Other lymphokines attract other immune cells—fresh macrophages, granulocytes, and other lymphocytes—to the site of the infection. Yet others direct the cells' activities once they arrive on the scene. Some subsets of T cells become killer (or cytotoxic) cells and set out to track down body cells infected by viruses. And when the infection has been brought under control, suppressor T cells draw the immune response to a close.

Humoral immunity chiefly involves B cells, although the cooperation of helper T cells is almost always necessary. B cells, like macrophages, take in and process circulating antigen. Unlike macrophages, however, a B cell can bind only that antigen that specifically fits its antibody-like receptor.

To enlist the help of a T cell, the B cell exhibits antigen fragments bound to its class II MHC molecules. This display attracts mature helper T cells (which may have been already activated by macrophages presenting the same antigen). The B cell and T cell interact, and the helper T cell secretes several lymphokines. These lymphokines set the B cell to multiplying, and soon there is a clone of identical B cells. The B cells differentiate into plasma cells and begin producing vast quantities of identical antigen-specific antibodies.

Released into the bloodstream, the antibodies lock onto matching antigens. The antigen-antibody complexes trigger the complement cascade or are removed from the circulation by clearing mechanisms in the liver and the spleen. The infection is overcome and, in response to suppressor influences wielded by yet other subsets of T cells, antibody production wanes.

Clinically, infections manifest themselves through the five classic symptoms of the *inflammatory response*: redness, warmth, swelling, pain, and loss of function. Redness and warmth develop when, under the influence of lymphokines and complement components, small blood vessels in the vicinity of the infection become dilated and carry more blood. Swelling results when the vessels, made leaky by yet other immune secretions, allow fluid and soluble immune substances to seep into the surrounding tissue, and immune cells to converge on the site.

A Billion Antibodies

Scientists were long puzzled by the opulence of the immune system's resources. The body apparently could recognize and mount unique responses to an endless variety of antigens, but how in the world could all that information be crammed into a limited number of genes?

The answer came as a surprise. A typical gene consists of a fixed segment of DNA, which directs the manufacture of a given protein molecule such as insulin. Antibody genes, in contrast, are assembled from bits and pieces of DNA scattered widely throughout the genetic material. As the B cell matures, it rearranges or shuffles these gene components, picking and choosing among hundreds of DNA segments, some for each of the antibody's variable (V), diversity (D), joining (J), and constant (C) regions. Intervening segments of DNA are cut out; the selected pieces are spliced together.

The new gene, and the antibody it encodes, are virtually unique. When the B cell containing this uniquely rearranged set of gene segments proliferates, all its descendants will make this unique antibody. Then, as the cells continue to multiply, numerous mutants arise; these allow for the natural selection of antibodies that provide better and better "fits" for the target antigen. The result of this entire process is that a limited number of genetically distinct B cells can respond to a seemingly unlimited range of antigens.

A similar mechanism was found to control a comparable structure on the T cell, the T cell's antigen receptor. The variable regions of T cell antigen receptors, like those of antibodies, are encoded by V, D, and J segments originally far apart, but which are brought together and fused into a single gene. With numerous candidates for each segment, the number of possible combinations becomes astronomical. However, in contrast to antibody genes, T cell receptor genes do not mutate as the T cells proliferate. This ensures that the self-tolerance imposed in the thymus will not be overthrown by the inadvertent generation of mutant T cell receptors that are anti-self.

A Web of Idiotypes

The unique and characteristic pocket on an antibody that recognizes a specific antigen, its variable region, can itself act as an antigen. More precisely, the variable region contains a number of antigen-like segments, and these are known collectively as an idiotype. Like any other antigen, an idiotype can trigger complementary antibody. This second-round antibody is known as an anti-idiotype. An anti-idiotype, in turn, can trigger an anti-anti-idiotype. Like a series of mirrored reflections, the process can go on and on.

Interactions between idiotypes and anti-idiotypes, it has been proposed, constitute a mechanism whereby the immune system regulates itself. According to the "network theory," not only antibodies but B cells and T cells carry, in their unique antigen-receptors, idiotypes. The B cells and T cells that proliferate in response to a certain antigen carry a complementary idiotype. Anti-idiotype B cells secrete anti-idiotype antibodies, which may neutralize the original idiotypes (antibodies), or bind to idiotypes on regulatory T cells. Alternatively, anti-idiotypes may trigger anti-anti-idiotypes, creating a spiraling response within the network—turning on, amplifying, and shutting down immune responses.

The concept of the idiotype is being put to practical use today in the development of experimental antigen-free vaccines (see Vaccines through Biotechnology).

Receptors for Recognizing Antigen

In order to recognize and respond to the antigens that are their specific targets, both B cells and T cells carry special receptor molecules on their surface. For the B cell this receptor is a prototype of the antibody the B cell is prepared to manufacture, anchored in its surface. When a B cell encounters a matching antigen in the blood or other body fluid, this antibody, like receptor allows the B cell to interact with it very efficiently.

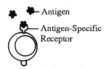

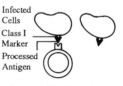

B cell's antigen-specific receptor, an antibody embedded on the cell's surface recognizes antigen in its natural state.

Helper T cell's antigen-specific receptor recognizes antigen that has been processed and presented along with a class II self marker by other immune system cells.

Cytotoxic T cell's antigen-specific receptor recognizes antigen that has been processed and presented along with a class I marker of self.

Figure 1.4. *Antigen Receptors.*

19

The T cell receptor is more complex. Structurally it is somewhat similar to an antibody, made of a pair of chemically linked chains with variable and constant regions. (But to work it needs the help of an associated set of signalling and anchoring cell surface molecules called T3.) Unlike a B cell, however, a T cell cannot recognize antigen in its natural state; the antigen must first be broken down, and the fragments bound to an MHC molecule, by an antigen-presenting cell.

Helper T cells (T4 cells) look for antigen bound to a class II MHC molecule, a combination displayed by macrophages and B cells. Most cytotoxic T cells (T8 cells), on the other hand, respond to antigen bound to MHC class I molecules which are found on almost all body cells.

The T cell receptor molecule thus forms a three-way complex with its specific foreign antigen and an MHC protein. This complicated arrangement assures that T cells, which affect other cells through either direct contact or bursts of secretions, act only on precise targets and at close range.

The major antigen receptor, named alpha/beta for its two chains, is found on most T4 and T8 cells. A second, more recently discovered antigen receptor also has two chains and is known as gamma/delta; it is found on a distinct subset of mature T cells. Like the alpha/beta receptor, the more primitive gamma/delta receptor works in conjunction with T3. The function of T cells that carry gamma/delta receptors is not known.

Immunity, Natural and Acquired

As long ago as the fifth century B.C., Greek physicians noted that people who had recovered from the plague would never get it again— they had acquired immunity. This is because, whenever T cells and B cells are activated, some of the cells become "memory" cells. Then, the next time that an individual encounters that same antigen, the immune system is primed to destroy it quickly.

The degree and duration of immunity depend on the kind of antigen, its amount, and how it enters the body. An immune response is also dictated by heredity; some individuals respond strongly to a given antigen, others weakly, and some not at all.

Infants are born with relatively weak immune responses. They have, however, a natural "passive" immunity, they are protected during the first months of life by means of antibodies they receive from their mothers. The antibody IgG, which travels across the placenta, makes them immune to the same microbes to which their mothers are immune. Children who are nursed also receive IgA from breast milk; it protects the digestive tract

Passive immunity can also be conveyed by anti-body-containing serum obtained from individuals who are immune to a specific infectious agent. Immune serum globulin or "gamma globulin" is sometimes given to protect travelers to countries where hepatitis is widespread. Passive immunity typically lasts only a few weeks.

"Active" immunity, mounting an immune response, can be triggered by both infection and vaccination. Vaccines contain microorganisms or parts of microorganisms that have been altered so they will produce an immune response but will not be able to induce full-blown disease. Some vaccines are made from microbes that have been killed. Others use microbes that have been changed slightly so they can no longer produce infection. They may, for instance, be unable to multiply. Some vaccines are made from a live virus that has been weakened, or attenuated, by growing it for many cycles in animals or cell cultures.

Recent research, benefiting from the biotechnology revolution, has focused on developing vaccines that use only part of the infectious agent. Such subunit vaccines, which are now available for meningitis, pneumonia, and hepatitis B, produce the desired immunity without stirring up separate and potentially harmful immune reactions to the many antigens carried, for instance, on a single bacterium.

Disorders of the Immune System

Allergy

The most common types of allergic reactions—hay fever, some kinds of asthma, and hives—are produced when the immune system responds to a false alarm. In a susceptible person, a normally harmless substance—grass pollen or house dust, for example—is perceived as a threat and is attacked.

Such allergic reactions are related to the antibody known as immunoglobulin E. Like other antibodies, each IgE antibody is specific; one reacts against oak pollen, another against ragweed. The role of IgE in the natural order is not known, although some scientists suspect that it developed as a defense against infection by parasitic worms.

The first time an allergy-prone person is exposed to an allergen, he or she makes large amounts of the corresponding IgE antibody.

21

These IgE molecules attach to the surfaces of mast cells (in tissue) or basophils (in the circulation). Mast cells are plentiful in the lungs, skin, tongue, and linings of the nose and intestinal tract.

When an IgE antibody sitting on a mast cell or basophil encounters its specific allergen, the IgE antibody signals the mast cell or basophil to release the powerful chemicals stored within its granules. These chemicals include histamine, heparin, and substances that activate blood platelets and attract secondary cells such as eosinophils and neutrophils. The activated mast cell or basophil also synthesizes new mediators, including prostaglandins and leukotrienes, on the spot.

It is such chemical mediators that cause the symptoms of allergy, including wheezing, sneezing, runny eyes, and itching. They can also produce anaphylactic shock, a life-threatening allergic reaction characterized by swelling of body tissues, including the throat, and a sudden fall in blood pressure.

Autoimmune Diseases

Sometimes the immune system's recognition apparatus breaks down, and the body begins to manufacture antibodies and T cells directed against the body's own constituents: cells, cell components, or specific organs. Such antibodies are known as autoantibodies, and the diseases they produce are called autoimmune diseases. (Not all autoantibodies are harmful; some types appear to be integral to the immune system's regulatory scheme.)

Autoimmune reactions contribute to many enigmatic diseases. For instance, autoantibodies to red blood cells can cause anemia, autoantibodies to pancreas cells contribute to juvenile diabetes, and autoantibodies to nerve and muscle cells are found in patients with the chronic muscle weakness known as myasthenia gravis. Autoantibody known as rheumatoid factor is common in persons with rheumatoid arthritis.

Persons with systemic lupus erythematosus (SLE), whose symptoms encompass many systems, have antibodies to many types of cells and cellular components. These include antibodies directed against substances found in the cell's nucleus—DNA, RNA, or proteins—which are known as antinuclear antibodies, or ANAs. These antibodies can cause serious damage when they link up with self antigens to form circulating immune complexes, which become lodged in body tissues and set off inflammatory reactions (see Immune Complex Diseases).

Autoimmune diseases affect the immune system at several levels. In patients with SLE, for instance, B cells are hyperactive while suppressor cells are underactive; it is not clear which defect comes first. Moreover, production of IL-2 is low, while levels of gamma interferon are high. Patients with rheumatoid arthritis, who have a defective suppressor T cell system, continue to make antibodies to a common virus, whereas the response normally shuts down after about a dozen days.

No one knows just what causes an autoimmune disease, but several factors are likely to be involved. These may include viruses and environmental factors such as exposure to sunlight, certain chemicals, and some drugs, all of which may damage or alter body cells so that they are no longer recognizable as self. Sex hormones may be important, too, since most autoimmune diseases are far more common in women than in men.

Heredity also appears to play a role. Autoimmune reactions, like many other immune responses, are influenced by the genes of the MHC. A high proportion of human patients with autoimmune disease have particular histocompatibility types. For example, many persons with rheumatoid arthritis display the self marker known as HLA-DR4.

Many types of therapies are being used to combat autoimmune diseases. These include corticosteroids, immunosuppressive drugs developed as anticancer agents, radiation of the lymph nodes, and plasmapheresis, a sort of "blood washing" that removes diseased cells and harmful molecules from the circulation.

Immune Complex Diseases

Immune complexes are clusters of interlocking antigens and antibodies. Under normal conditions immune complexes are rapidly removed from the bloodstream by macrophages in the spleen and Kupffer cells in the liver. In some circumstances, however, immune complexes continue to circulate. Eventually they become trapped in the tissues of the kidneys, lung, skin, joints, or blood vessels. Just where they end up probably depends on the nature of the antigen, the class of antibody—IgG, for instance, instead of IgM—and the size of the complex. There they set off reactions that lead to inflammation and tissue damage.

Immune complexes work their damage in many diseases. Sometimes, as is the case with malaria and viral hepatitis, they reflect

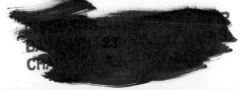

persistent low-grade infections. Sometimes they arise in response to environmental antigens, such as the moldy hay that causes the disease known as farmer's lung. Frequently, immune complexes develop in autoimmune disease (see above), where the continuous production of autoantibodies overloads the immune complex removal system.

Immunodeficiency Diseases

Lack of one or more components of the immune system results in immunodeficiency disorders. These can be inherited, acquired through infection or other illness, or produced as an inadvertent side effect of certain drug treatments.

People with advanced cancer may experience immune deficiencies as a result of the disease process or from extensive anticancer therapy. Transient immune deficiencies can develop in the wake of common viral infections, including influenza, infectious mononucleosis, and measles. Immune responsiveness can also be depressed by blood transfusions, surgery, malnutrition, and stress.

Some children are born with defects in their immune systems. Those with flaws in the B cell components are unable to produce antibodies (immunoglobulins). These conditions, known as agammaglobulinemias or hypogammaglobulinemias, leave the children vulnerable to infectious organisms; such disorders can be combatted with injections of immunoglobulins.

Other children, whose thymus is either missing or small and abnormal, lack T cells. The resultant disorders have been treated with thymic transplants.

Very rarely, infants are born lacking all the major immune defenses; this is known as severe combined immunodeficiency disease (SCID). Some children with SCID have lived for years in germ-free rooms and "bubbles." A few SCID patients have been successfully treated with transplants of bone marrow (see Bone Marrow Transplants).

The devastating immunodeficiency disorder known as the acquired immunodeficiency syndrome (AIDS) was first recognized in 1981. Caused by a virus (the human immunodeficiency virus, or HIV) that destroys T4 cells and that is harbored in macrophages as well as T4 cells, AIDS is characterized by a variety of unusual infections and otherwise rare cancers. The AIDS virus also damages tissue of the brain and spinal cord, producing progressive dementia.

AIDS infections are known as "opportunistic" because they are produced by commonplace organisms that do not trouble people whose

immune systems are healthy, but which take advantage of the "opportunity" provided by an immune defense in disarray. The most common infection is an unusual and life-threatening form of pneumonia caused by a one-celled organism (a protozoan) called Pneumocystis carinii. AIDS patients are also susceptible to unusual lymphomas and Kaposi's sarcoma, a rare cancer that results from the abnormal proliferation of endothelial cells that line blood vessels.

Some persons infected with the AIDS virus develop a condition known as AIDS-related complex, or ARC, characterized by fatigue, fever, weight loss, diarrhea, and swollen lymph glands. Yet other persons who are infected with the AIDS virus apparently remain well; however, even though they develop no symptoms, they can transmit the virus to others.

AIDS is a contagious disease, spread by intimate sexual contact, by direct inoculation of the virus into the bloodstream, or from mother to child during pregnancy. Most of the AIDS cases in the United States have been found among homosexual and bisexual men with multiple sex partners, and among intravenous drug abusers. Others have involved men who received untreated blood products for hemophilia; persons who received transfusions of inadvertently contaminated blood primarily before the AIDS virus was discovered and virtually eliminated from the nation's blood supply with a screening test; the heterosexual partners of persons with AIDS; and children born to infected mothers.

There is presently no cure for AIDS, although the antiviral agent zidovudine (AZT) appears to hold the virus in check, at least for a time. Many other anti-retroviral drugs are being tested, as are agents to bolster the immune system and agents to prevent or treat opportunistic infections. Research on vaccines to prevent the spread of AIDS is also under way.

Cancers of the Immune System

Cells of the immune system, like those of other body systems can proliferate uncontrollably; the result is cancer. Leukemias are caused by the proliferation of white blood cells, or leukocytes. The uncontrolled growth of antibody-producing (plasma) cells can lead to multiple myeloma. Cancers of the lymphoid organs, known as lymphomas, include Hodgkin's disease. These disorders can be treated—some of them very successfully—by drugs and/or irradiation.

Immunology and Transplants

Since organ transplantation was introduced over a quarter of a century ago, it has become a widespread remedy for life-threatening disease. Several thousand kidney transplants are performed each year in the United States alone. In addition, physicians have succeeded in transplanting the heart, lungs, liver, and pancreas.

The success of a transplant—whether it is accepted or rejected—depends on the stubbornness of the immune system. For a transplant to "take," the body of the recipient must be made to suppress its natural tendency to get rid of foreign tissue.

Scientists have tackled this problem in two ways. The first is to make sure that the tissue of the donor and the recipient are as similar as possible. Tissue typing, or *histocompatibility testing*, involves matching the markers of self on body tissues; because the typing is usually done on white blood cells, or leukocytes, the markers are referred to as human leukocyte antigens (HLA). Each cell has a double set of six major antigens, designated HLA-A, B, C, and three types of HLA-D-DR, DP, and DQ. (HLA-A, B, and C are the same as the class I antigens encoded by the genes of the major histocompatibility complex; HLA-D region molecules are the class II MHC antigens.)

Each of the HLA antigens exists, in different individuals, in as many as 20 varieties, so that the number of possible HLA types reaches about 10,000. Histocompatibility testing relies on antibodies to determine if a potential organ donor and recipient share two or more HLA antigens, and thus are likely to make a good "match." The best matches are identical twins; next best are close relatives, especially brothers and sisters.

The second approach to taming rejection is to lull the recipient's immune system. This can be achieved through a variety of powerful immunosuppressive drugs. Steroids suppress lymphocyte function; the drug cyclosporine holds down the production of the lymphokine interleukin-2, which is necessary for T cell growth. When such measures fail, the graft may yet be saved with a new treatment: OKT3 is a monoclonal antibody that seeks out the T3 marker carried on all mature T cells. By either destroying T cells or incapacitating them, OKT3 can bring an acute rejection crisis to a halt.

Not surprisingly, any such all-out assault on the immune system leaves a transplant recipient susceptible to both opportunistic infections and lymphomas. Although such patients need careful medical follow-up, many of them are able to lead active and essentially normal lives.

Bone Marrow Transplants

When the immune response is severely depressed—as the result of inherited defects, cancer therapy, or AIDS—one possible remedy is a transfer of healthy bone marrow. Bone marrow transplants are also used to treat patients with cancers of the blood, the blood-forming organs, and the lymphoid system: the leukemias and lymphomas.

Once in the circulation, transplanted bone marrow cells travel to the bones where the immature cells grow into functioning B and T cells. Like other transplanted tissue, however, bone marrow from a donor must carry self markers that closely match those of the person intended to receive it. This match is essential not only to prevent the transplant from being rejected, but also to fend off a life-threatening situation known as graft-versus-host disease. In graft-versus-host disease, mature T cells from the donor attack and destroy the tissues of the recipient.

To prevent graft-versus-host disease, scientists have developed techniques to "cleanse" the donor marrow of potentially dangerous mature T cells. These include chemicals and, more recently, a monoclonal antibody (OKT3) that specifically recognizes and eliminates mature T cells.

For cancer patients who face immunosuppressive therapy but who have no readily matched donor, doctors have used "autologous" transplants: the person's bone marrow is removed, frozen, and stored until therapy is complete; then the cells are thawed and reinfused.

But a Fetus Is Not Rejected

A fetus, which carries foreign antigens from its father as well as immunologically compatible self antigens from its mother, might be expected to trigger a graft rejection. But the uterus is an "immunologically privileged" site where immune responses are subdued. One source of protection appears to be a substance produced by the fetus, perhaps in response to antibodies from the mother: The substance promotes the development of special white blood cells in the uterus, and these cells release a factor that blocks the actions of IL-2. Another substance, produced by the uterus, helps disguise antigens on the fetal surface of the placenta, shielding them from the mother's immune defenses.

Immunity and Cancer

The immune system provides one of the body's main defenses against cancer. When normal cells turn into cancer cells, some of the antigens on their surface change. These new or altered antigens flag immune defenders, including cytotoxic T cells, natural killer cells, and macrophages.

According to one theory, patrolling cells of the immune system provide continuing bodywide surveillance, spying out and eliminating cells that undergo malignant transformation. Tumors develop when the surveillance system breaks down or is overwhelmed. Some tumors may elude the immune defenses by hiding or disguising their tumor antigens. Alternatively, tumors may survive by encouraging the production of suppressor T cells; these T cells act as the tumor's allies, blocking cytotoxic T cells that would normally attack it.

Blood tests show that people can develop antibodies to many types of tumor antigens (although the antibodies may not actually be effective in fighting the tumor). Skin testing (similar to skin testing for tuberculosis) has demonstrated that tumors provoke cellular immunity as well. Furthermore, studies indicate that cancer patients have a better prognosis when their tumors are infiltrated with many immune cells. Immune responses may underlie the spontaneous disappearance of some cancers.

Tests using antibodies derived from batches of human serum can detect various tumor-associated antigens—including carcinoembryonic antigen (CEA) and alphafetoprotein (AFP)—in blood samples. Because such antigens develop not only in cancer but in other diseases as well, the antibody tests are not useful for cancer screening in the general population. They are, however, valuable in monitoring the course of disease and the effectiveness of treatment in patients known to have cancer.

More recently, scientists have developed monoclonal antibodies (see Hybridoma Technology) that are targeted specifically at tumor antigens. Linked to radioactive substances, these antibodies can be used to track down and reveal hidden cancer metastases within the body. Monoclonal antitumor antibodies are also being used experimentally to treat cancer, either in their native form or as immunotoxins, linked to natural toxins, anticancer drugs, or radioactive substances.

Other efforts to attack cancer through the immune system center on stimulating or replenishing the patient's immune responses with substances known as biological response modifiers. Among these are interferons (now obtained through genetic engineering) and interleukins. In some cases biological response modifiers are injected directly into the patient; in other cases they are used in the laboratory to transform some of the patient's own lymphocytes into tumor-hungry cells known as lymphokine-activated killer (LAK) cells and tumor-infiltrating lymphocytes (TILS), which are then injected back into the patient. Researchers are even using structures from the tumor cells themselves to construct custom-made anticancer "vaccines."

The Immune System and the Nervous System

A new field of research, known as psychoneuroimmunology, is exploring how the immune system and the brain may interact to influence health. For years stress has been suspected of increasing susceptibility to various infectious diseases or cancer. Now evidence is mounting that the immune system and the nervous system may be inextricably interconnected. Research has shown that a wide range of stresses, from losing a spouse to facing a tough examination, can deplete immune resources, causing levels of B and T cells to drop, natural killer cells to become less responsive, and fewer IgA antibodies to be secreted in the saliva.

Biological links between the immune system and the central nervous system exist at several levels. One well-known pathway involves the adrenal glands, which, in response to stress messages from the brain, release corticosteroid hormones into the blood. In addition to helping a person respond to emergencies by mobilizing the body's energy reserves, these "stress hormones" decrease antibodies and reduce lymphocytes in both number and strength.

More recently it has become apparent that hormones and neuropeptides (hormone-like chemicals released by nerve cells), which convey messages to other cells of the nervous system and organs throughout the body, also "speak" to cells of the immune system. Macrophages and T cells carry receptors for certain neuropeptides; natural killer cells, too, respond to them. Even more surprising, some macrophages and activated lymphocytes actually manufacture typical neuropeptides. At the same time, some lymphokines secreted by activated lymphocytes, such as interferon and the interleukins, can transmit information to the nervous system. Hormones produced by the thymus, too, act on cells in the brain.

In addition, the brain may directly influence the immune system by sending messages down nerve cells. Networks of nerve fibers have been found that connect to the thymus gland, spleen, lymph nodes, and bone marrow. Moreover, experiments show that immune function can be altered by actions that destroy specific brain areas.

The image that is emerging is of closely interlocked systems facilitating a two-way flow of information, primarily through the language of hormones. Immune cells, it has been suggested, may function in a sensory capacity, detecting the arrival of foreign invaders and relaying chemical signals to alert the brain. The brain, for its part, may send signals that guide the traffic of cells through the lymphoid organs.

Frontiers in Immunology

Hybridoma Technology

Through a stratagem known as hybridoma technology, scientists are now able to obtain, in quantity, substances secreted by cells of the immune system—both antibodies and lymphokines. The ready supply of these materials has not only revolutionized immunology but has also created a resounding impact throughout medicine and industry.

A hybridoma is created by fusing two cells, a secreting cell from the immune system and a long-lived cancerous immune cell, within a single membrane. The resulting hybrid cell can be cloned, producing many identical offspring. Each of these daughter clones will secrete, over a long period of time, the immune cell product. A B-cell hybridoma secretes a single specific antibody.

Such monoclonal antibodies, as they are known, have opened remarkable new approaches to preventing, diagnosing, and treating disease. Monoclonal antibodies are used, for instance, to distinguish subsets of B cells and T cells. This knowledge is helpful not only for basic research but also for identifying different types of leukemias and lymphomas and allowing physicians to tailor treatment accordingly. Quantitating the numbers of B cells and helper T cells is all-important in immune disorders such as AIDS. Monoclonal antibodies are being used to track cancer antigens and, alone or linked to anti-cancer agents, to attack cancer metastases. The monoclonal antibody known as OKT3 is saving organ transplants threatened with rejection, and preventing bone marrow transplants from setting off graft-versus-host disease.

Monoclonal antibodies are essential to the manufacture of genetically engineered proteins (see Genetic Engineering); they single out the desired protein product so it can be separated from the jumble of molecules surrounding it. Monoclonal antibodies are also the key to developing new types of vaccines (see Vaccines through Biotechnology).

With growing experience, scientists have devised several sophisticated variants on the monoclonal antibody. For instance, they have created some monoclonal antibodies of human rather than mouse origin; human monoclonal antibodies can be used for therapy without risking an immune reaction to mouse proteins. They have also succeeded in "humanizing" mouse antibodies by splicing the mouse genes for the highly specific antigen-recognizing portion of the antibody into the human genes that encode the rest of the antibody molecule.

Other monoclonal antibodies have been designed to behave like enzymes; these so-called catalytic antibodies or abzymes speed up, or catalyze, selected chemical reactions by binding to a chemical reactant and holding it in a highly unstable "transition state." By in fact cutting the proteins they bind to, such antibodies may be useful for such things as dissolving blood clots or destroying tumor cells. Yet other researchers, by fusing two hybridoma cells that produce two different antibodies, have created hybrid hydridomas that secrete artificial antibodies made up of two nonidentical halves: While one arm of the bispecific antibody binds to one antigen, the second arm binds to another. One may bind to a marker molecule, for instance, and the second to a target cell, creating an entirely new way to stain cells. Or, one arm of a chimeric antibody may bind to a killer cell while the other locks to a tumor cell, creating a lethal bridge between the two.

The SCID Mouse

Research in immunology took a giant step forward with the development and manipulation of the SCID mouse. Lacking an enzyme necessary to fashion a functional immune system of their own, SCID mice, like their human counterparts with Severe Combined Immunodeficiency Disease (see Immunodeficiency Diseases), are helpless not only to fight infection but also to reject transplanted tissue.

In the late 1980s, scientists transformed the SCID mouse into an in vivo model of the human immune system. One group of researchers painstakingly transplanted a human fetal thymus gland and lymph nodes into the adult SCID mouse, then injected them with embryonic human immune cells. Some of these cells traveled to the human thymus, where they matured into T cells; others developed into working B cells and macrophages, circulating through the lymph nodes. A second group of researchers implanted mature human T cells in the SCID mouse. Such systems amount to a living test tube, making it possible to study the effects of drugs and of viruses, including HIV, in an intact mammalian immune system.

Genetic Engineering

Genetic engineering, more formally known as recombinant DNA technology, allows scientists to pluck genes (segments of DNA) from one type of organism and combine them with genes of a second organism. In this way, relatively simple organisms such as bacteria or yeast, or even mammalian cells in culture (and, in research programs, mammals such as goats and sheep), can be induced to make quantities of human proteins, including hormones such as insulin as well as lymphokines and monokines. Microorganisms can also be made to manufacture proteins from infectious agents such as the hepatitis virus or the AIDS virus, for use in vaccines.

Another facet of recombinant DNA technology involves gene therapy: replacing defective or missing genes with normal genes. The first approved gene therapy trials involved children with severe combined immunodeficiency disease, or SCID (see Immunodeficiency Diseases), which is caused by lack of an enzyme due to a single abnormal gene. The missing gene is introduced into a harmless virus, then mixed with progenitor cells from the patient's bone marrow. When the virus splices its genes into those of the bone marrow cells, it simultaneously inserts the gene for the missing enzyme. Injected back into the patient, the treated marrow cells produce the missing enzyme and revitalize the immune defenses. Researchers are also investigating the use of gene therapy for such diverse conditions as hemophilia, Parkinson's disease, diabetes, a hereditary form of dangerously high cholesterol, and AIDS.

An increasingly important target for gene therapy is cancer. In pioneering experiments, scientists are removing the immune cell known as the tumor-infiltrating lymphocyte or TIL (see Immunity and Cancer), or tumor cells themselves, inserting a gene that boosts the cells' ability to make quantities of a natural anticancer product such as tumor necrosis factor (TNF) or interleukin-2, and then growing the restructured cells in quantity in the laboratory. When the altered cells are returned to the patient, they seek out the tumor and deliver large doses of the anticancer chemical. They also appear to mobilize, in some unknown way, additional antitumor defenses.

On the horizon are anticancer vaccines made by manipulating genes. Intended to protect cancer patients against a recurrence, these vaccines can incorporate genes for immunogenic tumor antigens or genes for histocompatibility antigens able to galvanize killer T cells, as well as genes for substances such as TNF or interleukin-2. Other anticancer strategies call for introducing genes that can shut down cancer-promoting oncogenes replace faulty cancer-restraining suppressor genes.

Genes can be packaged, for delivery, in a variety of ways: inserted into the genetic material of such carriers as the familiar vaccinia virus (see Vaccines through Biotechnology) or inactivated retroviruses, grafted onto a protein carrier that magnifies the immune response (an adjuvant), or tucked into fat globules known as liposomes.

The Stem Cell

Scientists have long sought the hematopoietic stem cell, the precursor cell that continuously replenishes the body's entire panoply of blood cells, both red and white. Stem cells represent a small portion of all bone marrow cells (perhaps one in 2,000), and they are even rarer in the bloodstream. In the mouse, implanting just a few purified stem cells can completely restore an immune system that has been experimentally destroyed.

Although the human stem cell has yet to be isolated and purified, scientists have discovered that progenitor cells capable of giving rise to an array of blood cells (if not of actually reproducing themselves) carry the cell surface marker CD34. These cells can be sorted out from marrow and blood with monoclonal antibodies that recognize CD34. In experimental programs, CD34 cells are being tested as long-lived vehicles for gene therapy and as an alternative to bone marrow transplants.

Immunoregulation

Research into the delicate and complex checks and balances that regulate the immune response is increasing knowledge of normal and abnormal immune functions. Someday it may be possible to treat diseases such as systemic lupus erythematosus by suppressing parts of the immune system that are overactive and stimulating those that are underactive. Blocking a mechanism such as co-stimulation, by paralyzing T cell responses, may make it possible to prevent graft rejection or to sideline autoimmune diseases, while boosting co-stimulation might help the body rid itself of cells that are infected or cancerous.

Vaccines Through Biotechnology

Through genetic engineering, scientists can isolate specific genes and insert them into DNA of certain microbes or mammalian cells; the microbes or cells become living factories, mass producing the desired antigen. Then, using another product of biotechnology, a monoclonal antibody that recognizes the antigen, the scientists can separate the antigen from all the other material produced by the microbe or cell. This technique has been used to produce immunogenic but safe segments of the hepatitis B virus and the malaria parasite.

In another approach, scientists have inserted genes for desired antigens into the DNA of the vaccinia virus, the large cowpox virus familiar for its role in smallpox immunization. When the re-engineered vaccinia virus is inoculated, it stimulates an immune reaction to both the vaccinia and the products of its passenger genes. These have included, in animal experiments, genes from the viruses that cause hepatitis B, influenza, rabies, and AIDS.

Instead of adding a gene, some scientists have snipped a key gene out of an infectious organism. Thus crippled, the microbe can produce immunity but not disease. This technique has been tried with a bacterium that causes the severe diarrheal disease cholera; such a vaccine is commercially available against a virus disease of pigs.

A totally different approach to vaccine development lies in chemical synthesis. Once scientists have isolated the gene that encodes an antigen, they are able to determine the precise sequence of amino acids that make up the antigen. They then pinpoint small key areas on the large protein molecule, and assemble it chemical by chemical. Wholly synthetic vaccines are being explored for malaria and for the major diarrheal diseases that are so devastating in developing countries.

Another pioneering vaccine strategy exploits anti-idiotype antibodies (see A Web of Idiotypes). The original antibody (or idiotype) provokes an anti-antibody (or anti-idiotype) that resembles the original antigen on the disease-causing organism. The anti-idiotype will not itself cause disease, but it can serve as a mock antigen, inducing the formation of antibodies that recognize and block the original antigen.

To make such a vaccine, scientists inject animals with a monoclonal antibody (idiotype) against a disease-causing microorganism, then harvest the anti-idiotypes produced in response.

Chapter 2

Inheritance

A number of the immune deficiency diseases are inherited, or passed on, in families. In the same manner, many of our physical and chemical characteristics are passed along from parents to children. Examples of these include the color of our eyes, our hair color, and the chemicals which determine our blood type. The messages which determine these, and the thousands of other characteristics which make an individual unique, are called genes. These genes are packaged on long, string-like structures called chromosomes. Every cell in the body contains all the chromosomes, and therefore all of the genes, necessary for life.

Each of our cells contains 23 pairs of chromosomes and therefore 23 sets of gene pairs. One of each pair of chromosomes is inherited from our mother while the other is inherited from our father. Since genes are on these chromosomes, we also inherit one gene (or message) for a certain characteristic (such as eye color) from our mother and one gene for the same characteristic from our father.

During egg and sperm production, the total number of 46 parental chromosomes (23 pairs) is divided in half. One chromosome of each pair, and only one, is normally passed on in each egg or sperm. When fertilization of the egg occurs, the 23 chromosomes contained in the egg combine with the 23 chromosomes in the sperm to restore the total number to 46. In this way, each parent contributes half of his/her genetic information to each offspring.

All of the chromosomes except the sex chromosomes are called autosomes and are numbered from 1-22 according to size. One pair of chromosomes determines the sex of the individual. The sex chromosomes are of two types, X and Y chromosomes. As shown in Figure 2.1, females have two X chromosomes, and males have an X and a Y. Half of all the sperm produced will contain an X, and the others will carry a Y. The sex of the baby is determined by which type of sperm fertilizes the egg.

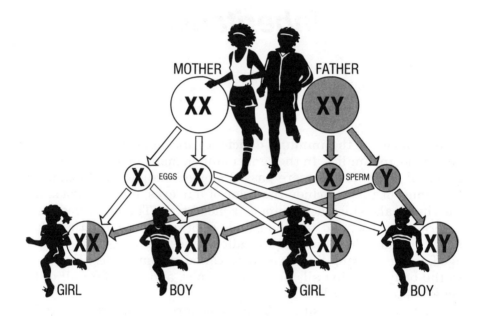

Figure 2.1. *The Sex Chromosones.*

Types of Inheritance

Different kinds of problems (or diseases) can result if an individual inherits genes along the chromosomes which do not work properly. Some diseases are genetic in origin and are therefore passed on in families. Laboratory studies can be helpful in establishing the possible role of genes or chromosomes in a particular disorder. In addition, family history information may help to identify a particular pattern of inheritance, as can comparisons to other families with similar problems.

Most of the immune deficiency diseases are inherited in one of two different modes of inheritance: autosomal recessive or X-Linked recessive. Consult the appropriate chapter or your physician to learn whether a particular immune deficiency disease is genetic, and if so, what form of inheritance is involved.

X-Linked Recessive

One type of single gene disorder involves those genes located on the X chromosome. Because women have two X chromosomes, they usually do not have problems when a gene on one X does not work properly. However, men have only one X, which is paired with their male-determining Y chromosome. Therefore, a non-functioning or abnormal gene on the X is expressed. This special type of recessive inheritance is called X-Linked recessive.

Examples of X-Linked recessive inheritance:

* X-Linked Agammaglobulinemia
* Severe Combined Immunodeficiency (one form)
* Chronic Granulomatous Disease (one form)

In this form of inheritance, a family history of several affected males may be found. The disease is passed on from females (mothers) to males (sons). While the males are affected with the disease, the carrier females are generally asymptomatic and healthy even though they carry the gene for the disease. The diagram in Figure 2.2 illustrates how this kind of inheritance operates in the usual situation. X-Linked agammaglobulinemia is used as the specific example.

Parents in the situation shown in Figure 2.2, can have four different types of children (with respect to X-Linked agammaglobulinemia). The X chromosome is diagrammed as an "X." An X chromosome which carries the gene for agammaglobulinemia is represented by an "^{A}X." A normal X chromosome is represented by an "X^N." A Y chromosome is represented by a "$Y°$." The mother can produce two kinds of eggs: one containing an X chromosome carrying the agammaglobulinemia gene (^{A}X) and one containing a normal X chromosome (X^N). The father can produce two kinds of sperm: one containing a normal X chromosome (X^N) and one containing a Y chromosome. If the egg containing the agammaglobulinemia X chromosome combines with (or is fertilized by) the sperm containing the normal X chromosome, then a daughter who is a carrier is produced; the gene for agammaglobulinemia is balanced out by the normal gene on the other X chromosome. If the egg containing the agammaglobulinemia X chromosome combines with the sperm containing the Y chromosome, then a male who is affected with agammaglobulinemia is produced; in this case there is no gene on the Y chromosome that corresponds to the agammaglobulinemia gene and only the agammaglobulinemia gene is active in the child. If the egg containing the normal X chromosome combines with the sperm containing the normal X chromosome then a normal female is produced; in this case the child does not carry the agammaglobulinemia gene. Finally, if the egg containing the normal X chromosome combines with the sperm containing the Y chromosome, then a normal male results.

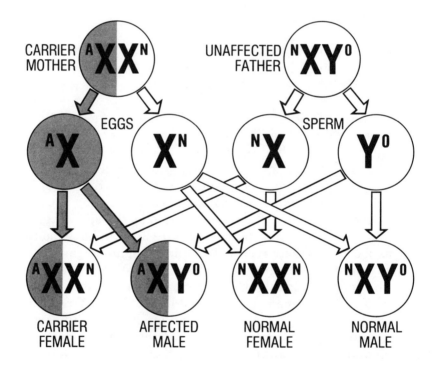

Figure 2.2. *X-Linked Recessive Inheritance.*

The chances for a given egg combining with a given sperm are completely random. According to the laws of probability, the chance for any pregnancy of a carrier female to result in each of these outcomes is as follows:

- carrier female has a 1 in 4 chance or 25 percent
- agammaglobulinemia male has a 1 in 4 chance or 25 percent
- normal female has a 1 in 4 chance or 25 percent
- normal male has a 1 in 4 chance or 25 percent

It should be noted that the outcome of one pregnancy is not influenced by the outcome of a previous pregnancy. Just as in coin-flipping, the fact that you get a "heads" on your first toss doesn't mean you will get a "tails" on the next. Similarly, if you have an agammaglobulinemia son with your first pregnancy you are not guaranteed to have an unaffected child with your second pregnancy; your chances of having an agammaglobulinemia son are still 1 in 4 (25 percent) with each pregnancy.

In some of the immune deficiency diseases, carrier females can be identified by laboratory tests; in other immune deficiency diseases carrier females can only be identified by the fact that they have had affected sons. Consult with your physician or genetic counselor to learn if carrier detection is available in your specific situation.

With earlier diagnosis and improved therapy, many young men with X-Linked disorders, such as agammaglobulinemia, are reaching adult life and having children of their own. The following diagram illustrates the kind of children they would have if they married a woman who did not carry the gene for agammaglobulinemia.

As can be seen in Figure 2.3 [on the next page], all of the daughters of an affected male would be carrier females and none of the sons would be affected.

Autosomal Recessive

If a disorder or disease can only be present if two abnormal genes (one from each parent) are present in the patient, then the disorder is inherited as an autosomal recessive disorder. If an individual inherits only one gene for the disorder, then he or she carries the gene for the disorder but does not have the disorder itself.

41

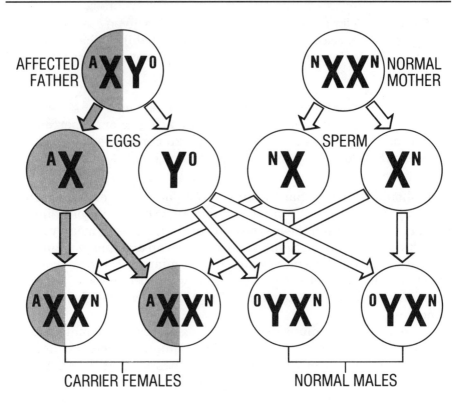

Figure 2.3. *Carrier Females.*

Examples of autosomal recessive inheritance:

- Severe Combined Immunodeficiency (one form)
- Chronic Granulomatous Disease (one form)

In this form of inheritance, affected brothers and sisters may be found. Males and females are affected with equal frequency. Both parents carry the gene for the disease although they themselves are healthy. Figure 2.4 illustrates how this kind of inheritance operates in the usual situation. One form of severe combined immunodeficiency disease (SCID)is used as the specific example.

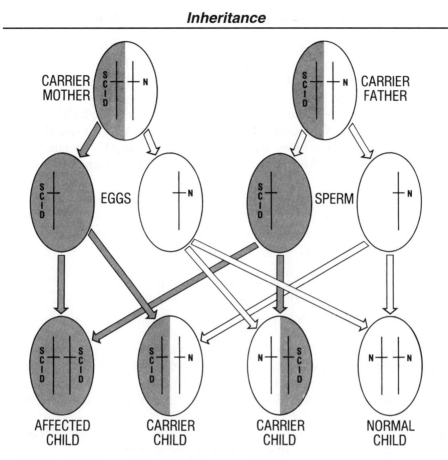

Figure 2.4. Severe Combined Immunodeficiency.

Illustrated in Figure 2.4, these parents can have three different types of children with respect to SCID. The chromosome carrying the gene for SCID is diagrammed as a vertical line with the initials SCID next to it. The normal chromosome is diagrammed as a vertical line with the initial N next to it. The mother can produce two kinds of eggs: one containing the SCID gene and one containing a normal chromosome. Similarly, the father can produce two kinds of sperm: one kind containing the chromosome carrying the SCID gene and the other containing the normal chromosome. If an egg containing the SCID chromosome combines with a sperm containing the SCID chromosome, then a child with the disease is produced; in this case the child has two genes for SCID and no normal genes to counteract them. If an egg containing the SCID gene combines with a sperm containing a normal chromosome then a carrier child results; in this case the gene for SCID is balanced by a normal gene and the child is well but still carries the gene for SCID.

Similarly, if an egg containing the normal chromosome combines with a sperm containing the chromosome carrying the SCID gene, a carrier child is also produced. Finally, if an egg containing the normal chromosome combines with a sperm containing the normal chromosome, a normal child who is neither a carrier nor has the disease is produced.

The chances for a given egg to combine with a given sperm are completely random. According to the laws of probability, the chance for any pregnancy of carrier parents to result in each of the following outcomes is as follows:

- affected child has a 1 in 4 chance or 25 percent
- carrier child has a in 4 chance or 50 percent
- normal child has a 1 in 4 chance or 25 percent

It should be noted that the outcome of one pregnancy is not influenced by the outcome of a previous pregnancy. Just as in coin-flipping, the fact that you get a "heads" on your first toss doesn't mean you will get a "tails" on your next. Similarly, if you have a child with SCID with your first pregnancy you are not guaranteed a normal or carrier child with your second pregnancy; your chances of having a child with SCID are still 25 percent or 1 in 4 with each pregnancy.

In some immune deficiency disorders, carrier parents can be identified by laboratory tests. Consult with your physician or genetic counselor to learn if carrier detection is available in your specific situation.

Reproductive Options

After the birth of a child with a special problem, many families face complicated decisions about future pregnancies. The risk of recurrence and the burden of the disorder are two important factors in those decisions. For instance, if a problem is unlikely to occur again, the couple may proceed with another pregnancy even if the first child's problem is serious. Or, if the risk of recurrence is high but good treatment is available, the couple may be willing to try again. On the other hand, when both the risk and the burden are high, the circumstances may seem unfavorable to some families. These decisions are personal, although important information can be gained from speaking to your pediatrician, immunologist, obstetrician or genetic counselor. In some situations, prenatal testing is available during an at-risk pregnancy. The specific procedures involved will vary depending on the particular diagnosis of concern. If an affected fetus is identified during the first or second trimester, the couple can then decide whether they wish to continue the pregnancy.

Some couples at risk for recessive disorders elect to use donor sperm through a process called artificial insemination. By using sperm from someone other than the father of the affected offspring, the risk is reduced substantially as the donor is unlikely to be a carrier for the same problem.

Some couples may choose to adopt a child as they do not wish to attempt another pregnancy themselves. Although this process can be frustrating and lengthy, many couples are successful in locating a baby or child to join their family.

Finally, the option of maintaining the current family size may seem best to some couples. Either because the possibility of having another similarly affected child is unacceptable or because the demands of the current family are high, expansion of the family may not be desired. Careful consideration of these options is important before decisions can be reached. In addition, periodic consultation with the medical staff can be helpful in keeping current with recent medical advances that could potentially provide more information for your family.

Chapter 3

Breast-Feeding Best Bet For Babies

New parents want to give their babies the very best. When it comes to nutrition, the best first food for babies is breast milk.

More than two decades of research have established that breast milk is perfectly suited to nourish infants and protect them from illness. Breast-fed infants have lower rates of hospital admissions, ear infections, diarrhea, rashes, allergies, and other medical problems than bottle-fed babies. "There are 4,000 species of mammals, and they all make a different milk. Human milk is made for human infants and it meets all their specific nutrient needs," says Ruth Lawrence, M.D., professor of pediatrics and obstetrics at the University of Rochester School of Medicine in Rochester, N.Y., and spokeswoman for the American Academy of Pediatrics.

The academy recommends that babies be breast-fed for six to 12 months. The only acceptable alternative to breast milk is infant formula. Solid foods can be introduced when the baby is 4 to 6 months old, but a baby should drink breast milk or formula, not cow's milk, for a full year.

"There aren't any rules about when to stop breast-feeding," says Lawrence. "As long as the baby is eating age-appropriate solid foods, a mother may nurse a couple of years if she wishes. A baby needs breast milk for the first year of life, and then as long as desired after that."

In 1993, 55.9 percent of American mothers breast-fed their babies in the hospital. Only 19 percent were still breast-feeding when their

FDA Consumer October 1995.

babies were 6 months old. Government and private health experts are working to raise those numbers.

The U.S. Food and Drug Administration is conducting a study on infant feeding practices as part of its ongoing goal to improve nutrition in the United States. The study is looking at how long mothers breast-feed and how they introduce formula or other foods.

Health experts say increased breast-feeding rates would save consumers money, spent both on infant formula and in health-care dollars. It could save lives as well.

"We've known for years that the death rates in Third World countries are lower among breast-fed babies," says Lawrence. "Breast-fed babies are healthier and have fewer infections than formula-fed babies."

Human Milk for Human Infants

The primary benefit of breast milk is nutritional. Human milk contains just the right amount of fatty acids, lactose, water, and amino acids for human digestion, brain development, and growth.

Cow's milk contains a different type of protein than breast milk. This is good for calves, but human infants can have difficulty digesting it. Bottle-fed infants tend to be fatter than breast-fed infants, but not necessarily healthier.

Breast-fed babies have fewer illnesses because human milk transfers to the infant a mother's antibodies to disease. About 80 percent of the cells in breast milk are macrophages, cells that kill bacteria, fungi and viruses. Breast-fed babies are protected, in varying degrees, from a number of illnesses, including pneumonia, botulism, bronchitis, staphylococcal infections, influenza, ear infections, and German measles. Furthermore, mothers produce antibodies to whatever disease is present in their environment, making their milk custom-designed to fight the diseases their babies are exposed to as well.

A breast-fed baby's digestive tract contains large amounts of *Lactobacillus bifidus*, beneficial bacteria that prevent the growth of harmful organisms. Human milk straight from the breast is always sterile, never contaminated by polluted water or dirty bottles, which can also lead to diarrhea in the infant.

Human milk contains at least 100 ingredients not found in formula. No babies are allergic to their mother's milk, although they may have a reaction to something the mother eats. If she eliminates it from her diet, the problem resolves itself.

Sucking at the breast promotes good jaw development as well. It's harder work to get milk out of a breast than a bottle, and the exercise strengthens the jaws and encourages the growth of straight, healthy teeth. The baby at the breast also can control the flow of milk by sucking and stopping. With a bottle, the baby must constantly suck or react to the pressure of the nipple placed in the mouth.

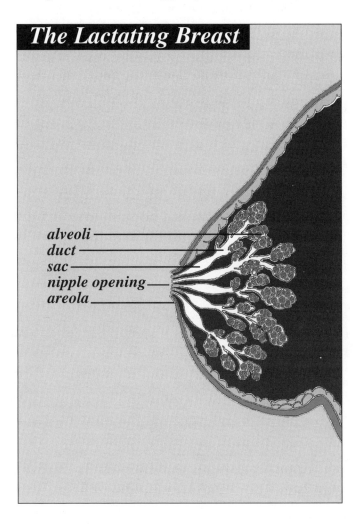

The Lactating Breast

alveoli
duct
sac
nipple opening
areola

Figure 3.1. *When the baby sucks, a hormone called oxytoxin starts the milk flowing from the alveoli, through the ducts (milk canals) into the sacs (milk pools) behind the areola, and finally into the baby's mouth.*

Nursing may have psychological benefits for the infant as well, creating an early attachment between mother and child. At birth, infants see only 12 to 15 inches, the distance between a nursing baby and its mother's face. Studies have found that infants as young as 1 week prefer the smell of their own mother's milk. When nursing pads soaked with breast milk are placed in their cribs, they turn their faces toward the one that smells familiar.

Many psychologists believe the nursing baby enjoys a sense of security from the warmth and presence of the mother, especially when there's skin-to-skin contact during feeding. Parents of bottle-fed babies may be tempted to prop bottles in the baby's mouth, with no human contact during feeding. But a nursing mother must cuddle her infant closely many times during the day. Nursing becomes more than a way to feed a baby; it's a source of warmth and comfort.

Benefits to Mothers

Breast-feeding is good for new mothers as well as for their babies. There are no bottles to sterilize and no formula to buy, measure and mix. It may be easier for a nursing mother to lose the pounds of pregnancy as well, since nursing uses up extra calories. Lactation also stimulates the uterus to contract back to its original size.

A nursing mother is forced to get needed rest. She must sit down, put her feet up, and relax every few hours to nurse. Nursing at night is easy as well. No one has to stumble to the refrigerator for a bottle and warm it while the baby cries. If she's lying down, a mother can doze while she nurses.

Nursing is also nature's contraceptive, although not a very reliable one. Frequent nursing suppresses ovulation, making it less likely for a nursing mother to menstruate, ovulate, or get pregnant. There are no guarantees, however. Mothers who don't want more children right away should use contraception even while nursing. Hormone injections and implants are safe during nursing, as are all barrier methods of birth control. The labeling on birth control pills says if possible, another form of contraception should be used until the baby is weaned.

Breast-feeding is economical also. Even though a nursing mother works up a big appetite and consumes extra calories, the extra food for her is less expensive than buying formula for the baby. Nursing saves money while providing the best nourishment possible.

When Formula's Necessary

There are very few medical reasons why a mother shouldn't breast-feed, according to Lawrence.

Most common illnesses, such as colds, flu, skin infections, or diarrhea, cannot be passed through breast milk. In fact, if a mother has an illness, her breast milk will contain antibodies to it that will help protect her baby from those same illnesses.

A few viruses can pass through breast milk, however. HIV, the virus that causes AIDS, is one of them. Women who are HIV positive should not breast-feed.

A few other illnesses such as herpes, hepatitis, and beta streptococcus infections can also be transmitted through breast milk. But that doesn't always mean a mother with those diseases shouldn't breast-feed, Lawrence says.

"Each case must be evaluated on an individual basis with the woman's doctor," she says.

Breast cancer is not passed through breast milk. Women who have had breast cancer can usually breast-feed from the unaffected breast. There is some concern that the hormones produced during pregnancy and lactation may trigger a recurrence of cancer, but so far this has not been proven. Studies have shown, however, that breast-feeding a child reduces a woman's chance of developing breast cancer later.

Silicone breast implants usually do not interfere with a woman's ability to nurse, but if the implants leak, there is some concern that the silicone may harm the baby. Some small studies have suggested a link between breast-feeding with implants and later development of problems with the child's esophagus. Further studies are needed in this area. But if a woman with implants wants to breast-feed, she should first discuss the potential benefits and risks with her child's doctor.

Possible Problems

For all its health benefits, breast-feeding does have some disadvantages. In the early weeks, it can be painful. A woman's nipples may become sore or cracked. She may experience engorgement more than a bottle-feeding mother, when the breasts become so full of milk they're hard and painful. Some nursing women also develop clogged milk ducts, which can lead to mastitis, a painful infection of the breast. While most nursing problems can be solved with home remedies, mastitis requires prompt medical care.

Another possible disadvantage of nursing is that it affects a woman's entire lifestyle. A nursing mother with baby-in-tow must wear clothes that enable her to nurse anywhere, or she'll have to find a private place to undress. She should eat a balanced diet and she might need to avoid foods that irritate the baby. She also shouldn't smoke, which can cause vomiting, diarrhea and restlessness in the baby, as well as decreased milk production.

Women who plan to go back to work soon after birth will have to plan carefully if they want to breast-feed. If her job allows, a new mother can pump her breast milk several times during the day and refrigerate or freeze it for the baby to take in a bottle later. Or, some women alternate nursing at night and on weekends with daytime bottles of formula.

In either case, a nursing mother is physically tied to her baby more than a bottle-feeding mother. The baby needs her for nourishment, and she needs to nurse regularly to avoid getting uncomfortably full breasts. But instead of feeling it's a chore, nursing mothers often cite this close relationship as one of the greatest joys of nursing. Besides, nursing mothers can get away between feedings if they need a break.

Finally, some women just don't feel comfortable with the idea of nursing. They don't want to handle their breasts, or they want to think of them as sexual, not functional. They may be concerned about modesty and the possibility of having to nurse in public. They may want a break from child care to let someone else feed the baby, especially in the wee hours of the morning.

If a woman is unsure whether she wants to nurse, she can try it for a few weeks and switch if she doesn't like it. It's very difficult to switch to breast-feeding after bottle-feeding is begun.

If she plans to breast-feed, a new mother should learn as much as possible about it before the baby is born. Obstetricians, pediatricians, childbirth instructors, nurses, and midwives can all offer information about nursing. But perhaps the best ongoing support for a nursing mother is someone who has successfully nursed a baby.

La Leche League, a national support organization for nursing mothers, has chapters in many cities that meet regularly to discuss breast-feeding problems and offer support.

"We encourage mothers to come to La Leche League before their babies are born," says Mary Lofton, a league spokeswoman. "On-the-job training is hard to do. It's so important to learn how to breast-feed beforehand to avoid problems."

Most La Leche League chapters allow women to come to a few meetings without charge. League leaders offer advice by phone as well. To find a convenient La Leche League chapter, call (1-800) LA-LECHE.

Tips for Breast-Feeding Success

It's helpful for a woman who wants to breast-feed to learn as much about it as possible before delivery, while she is not exhausted from caring for an infant around-the-clock. The following tips can help foster successful nursing:

- **Get an early start:** Nursing should begin within an hour after delivery if possible, when an infant is awake and the sucking instinct is strong. Even though the mother won't be producing milk yet, her breasts contain colostrum, a thin fluid that contains antibodies to disease.

- **Proper positioning:** The baby's mouth should be wide open, with the nipple as far back into his or her mouth as possible. This minimizes soreness for the mother. A nurse, midwife, or other knowledgeable person can help her find a comfortable nursing position.

- **Nurse on demand:** Newborns need to nurse frequently, at least every two hours, and not on any strict schedule. This will stimulate the mother's breasts to produce plenty of milk. Later, the baby can settle into a more predictable routine. But because breast milk is more easily digested than formula, breast-fed babies often eat more frequently than bottle-fed babies.

- **No supplements:** Nursing babies don't need sugar water or formula supplements. These may interfere with their appetite for nursing, which can lead to a diminished milk supply. The more the baby nurses, the more milk the mother will produce.

- **Delay artificial nipples:** It's best to wait a week or two before introducing a pacifier, so that the baby doesn't get confused. Artificial nipples require a different sucking action than real ones. Sucking at a bottle could also confuse some babies in the early days. They, too, are learning how to breast-feed.

- **Air dry:** In the early postpartum period or until her nipples toughen, the mother should air dry them after each nursing to prevent them from cracking, which can lead to infection. If her nipples do crack, the mother can coat them with breast milk or other natural moisturizers to help them heal. Vitamin E oil and lanolin are commonly used, although some babies may have allergic reactions to them. Proper positioning at the breast can help prevent sore nipples. If the mother's very sore, the baby may not have the nipple far enough back in his or her mouth.

- **Watch for infection:** Symptoms of breast infection include fever and painful lumps and redness in the breast. These require immediate medical attention.

- **Expect engorgement:** A new mother usually produces lots of milk, making her breasts big, hard and painful for a few days. To relieve this engorgement, she should feed the baby frequently and on demand until her body adjusts and produces only what the baby needs. In the meantime, the mother can take over-the-counter pain relievers, apply warm, wet compresses to her breasts, and take warm baths to relieve the pain.

- **Eat right, get rest:** To produce plenty of good milk, the nursing mother needs a balanced diet that includes 500 extra calories a day and six to eight glasses of fluid. She should also rest as much as possible to prevent breast infections, which are aggravated by fatigue.

Medicines and Nursing Mothers

Most medications have not been tested in nursing women, so no one knows exactly how a given drug will affect a breast-fed child. Since very few problems have been reported, however, most over-the-counter and prescription drugs, taken in moderation and only when necessary, are considered safe. Even mothers who must take daily medication for conditions such as epilepsy, diabetes, or high blood pressure can usually breast-feed. They should first check with the child's pediatrician, however. To minimize the baby's exposure, the mother can take the drug just after nursing or before the child sleeps. In the January 1994 issue of *Pediatrics*, the American Academy of Pediatrics included the following in a list of drugs that are usually compatible with breast-feeding:

- acetaminophen
- many antibiotics
- antiepileptics (although one, Primidone, should be given with caution)
- most antihistamines
- alcohol in moderation (large amounts of alcohol can cause drowsiness, weakness, and abnormal weight gain in an infant)
- most antihypertensives
- aspirin (should be used with caution)
- caffeine (moderate amounts in drinks or food)
- codeine
- decongestants
- ibuprofen
- insulin
- quinine
- thyroid medications

Drugs That Are Not Safe While Nursing

Some drugs can be taken by a nursing mother if she stops breast-feeding for a few days or weeks. She can pump her milk and discard it during this time to keep up her supply, while the baby drinks previously frozen milk or formula.

Radioactive drugs used for some diagnostic tests like Gallium-69, Iodine-125, Iodine-131, or Technetium-99m can be taken if the woman stops nursing temporarily.

Drugs that should never be taken while breast-feeding include:

- Bromocriptine (Parlodel): A drug for Parkinson's disease, it also decreases a woman's milk supply.
- Most Chemotherapy Drugs for Cancer: Since they kill cells in the mother's body, they may harm the baby as well.
- Ergotamine (for migraine headaches): Causes vomiting, diarrhea, convulsions in infants.
- Lithium (for manic-depressive illness): Excreted in human milk.
- Methotrexate (for arthritis): Can suppress the baby's immune system.

- Drugs of Abuse: Some drugs, such as cocaine and PCP, can intoxicate the baby. Others, such as amphetamines, heroin and marijuana, can cause a variety of symptoms, including irritability, poor sleeping patterns, tremors, and vomiting. Babies become addicted to these drugs.

- Tobacco Smoke: Nursing mothers should avoid smoking. Nicotine can cause vomiting, diarrhea and restlessness for the baby, as well as decreased milk production for the mother. Maternal smoking or passive smoke may increase the risk of sudden infant death syndrome (SIDS) and may increase respiratory and ear infections.

—by Rebecca D. Williams

Rebecca D. Williams is a writer in Oak Ridge, Tenn.

Chapter 4

How Breast Milk Protects Newborns

Some of the molecules and cells in human milk actively help infants stave off infection.

Doctors have long known that infants who are breast-fed contract fewer infections than do those who are given formula. Until fairly recently, most physicians presumed that breast-fed children fared better simply because milk supplied directly from the breast is free of bacteria. Formula, which must often be mixed with water and placed in bottles, can become contaminated easily. Yet even infants who receive sterilized formula suffer from more meningitis and infection of the gut, ear, respiratory tract and urinary tract than do breast-fed youngsters.

The reason, it turns out, is that mother's milk actively helps newborns avoid disease in a variety of ways. Such assistance is particularly beneficial during the first few months of life, when an infant often cannot mount an effective immune response against foreign organisms. And although it is not the norm in most industrial cultures, UNICEF and the World Health Organization both advise breast-feeding to "two years and beyond." Indeed, a child's immune response does not reach its full strength until age five or so.

All human babies receive some coverage in advance of birth. During pregnancy, the mother passes antibodies to her fetus through the placenta. These proteins circulate in the infant's blood for weeks to months after birth, neutralizing microbes or marking them for destruction by phagocytes—immune cells that consume and break down bacteria, viruses and cellular debris. But breast-fed infants gain extra protection from antibodies, other proteins and immune cells in human milk.

Once ingested, these molecules and cells help to prevent microorganisms from penetrating the body's tissues. Some of the molecules bind to microbes in the hollow space (lumen) of the gastrointestinal tract. In this way, they block microbes from attaching to and crossing through the mucosa—the layer of cells, also known as the epithelium, that lines the digestive tract and other body cavities. Other molecules lessen the supply of particular minerals and vitamins that harmful bacteria need to survive in the digestive tract. Certain immune cells in human milk are phagocytes that attack microbes directly. Another set produces chemicals that invigorate the infant's own immune response.

Breast Milk Antibodies

Antibodies, which are also called immunoglobulins, take five basic forms, denoted as IgG, IgA, IgM, IgD and IgE. All have been found in human milk, but by far the most abundant type is IgA, specifically the form known as secretory IgA, which is found in great amounts throughout the gut and respiratory system of adults. These antibodies consist of two joined IgA molecules and a so-called secretory component that seems to shield the antibody molecules from being degraded by the gastric acid and digestive enzymes in the stomach and intestines. Infants who are bottle-fed have few means for battling ingested pathogens until they begin making secretory IgA on their own, often several weeks or even months after birth.

The secretory IgA molecules passed to the suckling child are helpful in ways that go beyond their ability to bind to microorganisms and keep them away from the body's tissues. First, the collection of antibodies transmitted to an infant is highly targeted against pathogens in that child's immediate surroundings. The mother synthesizes antibodies when she ingests, inhales or otherwise comes in contact with a disease-causing agent. Each antibody she makes is specific to that agent; that is, it binds to a single protein, or antigen, on the agent and will not waste time attacking irrelevant substances. Because the mother makes antibodies only to pathogens in her environment, the baby receives the protection it most needs against the infectious agents it is most likely to encounter in the first weeks of life.

Second, the antibodies delivered to the infant ignore useful bacteria normally found in the gut. This flora serves to crowd out the growth of harmful organisms, thus providing another measure of resistance. Researchers do not yet know how the mother's immune system knows to make antibodies against only pathogenic and not normal bacteria, but whatever the process may be, it favors the establishment of "good bacteria" in a baby's gut.

Secretory IgA molecules further keep an infant from harm in that, unlike most other antibodies, they ward off disease without causing inflammation—a process in which various chemicals destroy microbes but potentially hurt healthy tissue. In an infant's developing gut, the mucosal membrane is extremely delicate, and an excess of these chemicals can do considerable damage. Interestingly, secretory IgA can probably protect mucosal surfaces other than those in the gut. In many countries, particularly in the Middle East, western South America and northern Africa, women put milk in their infants' eyes to treat infections there. I do not know if this remedy has ever been tested scientifically, but there are theoretical reasons to believe it would work. It probably does work at least some of the time, or the practice would have died out.

An Abundance of Helpful Molecules

Several molecules in human milk besides secretory IgA prevent microbes from attaching to mucosal surfaces. Oligosaccharides, which are simple chains of sugars, often contain domains that resemble the binding sites through which bacteria gain entry into the cells lining the intestinal tract. Thus, these sugars can intercept bacteria, baby excretes. In addition, human milk contains large molecules called mucins that include a great deal of protein and carbohydrate. They, too, are capable of adhering to bacteria and viruses and eliminating them from the body.

The molecules in milk have other valuable functions as well. Each molecule of a protein called lactoferrin, for example, can bind to two atoms of iron. Because many pathogenic bacteria thrive on iron, lactoferrin halts their spread by making iron unavailable. It is especially effective at stalling the proliferation of organisms that often cause serious illness in infants, including *Staphylococcus aureus*. Lactoferrin also disrupts the process by which bacteria digest carbohydrates, further limiting their growth. Similarly, B^{12} binding protein, as its name suggests, deprives microorganisms of vitamin B^{12}.

Bifidus factor, one of the oldest known disease-resistance factors in human milk, promotes the growth of a beneficial organism named *Lactobacillus bifidus*. Free fatty acids present in milk can damage the membranes of enveloped viruses, such as the chicken pox virus, which are packets of genetic material encased in protein shells. Interferon, found particularly in colostrum—the scant, sometimes yellowish milk a mother produces during the first few days after birth—also has strong antiviral activity. And fibronectin, present in large quantities in colostrum, can make certain phagocytes more aggressive so that they will ingest microbes even when the microbes have not been tagged by an antibody. Like secretory IgA, fibronectin minimizes inflammation; it also seems to aid in repairing tissue damaged by inflammation.

Component	Action
White Blood Cells	
B lymphocytes	Give rise to antibodies targeted against specific microbes.
Macrophages	Kill microbes outright in the baby's gut, produce lysozyme and activate other components of the immune system.
Neutrophils	May act as phagocytes, injesting bacteria in baby's digestive system.
T lymphocytes	Kill infected cells directly or send out chemical messages to mobilize other defenses. They proliferate in the presence of organisms that cause serious illness in infants. They also manufacture compounds that can strengthen a child's own immune response.

Table 4.1a. *Immune Benefits of Breast Milk*

Molecules	
Antibodies of secretory IgA class	Bind to microbes in baby's digestive tract and thereby prevent them from passing through walls of the gut into body's tissues.
B_{12} binding protein	Reduces amount of vitamin B_{12}, which bacteria need in order to grow.
Bifidus factor	Promotes growth of *Lactobacillus bifidus,* a harmless bacterium, in baby's gut. Growth of such nonpathogenic bacteria helps to crowd out dangerous varieties.
Fatty acids	Disrupt membranes surrounding certain viruses and destroy them.
Fibronectin	Increases antimicrobial activity of macrophages; helps to repair tissues that have been damaged by immune reactions in baby's gut.
Gamma-interferon	Enhances antimicrobial activity of immune cells.
Hormones and growth factors	Stimulate baby's digestive tract to mature more quickly. Once the initially "leaky" membranes lining the gut mature, infants become less vulnerable to microorganisms.
Lactoferrin	Binds to iron, a mineral many bacteria need to survive. By reducing the available amount of iron, lactoferrin thwarts growth of pathogenic bacteria.
Lysozyme	Kills bacteria by disrupting their cell walls.
Mucins	Adhere to bacteria and viruses, thus keeping such microorganisms from attaching to mucosal surfaces.
Oligosaccharides	Bind to microorganisms and bar them from attaching to mucosal surfaces.

Table 4.1b. Immune Benefits of Breast Milk

Cellular Defenses

As is true of defensive molecules, immune cells are abundant in human milk. They consist of white blood cells, or leukocytes, that fight infection themselves and activate other defense mechanisms. The most impressive amount is found in colostrum. Most of the cells are neutrophils, a type of phagocyte that normally circulates in the bloodstream. Some evidence suggests that neutrophils continue to act as phagocytes in the infant's gut. Yet they are less aggressive than blood neutrophils and virtually disappear from breast milk six weeks after birth. So perhaps they serve some other function, such as protecting the breast from infection.

The next most common milk leukocyte is the macrophage, which is phagocytic like neutrophils and performs a number of other protective functions. Macrophages make up some 40 percent of all the leukocytes in colostrum. They are far more active than milk neutrophils, and recent experiments suggest that they are more motile than are their counterparts in blood. Aside from being phagocytic, the macrophages in breast milk manufacture lysozyme, increasing its amount in the infant's gastrointestinal tract. Lysozyme is an enzyme that destroys bacteria by disrupting their cell walls.

In addition, macrophages in the digestive tract can rally lymphocytes into action against invaders. Lymphocytes constitute the remaining 10 percent of white cells in the milk. About 20 percent of these cells are B lymphocytes, which give rise to antibodies; the rest are T lymphocytes, which kill infected cells directly or send out chemical messages that mobilize still other components of the immune system. Milk lymphocytes seem to behave differently from blood lymphocytes. Those in milk, for example, proliferate in the presence of *Escherichia coli*, a bacterium that can cause life-threatening illness in babies, but they are far less responsive than blood lymphocytes to agents posing less threat to infants. Milk lymphocytes also manufacture several chemicals—including gamma-interferon, migration inhibition factor and monocyte chemotactic factor—that can strengthen an infant's own immune response.

Added Benefits

Several studies indicate that some factors in human milk may induce an infant's immune system to mature more quickly than it would were the child fed artificially. For example, breast-fed babies produce higher levels of antibodies in response to immunizations.

Also, certain hormones in milk (such as cortisol) and smaller proteins (including epidermal growth factor, nerve growth factor, insulin-like growth factor and somatomedin C) act to close up the leaky mucosal lining of the newborn, making it relatively impermeable to unwanted pathogens and other potentially harmful agents. Indeed, animal studies have demonstrated that postnatal development of the intestine occurs faster in animals fed their mother's milk. And animals that also receive colostrum, containing the highest concentrations of epidermal growth factor, mature even more rapidly.

Other unknown compounds in human milk must stimulate a baby's own production of secretory IgA, lactoferrin and lysozyme. All three molecules are found in larger amounts in the urine of breast-fed babies than in that of bottle-fed babies. Yet breast-fed babies cannot absorb these molecules from human milk into their gut. It would appear that the molecules must be produced in the mucosa of the youngsters' urinary tract. In other words, it seems that breast-feeding induces local immunity in the urinary tract.

In support of this notion, recent clinical studies have demonstrated that the breast-fed infant has a lower risk of acquiring urinary tract infections. Finally, some evidence also suggests that an unknown factor in human milk may cause breast-fed infants to produce more fibronectin on their own than do bottle-fed babies.

All things considered, breast milk is truly a fascinating fluid that supplies infants with far more than nutrition. It protects them against infection until they can protect themselves.

Further Reading

Mucosal Immunity: the Immunology of Breast Milk. H. B. Slade and S. A. Schwartz in *Journal of Allergy and Clinical Immunology,* Vol. 80, No. 3, pages 348-356; September 1987.

Immunology of Milk and the Neonate. Edited by J. Mestecky et al. Plenum Press, 1991.

Breastfeeding and Health in the 1980 S: a Global Epidemiologic Review. Allan S. Cunningham in *Journal of Pediatrics*, Vol. 118, No. 5, pages 659-666; May 1991.

The Immune System of Human Milk: Antimicrobial, Antiinflammatory and Immunomodulating Properties. A. S. Goldman in *Pediatric Infectious Disease Journal*, Vol. 12, No. 8, pages 664-671; August 1993.

Host-resistance Factors and Immunologic Significance of Human Milk. In *Breastfeeding: A Guide for the Medical Profession*, by Ruth A. Lawrence. Mosby Year Book, 1994.

—by Jack Newman.

Jack Newman founded the breast-feeding clinic at the Hospital for Sick Children in Toronto in 1984 and serves as its director. He has more recently established similar clinics at Doctors Hospital and St. Michael's Hospital, both in Toronto. Newman received his medical degree in 1970 from the University of Toronto, where he is now an assistant professor. He completed his postgraduate training in New Zealand and Canada. As a consultant for UNICEF, he has worked with pediatricians in Africa. He has also practiced in New Zealand and in Central and South America.

Part Two

Immunodeficiency Diseases and Disorders

Chapter 5

Immunodeficiency Diseases

The potential for error exists in any complicated system of nature. Errors of the immune system occur more frequently than a casual estimate might suppose. These errors are termed immunodeficiency diseases and afflict, in varying degrees, approximately 1 in every 500 U.S. citizens. Immunodeficiencies can be inherited or acquired. The most dramatic heritable disease is severe combined immunodeficiency (SCID), which is responsible for the "boy in the bubble" syndrome. Children who have SCID are born without an adequately functioning immune system and thus must remain in a controlled environment because exposure to any pathogenic organism would result in death.

Immunodeficiency also can result secondarily from disease. For example, AIDS is caused by infection of the immune cells with the human immunodeficiency virus (HIV). HIV infection cripples the immune system and leaves the afflicted individual defenseless against pathogens. Other types of acquired immunodeficiencies can result from malnutrition, infection, drug therapies, and, it has been speculated, stress.

Although immunodeficiency diseases have unfortunate consequences, they also have provided scientists an opportunity to study many important aspects of the immune system. For example, by studying these diseases, immunologists have learned about the functions of immune system components as well as the devastating effects of their absence. Significant progress has been made in the effort to

Excerpted from NIH Pub No. 91-2414.

cure immunodeficiency diseases. Advances in therapies include better therapeutic drugs, bone marrow transplantation, synthetic substitutes for substances normally produced by the body, and the advent of gene-replacement therapy. Continued study is needed to produce full understanding of the cause and inheritance of these diseases; to perfect drug- and gene-product replacement therapies; to perfect bone marrow transplantation; and to continue advances in gene therapy.

Overview

We inhabit our world with an almost infinite variety of other organisms, and our survival therefore depends on the integrity of a sophisticated immune system that can recognize and eliminate infectious organisms and their toxic products. Although we still have much to learn about our immune system, we know that it is composed of many different types of specialized cells, which must closely coordinate their functions with each other. To ensure this coordination, each cell type uses special sets of genes to encode essential components of the immune system, including:

1. millions of receptors that recognize different foreign antigens;

2. intricate sets of interacting molecules that are required for communication between the different cells;

3. well-coordinated enzyme systems that are responsible for extracellular destruction of microorganisms; and

4. molecules that construct elaborate traps for cellular ingestion and digestion of invading bacteria, viruses, fungi, parasites, and other pathogens.

Because the immune system is complex and vital to human well-being, defects in one or more of its components occur frequently and can produce a wide spectrum of serious illnesses (Table 5.1). These immune system disorders, known as immunodeficiency diseases, affect large numbers of people. It is estimated that more than 1 in 500 U.S. citizens are born with an immune system defect. Many more individuals will acquire a transient or permanent immunodeficiency, which may have devastating consequences.

Figure 5.1. *Cells of the Immune System.*

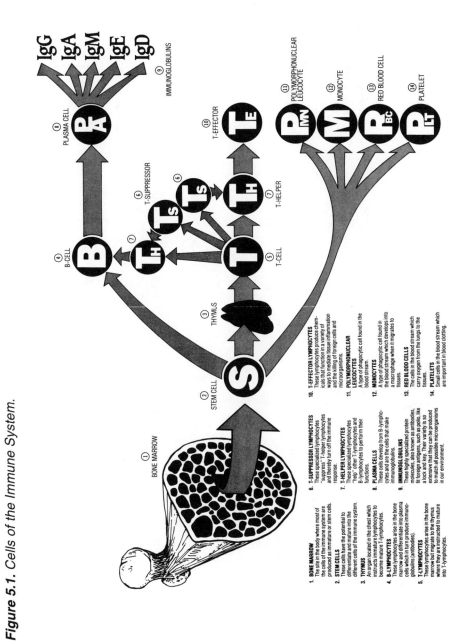

1. **BONE MARROW**
   The site in the body where most of the cells of the immune system are produced as immature or stem cells.

2. **STEM CELLS**
   These cells have the potential to differentiate and mature into the different cells of the immune system.

3. **THYMUS**
   An organ located in the chest which instructs immature lymphocytes to become mature T-lymphocytes.

4. **B-LYMPHOCYTES**
   These lymphocytes arise in the bone marrow and differentiate into plasma cells which in turn produce immuno-globulins (antibodies).

5. **T-LYMPHOCYTES**
   These lymphocytes arise in the bone marrow but migrate to the thymus where they are instructed to mature into T-lymphocytes.

6. **T-SUPPRESSOR LYMPHOCYTES**
   These specialized lymphocytes "suppress" T-helper lymphocytes and thereby turn off the immune response.

7. **T-HELPER LYMPHOCYTES**
   These specialized lymphocytes "help" other T-lymphocytes and B-lymphocytes to perform their functions.

8. **PLASMA CELLS**
   These cells develop from B-lympho-cytes and are the cells that make immunoglobulins.

9. **IMMUNOGLOBULINS**
   These highly specialized protein molecules, also known as antibodies, fit foreign antigens, such as polio, like a lock and key. Their variety is so extensive that they can be produced to match all possible microorganisms in our environment.

10. **T-EFFECTOR LYMPHOCYTES**
    These lymphocytes produce chem-icals that function in a variety of ways to mediate tissue inflammation and the killing of foreign cells and microorganisms.

11. **POLYMORPHONUCLEAR LEUCOCYTES**
    A type of phagocytic cell found in the blood stream.

12. **MONOCYTES**
    A type of phagocytic cell found in the blood stream which develops into a macrophage when it migrates to tissues.

13. **RED BLOOD CELLS**
    The cells in the blood stream which carry oxygen from the lungs to the tissues.

14. **PLATELETS**
    Small cells in the blood stream which are important in blood clotting.

Table 5.1. Some examples of antibody deficiency disorders.

Disorder	Functional Deficiencies	Presumed Cellular Level of Defect
X-linked agammaglobulinemia	Antibody	Pre-B cell
Common variable (acquired) hypogammaglobulinemia	Antibody	B lymphocyte
Selective IgA deficiency	IgA antibody	IgA B lymphocyte
Secretory component deficiency	Secretory IgA	Mucosal epithelium
Selective IgM deficiency	IgM antibody	T helper cells
Immunodeficiency with elevated IgM	IgG and IgA antibodies	IgG, IgA B lymphocytes; "switch" T cells
Transient hypogammaglobulinemia of infancy	None; immunoglobulins low but antibodies present	Unknown
Antibody deficiency with near-normal immunoglobulins	Antibody	Unknown; ?B cell
X-linked lymphoproliferative disease	Anti-EBNA antibody	B cell; ?also T cell

These statistics emphasize the need to learn more about immunodeficiency diseases, including ways to treat and, ultimately, to prevent them. Although this task is particularly urgent for overtly affected individuals, research also will benefit persons who are not obviously affected. By studying patients who have recognized defects in their immune systems, investigators have learned how immune system components work in the elaborate composite as well as how they affect health and disease. For example, scientists have discovered that susceptibility to health problems such as cancers and autoimmune diseases may, in fact, reflect underlying immunodeficiencies that were previously unsuspected.

Deficiencies of immune responsiveness can occur as either primary or secondary disorders. The primary immunodeficiency diseases are inherited defects of the immune system that usually lead to manifest infection susceptibility soon after birth. However, some inherited defects may not become apparent until later in life. The secondary immunodeficiencies may be acquired as a consequence of treatment with immunosuppressive agents, nutritional deficiencies, and infections with certain viral agents, such as HIV-1 and HIV-2. Immune system defects are characterized by frequent or unusually severe infections that vary according to the nature of the defect. Autoimmune disorders and malignancies also occur more frequently in individuals with immunodeficiency diseases.

Immunodeficiency diseases may involve either specific or nonspecific components of the immune system. Defects of phagocytic white blood cells and deficiencies of serum complement components are examples of disorders that affect nonspecific immunity. Defects of specific immunity, both cellular and humoral, involve altered development and function of either thymus-derived T cells or bone marrow-derived B cells. Scientists are making progress in defining a wide assortment of defects in the immune system and in devising treatment for these diseases.

Immunologists have made considerable advances in elucidating the cellular and molecular abnormalities that underlie the recognized primary immunodeficiencies. However, the fundamental biological errors responsible for most of these diseases remain unknown. Exceptions include an understanding of two defects that are accompanied by purine salvage pathway enzyme deficiencies:

1. adenosine deaminase (ADA) deficiency, which occurs in some cases of autosomal recessive SCID; and

Table 5.2. *Some examples of cellular and combined immunodeficiency.*

Disorder	Deficiencies	Level of Defect
DiGeorge's syndrome	T cellular; some antibody	Dysmorphogenesis of 3rd and 4th branchial pouches
Nezelof's syndrome (including with PNP deficiency)	T cellular; some antibody	Unknown; ?thymus; ?T cell; metabolic defects
Severe combined immunodeficiency syndromes (autosomal recessive); ADA deficiency; X-linked recessive; defective expression of HLA antigens; reticular dysgenesis	Antibody and T cellular; phagocytic in reticular dysgenesis	Unknown; metabolic defect(s) ?T cell; ?stem cell; ?thymus; regulatory gene defects
Wiskott-Aldrich syndrome	Antibody, T cellular	Many; defective expression of CD43
Ataxia telangiectasia	Antibody; T cellular	B lymphocyte; helper T
Cartilage-hair hypoplasia	T cellular	G1 cycle of many cells
Immunodeficiency with thymoma	Antibody; some T cellular	B lymphocyte; excessive T suppressor cells
Hyperimmunoglobulinemia E	Specific immune responses; excessive IgE	Unknown
Leukocyte adhesion (CD11/18) deficiency	Cytotoxic lymphocytic, phagocytic cells	95 kD MW beta chain of LFA-1, CR3 and p150,95

2. purine nucleoside phosphorylase (PNP) deficiency, which occurs in some patients with Nezelof's syndrome.

Scientists are beginning to identify the bases of other immunodeficiency diseases (Table 5.2). For example, the molecular basis of CD11/CD18 (or leukocyte adhesion) deficiency now is attributed to the defective synthesis of a common beta chain that is shared by three leukocyte surface glycoproteins. Defective synthesis of an X-box binding protein, which normally binds to a human leukocyte antigen (HLA) DR promoter, has been identified recently as the basis for HLA class II antigen deficiency. Scientists have obtained complementary DNA clones for all of the complement components and have identified deletions and point mutations for the C1 inhibitor gene in hereditary angioneurotic edema (HANE).

In addition, the gene that encodes the heavy chain of cytochrome b_{245} has been cloned and found to be abnormal in X-linked chronic granulomatous disease. Scientists also are beginning to explore the molecular bases of a newly recognized group of lymphocyte activation defects. The bases for these defects vary according to type and appear to include defective expression of the TcR-CD3 complex, failure of signal transduction, and failure of IL-2 production. Finally, the abnormal genes that are responsible for X-linked agammaglobulinemia, X-linked SCID, and Wiskott-Aldrich syndrome are being localized to certain other regions of the X chromosome. Nevertheless, much remains to be learned about the cellular and molecular bases of these and, indeed, a majority of the primary immunodeficiencies.

During the past decade, major advances have been made in developing therapies for immunodeficiency diseases. Among the most important advances are:

1. the development of several safe and effective forms of intravenous immunoglobulin (IVIG) for treating antibody-deficient individuals;

2. techniques for removing mature T cells from bone marrow cell suspensions, thereby permitting mismatched marrow transplantation in T cell-deficient patients;

3. development of new antibiotics that are effective against opportunistic infectious agents;

4. enzyme replacement therapy for ADA deficiency; and

5. recombinant cytokines for treating a variety of immunodeficiencies.

The promise for even greater accomplishment in treating immunodeficiency diseases lies in the rapidly evolving understanding of the primary causes for these diseases and in the infinite potential of molecular biological approaches to therapy. Continued progress will require the support of research conducted by clinical scientists who care for patients with immunodeficiencies, study these rare patients at a cellular level, and evaluate innovative therapies. Furthermore, these efforts must be combined with the work of basic scientists who investigate the molecular aberrations associated with immunodeficiency diseases.

Identification of Faulty Genes And Gene Products

To develop targeted therapies for immunodeficiencies, scientists need to identify the faulty genes and gene products for each primary immunodeficiency disease. This effort will require the coordinated use of family studies, modern molecular biology, and studies of cell function and specific protein products. Potentially helpful strategies include:

1. studying large numbers of individuals from families that carry the gene defect, thus increasing the chances of linking the gene defect to the closest restriction fragment length polymorphisms (RFLPs);

2. identifying individuals who have a chromosomal deletion that includes the defective gene, thus allowing identification of the missing pieces of DNA; and

3. identifying cell types in which the defective gene is normally exposed, thus permitting the investigator to determine whether messages from the candidate gene are expressed.

Successful approaches to identifying faulty genes and gene products probably will combine all of these strategies in a cooperative venture among patients, their families, and clinical scientists.

Research Opportunity:

- Identify the faulty genes and gene products for each primary immunodeficiency disease through the coordinated use of family studies, modern molecular biology, and studies of cell function and specific protein products.

Gene Therapy and Replacement Therapy

Scientists have begun to develop therapies using genes and gene products such as enzymes, antibodies, and cytokines. However, a variety of problems must be solved before gene therapy is feasible. Research now must focus on methods for stable integration of the normal gene with high efficiency into the DNA of a self-renewing cell population, preferably a precursor cell pool. Scientists then must determine how to transcribe and translate the gene to generate adequate but nontoxic concentrations of the gene product. ADA is an attractive candidate for gene therapy because cells tolerate a wide range of concentrations of this enzyme. Preliminary work suggests that it may be possible to replace a defective form of the gene encoding ADA with a normal gene by homologous recombination. This approach would allow the normal gene to be regulated by the appropriate endogenous promoters and enhancers.

In addition to continuing efforts toward gene therapy, researchers must further develop replacement therapy with gene products. Scientists currently are replacing missing enzymes, antibodies, and cytokines with the use of modified natural proteins or recombinant molecules. However, with the exception of missing blood serum antibodies, few immunodeficiencies are being addressed by replacement therapy.

Research Opportunities:

- Perfect therapies with genes and gene products such as enzymes, antibodies, and cytokines.

- Further develop techniques of replacement therapy with gene products.

Bone Marrow Transplantation

Studies of bone marrow transplantation provide another arena for developing therapies for immunodeficiency diseases. Marrow transplants have proven capable of permanently correcting many genetic immunodeficiencies, particularly those in infants with SCID. More important, studies following the transplantation of T cell-depleted marrow stem cells into infants with SCID offer an otherwise unavailable opportunity to study the normal development of the human immune system. Infant SCID patients who have had stem cell transplants provide more effective models for certain studies than do other marrow transplant recipients, including SCID mice transplanted with human lymphoid tissues and cells. They are particularly effective for studying the development of human T cell and B cell functions, mechanisms of tolerance induction, and mechanisms of acquiring MHC restriction.

Research Opportunities:

- Conduct further studies on the use of bone marrow transplantation for treating immunodeficiency diseases.

- Use infants with SCID who have had stem cell transplants as models for studying the normal development of the human immune system.

Biology of the Immune System

Scientists presently do not have sufficient knowledge to understand all of the defects that can affect the immune system. Therefore, future research must include further fundamental studies of the biology of the immune system at the levels of the molecule, the cell, and the whole. The biology of the immune system is often abnormal for one component but normal for all others. Thus, both in vitro and in vivo studies in patients with genetically determined immunodeficiencies are particularly informative, because they can demonstrate clearly the interactive as well as individual role of the particular component.

Research Opportunity:

- Continue basic studies of the biology of the immune system at the molecular, cellular, and whole organism levels. In particular, conduct in vitro and in vivo studies in patients with genetic immunodeficiencies.

AIDS

The recognition of AIDS in 1980 focused concern on a major new immunodeficiency disease. It is predicted that the vast majority of individuals who are infected with HIV will ultimately succumb to the infection and its complications. In spite of this grim reality, remarkable progress has been made in understanding AIDS and HIV infection. Scientists have accumulated extensive knowledge in areas ranging from the most basic molecular analysis of the virus to programs aimed at developing new treatments and vaccines. Broad educational, social, and legal programs have been implemented to protect society at large, to safeguard the rights of the individual, and to educate various segments of the public about the ways that HIV can and cannot be transmitted.

During the past 10 years, advances in fields such as virology, immunology, and molecular and cell biology have provided powerful tools for the study of HIV infection. Scientists now are applying these new techniques to the expeditious development of active therapies and preventive vaccines for this deadly virus infection.

Continued basic research is needed to elucidate how HIV attacks the immune system. A particularly urgent application of this information is the development of a vaccine that can prevent HIV infection. HIV vaccine research needs to be expanded to include vaccines that are designed to provide for protection by targeting critical sites on the virus, such as the site that allows glycoprotein gp120 to bind to T cells. Other approaches should include the use of vaccines with broad immunogenicity, such as a whole killed virus or a series of sequences designed to induce both antibody and cell-mediated immunity.

Research Opportunities:

- Investigate how HIV attacks the immune system.

- Expand HIV vaccine research to include both site-specific and broad immunogenic designs.

Bibliography

Barrett, D.J.; Ammann, A.J.; Wara, D.W.; Cowan, M.J.; Fisher, R.J.; Stiehm, E.R. Clinical and immunologic spectrum of the Di-George syndrome. *Journal of Clinical Laboratory Immunology* 6: 1-6, 1981.

Buckley, R.H. Bone marrow transplantation in treatment of severe primary T cell immunodeficiency: recent advances. *Pediatric Annals* 16: 412-421, 1987.

Chatila T.; Wong, R.; Young, M.; Terhorst, C; Geha, R.S. An immunodeficiency characterized by defective signal transducin in T lymphocytes. *New England Journal of Medicine* 320: 696-702, 1989.

Fauci, A.S. The human immunodeficiency virus: infectivity and mechanisms of pathogenesis. *Science* 239: 617-622, 1988.

Markert, M.L.; Hershfield, M.S.; Wiginton, D.A.; States, J.C.; Ward, F.E.; Bigner, S.H.; Buckley, R.H.; Kaufman, R.E.; Hutton, J.J. Identification of a deletion in the adenosine deaminase gene in a child with severe combined immunodeficiency. *Journal of Immunology* 138: 3203-3206, 1987.

Rosen, F.S.; Cooper, M.D.; Wedgewood, R. The primary immunodeficiencies. *New England Journal of Medicine* 311: 235-242, 300310, 1984.

Ross, S.C.; Densen, P. Complement deficiency states and infection: epidemiology, pathogenesis and consequences of Neisseria and other infections in an immune deficiency. *Medicine* 63: 243-212, 1984.

Tiller, T.L.; Buckley, R.H. Transient hypogammaglobulinemia of infancy: review of the literature, clinical and immunologic features of 11 new cases and long-term follow-up. *Journal of Pediatrics* 92: 347-353, 1978.

Chapter 6

X-Linked Agammaglobulinemia

Most X-Linked Agammaglobulinemia patients have pre-B-lymphocytes, but very few of these go on to become B-lymphocytes. Thus, the basic defect in X-Linked Agammaglobulinemia is a failure of pre-B-lymphocytes to mature into B-lymphocytes. The specific defect which causes this failure to produce mature B-lymphocytes is not known, but the defect appears to be within the B-lymphocyte itself.

Definition

X-Linked Agammaglobulinemia was first described in 1952 by Dr. Ogden Bruton. This disease, sometimes called Bruton's Agammaglobulinemia or Congenital Agammaglobulinemia, was the first immunodeficiency disease to be identified. X-Linked Agammaglobulinemia is an inherited immunodeficiency disease in which patients lack the ability to produce antibodies, proteins that make up the gamma globulin or immunoglobulin fraction of blood plasma. Antibodies are an integral part of the body's defense mechanism against certain microorganisms (bacteria, viruses).

Microorganisms are constantly coming in contact with body surfaces. They are in the food we eat and in the air we breathe. When microorganisms such as bacteria enter the body and land on a mucosal surface, antibody molecules stick to the surface of the microorganism.

Antibody bound to the surface of a microorganism can have one or more effects which are beneficial to the person. For example, some microorganisms must attach to body cells before they can cause an infection, but antibody coated microorganisms are often not "sticky" enough to attach. Antibody attached to the surface of some microorganisms will cause the activation of other body defenses (such as a group of blood proteins called serum complement) which can directly kill the bacteria or viruses. Antibody coated bacteria are much easier for white blood cells (phagocytes) to ingest and kill than bacteria which are not coated with antibody. All of these actions prevent microorganisms from invading body tissues where they may cause serious infections.

Antibodies are important in the recovery from infections, and also protect against getting certain infections more than once. There are antibodies specifically designed to combine with each and every microorganism much like a lock and key. Once the antibodies combine with the microorganism, the microorganism is neutralized and the infection controlled. The basic defect in X-Linked Agammaglobulinemia is an inability of the patient to produce antibodies.

Antibodies are proteins which are produced by specialized cells in the body, the plasma cells (see chapter on Understanding the Immune System). The development of plasma cells proceeds in an orderly fashion from stem cells located in the bone marrow. The stem cells give rise to immature lymphocytes, called pre-B-lymphocytes. Pre-B-lymphocytes then give rise to B-lymphocytes, which on contact with a foreign substance (called an antigen), mature into the plasma cells which produce and secrete antibodies.

Most X-Linked Agammaglobulinemia patients have pre-B-lymphocytes, but very few of these go on to become B-lymphocytes. Thus, the basic defect in X-Linked Agammaglobulinemia is a failure of pre-B-lymphocytes to mature into B-cells. The specific defect which causes this failure to produce mature B-lymphocytes is not known, but the defect appears to be within the B-cell itself.

Clinical Presentation

Patients with X-Linked Agammaglobulinemia are prone to develop infections because they lack antibodies. The infections frequently occur at or near the surfaces of mucous membranes, such as the middle ear, sinuses and lungs, but in some instances can also involve the bloodstream or internal organs. Thus, patients with X-Linked

Agammaglobulinemia may have infections which involve the sinuses (sinusitis), the eyes (conjunctivitis), the ears (otitis), the nose (rhinitis), the airways to the lung (bronchitis) or the lung itself (pneumonia). They also may have recurrent gastrointestinal tract infections which can cause diarrhea (gastroenteritis). In patients without antibodies, any of these infections may also penetrate the mucosal surface, invade the bloodstream, and spread to other organs deep within the body.

Infections in X-Linked Agammaglobulinemia patients are usually caused by microorganisms which are killed or inactivated very effectively by antibodies in normal people. The most common bacteria which cause infection are the pneumococcus, the streptococcus, the staphylococcus and Hemophilus influenzae. Viruses may also cause disease. X-Linked Agammaglobulinemia patients are particularly susceptible to the common viruses which cause diarrhea and those which cause respiratory infections such as colds and the "flu."

Diagnosis

When a patient is suspected of having X-Linked Agammaglobulinemia, the diagnosis is established by several tests. The amounts of immunoglobulins (IgG, IgM, and IgA) in the blood are measured. In X-Linked Agammaglobulinemia, all of the immunoglobulins will be markedly reduced or absent. It is difficult to provide exact numbers for normal immunoglobulin levels because they vary with the age of the child. Since even normal babies make only small quantities of immunoglobulin in the first few months of life, it is important to remember that it may be difficult to distinguish a very young baby (less than 6 months old) with X-Linked Agammaglobulinemia from a normal baby by only testing blood levels of immunoglobulins. In some cases, tests may also be performed to see how well the patient's immunoglobulins function as antibodies. For example, the patient's blood may be tested to determine if he has responded with antibodies to the usual childhood immunizations (for example, tetanus, diphtheria, pertussis), or the child may be immunized with these killed vaccines and then tested. Finally, the blood may be tested to determine if the patient has B-lymphocytes.

Inheritance

X-Linked Agammaglobulinemia is a genetic disease and as such can be inherited or passed on in a family. It is inherited as an X-linked recessive trait. A complete explanation of how X-linked recessive traits are inherited is beyond the scope of this chapter, but can be found in the chapter on Inheritance. It is important to understand the type of inheritance so that families can understand why a child has been affected, the risk that subsequent children may be affected, and the implications for other members of the family.

Under certain circumstances it is possible to test the female siblings (sisters) of an X-Linked Agammaglobulinemia patient to determine if they are carriers of the disease. Carriers of X-Linked Agammaglobulinemia have no symptoms, but have a 50 percent chance of transmitting the disease to their sons (see chapter on Inheritance). In some instances, it is also possible to determine if a fetus of a carrier female will be born with X-Linked Agammaglobulinemia. At the present time, these tests are being performed in only a few research laboratories but should soon be more widely available.

Treatment

At the present time, there is no way to cure patients who have X-Linked Agammaglobulinemia. The defective gene cannot be repaired or replaced, nor can maturation of pre-B-lymphocytes to B-lymphocytes and plasma cells be induced. However, patients with X-Linked Agammaglobulinemia can be given some of the antibodies that they are lacking. The antibodies are supplied in the form of gamma globulins (or immunoglobulins).

As discussed previously, once B-lymphocytes mature and become plasma cells which produce antibodies, the antibodies are released into the bloodstream. In order to prepare antibodies which can be given to agammaglobulinemia patients, blood is collected from large numbers of healthy normal individuals. The red and white blood cells are removed, and the gamma globulin fraction of the serum is separated by a series of chemical purification steps. The purified gamma globulin fraction contains antibodies, primarily of the IgG class. Until a few years ago, the gamma globulin preparations could only be given to patients by injection into the muscle (intramuscularly). Recently, however, preparations of gamma globulins have been produced that can be safely given directly into the bloodstream (intravenously). (See also chapter on Specific Medical Therapy.)

The gamma globulin preparations contain antibodies which substitute for the antibodies which the X-Linked Agammaglobulinemia patient can not make himself. They contain antibodies to wide varieties of microorganisms. Gamma globulin is particularly effective in preventing the spread of infections into the bloodstream and to deep body tissues or organs.

Recurrent or chronic infections, both bacterial and viral, occur in some patients with X-Linked Agammaglobulinemia despite the use of gamma globulin. In these patients, it may be necessary to obtain specimens of sputum, stool, or occasionally the infected tissue itself. These specimens are cultured in the laboratory in order to identify exactly which microorganisms are responsible for causing the infection. The culture results will guide the specific course of therapy, which may include antibiotics.

Finally, patients with X-Linked Agammaglobulinemia should not receive any live viral vaccines, such as live polio, or the measles, mumps, rubella (MMR) vaccine. Although uncommon, it is possible that live vaccines in agammaglobulinemia patients can transmit the diseases which they were designed to prevent.

Expectations

Most X-Linked Agammaglobulinemia patients who are receiving gamma globulin on a regular basis will be able to lead relatively normal lives. They do not need to be isolated. Infections may require some extra attention from time to time, but children with X-Linked Agammaglobulinemia can participate in all regular school and extra-curricular activities. A full active lifestyle is to be encouraged.

Chapter 7

Selective IgA Deficiency

Individuals with Selective IgA Deficiency have the B-lymphocytes which normally produce IgA. However, apparently the B-lymphocytes are unable to change into IgA producing plasma cells. It is possible that there are a variety of causes for Selective IgA Deficiency and that the cause may be different from patient to patient.

Definition

Selective IgA Deficiency is the total absence or severe deficiency of the IgA class of immunoglobulins in the blood serum and secretions. In order to understand Selective IgA Deficiency, it is first necessary to review some basic information about the human immune system.

In blood, there are five types (classes) of immunoglobulins or antibodies; IgG, IgA, IgM, IgD, IgE. The immunoglobulin class present in the largest amounts in blood is IgG, followed by IgM and IgA. IgD and IgE are present in very small amounts in the blood. Of these immunoglobulin classes, it is primarily IgM and IgG that protect the bloodstream, body tissues, and internal organs from infection. It is also important that the body be protected at surfaces which come in close contact with the environment. These sites are the mucosal surfaces: the mouth and nose, the lungs, the throat, the gastrointestinal tract, the eyes, and the genitalia. In contrast to the other classes of antibodies, it is primarily the IgA antibody which is transported to secretions and which protects these mucosal surfaces from infection. These mucosal surfaces are also protected to some degree by the other antibody classes; IgG, IgM and IgE are also found at these sites in secretions but not in the same amount as is IgA. This is why IgA is known as the secretory antibody.

IgA has some special chemical characteristics. It is present in the secretions as two antibody molecules attached by a component called the J chain ("J" for "joining"). In order for these antibodies to be secreted, they must also be attached to another molecule called secretory component. The IgA unit that offers protection for the mucosal surfaces is, therefore, actually composed of two IgA molecules joined by the J chain and attached to the secretory piece.

Certain individuals do not produce IgA. They do, however, produce all the other antibody classes normally. In addition, the function of their T-cells, phagocytic cells and complement system are all normal or near normal. Hence, the condition is known as Selective IgA Deficiency.

The cause or causes of Selective IgA Deficiency are unknown. Individuals with Selective IgA Deficiency have B-lymphocytes which appear to be normal, but are unable to change into IgA producing plasma cells. It is possible that there are a variety of causes for Selective IgA Deficiency and that the cause may be different from patient to patient.

Clinical Features

Selective IgA Deficiency is the most common of the immunodeficiency diseases. Some studies have indicated that as many as one in every five hundred people have Selective IgA Deficiency. It is probable that many of these individuals have relatively mild clinical illnesses, are therefore not sick enough to be seen by a doctor, and would not normally be found to have IgA deficiency. Thus, there are large numbers of individuals with Selective IgA Deficiency who are relatively healthy and free of symptoms. In contrast, there are also a large number of individuals with Selective IgA Deficiency who have significant illnesses. To this date, it is not understood why some individuals with IgA deficiency have almost no illness at all while others will be sick. Recent studies however, suggest that some patients with IgA deficiency may be missing a fraction of their IgG (the IgG2 subclass) and this may explain why some patients with IgA deficiency are more susceptible to infection than others.

One of the most common presentations of IgA deficiency is recurrent infections. This is understandable in view of the fact that IgA protects mucosal surfaces from infections. Recurrent ear infections, sinusitis, and pneumonia are some of the more common presentations. Often these infections may become chronic, the infection may not completely clear with treatment, and patients may have to remain on antibiotics for longer than usual.

Another of the common presentations of IgA deficiency are allergies. The types of allergies may be quite varied. Asthma is one of the common allergic diseases that may occur with Selective IgA Deficiency. It has been suggested that asthma in this situation tends to be more severe and may not respond as well to therapy as does asthma in normal individuals. Another type of allergy that may be associated with IgA deficiency is food allergy, in which patients may have reactions to certain foods. Symptoms associated with this may be diarrhea or abdominal cramping. It is not certain whether there is an increased incidence of allergic rhinitis (hay fever) or eczema in Selective IgA Deficiency.

There is another unusual, but important, form of allergy that can also occur in IgA deficiency. In people whose blood contains no IgA, the IgA itself is recognized by the body as a foreign protein. Since antibodies are normally made against foreign proteins, some people with Selective IgA Deficiency will make an IgG or IgE antibody against IgA. In this situation, if an IgA deficient person who has antibodies against IgA receives a blood product which has IgA in it, a massive allergic reaction can result. It is important, therefore, that any patient with Selective IgA Deficiency be aware of the potential risk in receiving blood products.

Another major problem in IgA deficiency is autoimmune disease. Autoimmune disease occurs when the patient produces antibodies to their own tissues. As a result, patients with autoimmune diseases can cause damage to some of their own organs or tissues. There are a variety of autoimmune diseases that are associated with Selective IgA Deficiency. Some of the more frequent diseases that have been observed included Rheumatoid Arthritis and Systemic Lupus Erythematosus. These autoimmune diseases may present in the form of sore and swollen joints of the hands or knees, a rash on the face, anemia (a low red blood cell count) or thrombocytopenia (a low platelet count). Other forms of autoimmune disease may affect the endocrine system, the blood forming organs, and the gastrointestinal system.

Diagnosis

The diagnosis of Selective IgA Deficiency is usually first suspected because of either chronic or recurrent infections, allergies, autoimmune diseases, or chronic diarrhea.

The diagnosis of Selective IgA Deficiency is usually established when appropriate blood tests are performed. The patient's blood serum demonstrates either a marked reduction or near absence of IgA. In contrast, the other classes of immunoglobulins (IgG, IgM, IgE and IgD) are normal as is their function as antibodies. An occasional patient may also have IgG2 subclass deficiency (see chapter on IgG Subclass Deficiency). In addition, the numbers and functions of T-cells are normal.

Several general tests which also may be important include a complete blood count, measurement of lung function, and a urinalysis. Other tests that may be specifically indicated in certain patients may include measurement of thyroid function, measurements of absorption of nutrients by the gastrointestinal tract, measurements of the kidney's function, and measurements for special antibodies directed against the body's own tissues.

Treatment

Unfortunately, the currently available preparations of gamma globulin do not contain IgA. Even if such products could be prepared, there is no method of causing IgA administered by injection to find its way to the mucous membranes which lack this immunoglobulin. Therefore, it is not possible to replace IgA in IgA deficient patients. An occasional patient who has IgA deficiency also has IgG2 subclass deficiency. In these cases the use of replacement gammaglobulin may be helpful in diminishing the frequency of infections (see also chapter on Specific Medical Therapy).

Treatment of the problems associated with Selective IgA Deficiency should be directed towards that particular problem. In patients who have chronic or recurrent infections, it is appropriate to administer antibiotics. The antibiotic therapy should ideally be directed at the specific organism causing the infection. It is not always possible to identify these organisms, however, and the use of broad spectrum antibiotics may be necessary. Certain patients who have chronic sinusitis or chronic bronchitis may need to stay on long term therapy with antibiotics. It is important that the doctor and the patient communicate closely so that appropriate decisions can be reached for this kind of therapy.

There are a variety of therapies for the treatment of autoimmune diseases. There are several anti-inflammatory drugs, such as aspirin, which help in the diseases which cause joint inflammation. Autoimmune diseases involving the blood system may require steroids in order to relieve the disease process. If autoimmune disease has resulted in an abnormality of the endocrine system, replacement therapy with hormones may be necessary. The treatment of the allergy associated with IgA deficiency is similar to that of treatment of allergies in general. It may be necessary to treat these problems especially aggressively in Selective IgA Deficiency. It is not known whether immunotherapy (allergy shots) is helpful in the allergies associated with Selective IgA Deficiency.

As a matter of precaution, it may also be desirable to test the blood for antibodies against IgA in the eventuality that a patient may need a blood transfusion.

The most important aspect of therapy in IgA deficiency, as it is in all the immunodeficiency diseases, is close communication between the family and the physician so that problems can be treated as soon as they arise.

Expectations

Although Selective IgA Deficiency is one of the milder forms of immunodeficiency, it may result in very severe disease in certain people. Therefore, it is difficult to predict the long term outcome in a given patient with Selective IgA Deficiency. In general, the prognosis in Selective IgA Deficiency depends on the prognosis of the associated diseases. It is important for physicians to continually assess and reevaluate patients with Selective IgA Deficiency for the existence of the associated diseases. The physician should be notified of anything unusual; especially fever, productive cough, skin rash or sore joints. The key to a good prognosis is good communication with the physician and the development of effective therapeutic strategies as soon as disease processes are recognized.

Chapter 8

Common Variable Immunodeficiency

Studies on the cells of the immune system in patients with Common Variable Immunodeficiency have shown that this disorder is not caused by a single defect. Some patients have few or non-functional B-lymphocytes, while others seem to lack the helper T-lymphocytes necessary for a normal antibody response. A third group seems to have excessive numbers of suppressor T-lymphocytes.

Definition

Common Variable Immunodeficiency is a disorder characterized by unusual infections and low levels of serum immunoglobulins (antibodies). It is a relatively common form of immunodeficiency—hence, the word "common"—and the degree and type of deficiency of serum immunoglobulins varies from patient to patient—hence, the word "variable." In some patients there is a decrease in just the IgG fraction of immunoglobulins, in others both IgG and IgA may be decreased, and still others all three major types (IgG, IgA and IgM) of immunoglobulins may be decreased. The clinical signs and symptoms also vary and may be severe in some, and mild in other patients. Frequent and unusual infections may first occur during infancy and childhood, during or after puberty, or even during the third or fourth decades of life.

©1987, 1993. Excerpted from *Patient and Family Handbook for the Primary Immune Deficiency Diseases.* Immune Deficiency Foundation. Reprinted with permission.

Most individuals with Common Variable Immunodeficiency present first with recurrent bacterial infections and, when tested show markedly decreased serum immunoglobulin levels and impaired antibody responses. Other names used for this disorder include "acquired" agammaglobulinemia, "adult onset" agammaglobulinemia, or "late onset" hypogammaglobulinemia. The term "acquired immunodeficiency" is now used to refer to a syndrome caused by the AIDS virus (HIV virus) and therefore should not be used for patients who have Common Variable Immunodeficiency or other forms of primary immunodeficiency diseases. These two disorders are quite different. The cause or causes of Common Variable Immunodeficiency are largely unknown. Studies on the cells of the immune system in patients with Common Variable Immunodeficiency have shown that this disorder is not caused by a single defect in the patient's lymphocytes. Some patients have few or non-functional B-lymphocytes. Others seem to lack the helper T-lymphocytes necessary for a normal antibody response; this may be due to an inability of their helper T-lymphocytes to produce certain proteins (called lymphokines) which are necessary for B-lymphocyte development. A third group seems to have excessive numbers of suppressor T-lymphocytes. Unlike X-Linked Agammaglobulinemia, Common Variable Immunodeficiency is not inherited in a single, well-defined pattern. In some families, more than one member may be affected, while in others the disease does not appear to be inherited.

Clinical Presentation

Both males and females can have Common Variable Immunodeficiency. Although some patients may have symptoms in the first few years of life, many patients may not develop symptoms until the second or third decade, or even later.

The presenting features of most patients with Common Variable Immunodeficiency are recurrent infections involving the ears, sinuses, nose, bronchi and lungs. If the infections are severe and occur repeatedly, permanent damage to the bronchial tree may occur and a chronic disease of the bronchi (breathing tubes) will develop causing widening and scarring of these structures, known as bronchi ectasis. The organisms commonly found are bacteria that are widespread in the population and that may often cause pneumonia (Hemophilus influenzae, pneumococci, and staphylococci). The purpose of treatment is to prevent the recurrent lung infections and the accompanying chronic damage to lung tissue. Regular cough in the morning which produces yellow or green sputum suggest the presence of chronic infection or bronchiectasis (widening and inflammation of the bronchi).

Patients with Common Variable Immunodeficiency may also develop enlarged lymph nodes in the neck area or in the chest. This process may be due to an infection with mycoplasma, a bacteria-like microorganism that is more difficult to detect than ordinary bacteria. Some adult patients with Common Variable Immunodeficiency may experience dysuria and/or urethral discharge due to an infection with chlamydia.

Some patients with Common Variable Immunodeficiency who do not receive adequate gamma globulin replacement may develop a painful inflammation of one or more joints, a condition called polyarthritis. In the majority of the cases, the joint fluid does not contain bacteria. However, to be certain that the arthritis is not caused by a treatable infection, the joint fluid may need to be removed by needle aspiration and studied for the presence of bacteria. The typical arthritis associated with hypogammaglobulinemia may involve knees, ankles, elbows and wrists, sometimes the shoulders, and rarely the finger joints. The symptoms of joint inflammation usually disappear from patients as soon as adequate gamma globulin therapy is instituted. In some patients, however, arthritis may occur even when on gamma globulin replacement.

Gastrointestinal complaints are frequently reported by patients with hypogammaglobulinemia. They may experience abdominal pain, bloating, nausea, vomiting, diarrhea and weight loss. Careful evaluation of the digestive organs may reveal malabsorption of fat and certain sugars. If a small sample (biopsy) of the bowel mucosa is obtained, very characteristic changes can be seen. In some patients with digestive problems, a small parasite called Giardia lamblia has been identified in these biopsies and sometimes can be found in the stool samples. Eradication of these parasites by medication may eliminate the gastrointestinal symptoms.

Not only do patients with Common Variable Immunodeficiency have a depressed antibody response and low levels of antibody in their blood (hypogammaglobulinemia), but some of the antibodies that they do produce may also attack their own tissues (autoantibodies). These autoantibodies may attack and cause destruction of certain blood cells (e.g. red cells, white cells or platelets), or they may cause other disorders.

Patients with Common Variable Immunodeficiency do not have physical abnormalities unless complications have developed. Lymphoid tissue (such as tonsils and lymph glands) may be small or barely identifiable; however, some patients with Common Variable Immunodeficiency may have an enlarged spleen and lymph nodes. If chronic lung disease has developed, the patient may have a reduced ability to exercise and decreased vital capacity (the maximum amount of air that can be taken into the lung voluntarily). Involvement of the gastrointestinal tract may, in some instances, interfere with normal growth and lead to weight loss.

Diagnosis

Common Variable Immunodeficiency may be suspected in children and adults who have a history of recurrent infections involving ears, sinuses, bronchi, and lungs. The diagnosis is confirmed by finding a low level of serum immunoglobulins, usually including IgG, IgA and IgM. The latter two immunoglobulin classes may be completely absent in some patients or near normal in others. Patients who have received complete immunizations against polio, measles, diphtheria and tetanus will have very low or absent antibody levels to these microorganisms. Experimental vaccines, available in specialized laboratories, may be helpful in determining exactly how much (quantity) and what kind (quality) of antibody an individual can produce. In some instances, these tests will help the physician to decide if the patient can benefit from gamma globulin injections.

The number of T-lymphocytes can also be enumerated and their function tested in samples of blood. Normally, approximately 5-10 percent of the blood lymphocytes are B-lymphocytes and 60-70 percent are T-lymphocytes. With special laboratory techniques, it is possible to determine if B-lymphocytes can produce antibody in a test tube (tissue culture), and if T-lymphocytes are able to help the B-cells in this task. One can also determine if a patient has too many suppressor T-lymphocytes which may interfere with normal antibody production.

Inheritance

Because of the non-uniform nature of Common Variable Immunodeficiency, no clear pattern of inheritance has been observed. In most instances the family history is negative. However, on occasion more than one family member or a sibling may be affected.

Treatment

The treatment of Common Variable Immunodeficiency is similar to that of other B-cell defects, including X-Linked Agammaglobulinemia. In the absence of a significant T-lymphocyte defect, gamma globulin injections almost always bring clinical improvement. Gamma globulin is extracted from a large pool of human plasma consisting mostly of IgG and containing all the important antibodies present in the normal population. For many years, the gamma globulin available had to be given intramuscularly because severe side effects occurred if it was injected directly into the veins. More recently, the immunoglobulin fraction obtained from large plasma pools has been modified by various methods so that it can be used for intravenous use. (See also chapter on Specific Medical Therapy.)

Those patients with chronic sinusitis or chronic lung disease may require long term treatment with broad spectrum antibiotics such as ampicillin, tetracycline, cephalosporin, trimethoprim/sulfamethoxazole and others. If mycoplasma or chlamydia infections are suspected, erythromycin or tetracycline may be indicated. If bronchiectasis has developed, physical therapy and daily postural drainage may be needed to remove the secretions and pus from the lungs and bronchi. Patients with gastrointestinal symptoms and malabsorption should be evaluated for the presence of Giardia lamblia, rotavirus and a variety of other infections. Most patients with immunodeficiency and arthritis respond favorably to adequate treatment with gamma globulin.

Expectations

Gamma globulin replacement combined with antibiotic therapy have greatly improved the outlook of patients with Common Variable Immunodeficiency. The aim of the treatment is to keep the patient from getting infections and to prevent the development of chronic lung disease. The outlook for patients with Common Variable Immunodeficiency depends to some extent on how much damage to their lungs and other organs has already occurred and how successfully infections can be prevented in the future by using gammaglobulin and antibiotic therapy.

Chapter 9

Severe Combined Immunodeficiency

There are at least three causes of SCID. In some patients the helper T-lymphocytes are absent or function poorly. In others, the thymus gland is absent or functions poorly. In another group the bone marrow stem cells from which the mature T- and B-lymphocytes develop are defective or absent.

Severe Combined Immunodeficiency (SCID, pronounced "skid") is a disease in which there is a severe defect (hence "severe") in both the T-lymphocyte and B-lymphocyte systems (hence "combined") causing a marked susceptibility to infections. Severe Combined Immunodeficiency Disease is generally considered to be the most serious of the primary immunodeficiency diseases. In the usual case, the onset of infections is in the first few months of life, the infections are severe and complicated, and the child quite ill.

There are at least three causes of SCID:

1.   The helper T-lymphocytes are absent or function poorly.

2.   The thymus gland is absent or functions poorly.

3.   The bone marrow stem cells from which the mature T- and B-lymphocytes develop are defective or absent.

Two kinds of lymphocytes must work together in order to develop a strong effective immune system capable of protecting an individual from infection (see chapter on Understanding the Immune System). These cells are the T-lymphocyte and the B-lymphocyte. A specialized type of T-lymphocyte, the helper T-lymphocyte helps both T- and B-lymphocytes to function normally in the immune response and thereby is critical in the defense against infection. If helper T-lymphocyte cells are absent or ineffective, neither the T-lymphocyte nor the B-lymphocyte systems function normally.

Another cause of SCID is an absence or poor function of the thymus gland. The thymus gland is the organ in which immature lymphocytes from the bone marrow mature and "learn" how to become helper T-lymphocytes, suppressor T-lymphocytes, or killer T-lymphocytes. If the thymus is not working properly, no mature T-lymphocytes are generated. As mentioned above, in the absence of T-lymphocytes, the immune system never functions normally. Not only does the T-lymphocyte system function poorly, but because there are no helper T-lymphocytes, the B-lymphocyte system also functions poorly.

Finally, the original source of the T- and B-lymphocytes may be defective. The mature T- and B-lymphocytes are derived from very immature cells of the bone marrow called stem cells. In some forms of SCID, bone marrow stem cells are missing.

The exact cause or causes of the deficiencies of the cell types mentioned above is usually not known. In general, one can only say that an error was made in the way the fetal development occurred. In some varieties of SCID, however, an important biochemical component (an enzyme) is missing from the lymphocytes. These varieties of SCID are known as enzyme deficiencies. A deficiency of the enzyme adenosine deaminase (ADA) is the cause of approximately 30 percent of the cases of SCID. Another closely related enzyme, purine nucleoside phosphorylase (PNP), causes a severe T-lymphocyte deficiency while the B-lymphocytes may be nearly normal. Each of these enzyme deficiencies causes immunodeficiency by allowing metabolic poisons to accumulate in the lymphocytes. Normally, these enzymes help the cell to clear the waste products it generates as the cell performs its functions. When these waste products are not removed, they poison the cells and the cells gradually die. In adenosine deaminase deficiency, both the T-lymphocytes and B-lymphocytes are affected. In purine nucleoside phosphorylase deficiency, the B-lymphocytes seem to be able to withstand the defect better than the T-lymphocytes. Since in some cases the enzyme deficiency is mild, and also because the process takes time, some children with adenosine deaminase deficiency or purine nucleoside phosphorylase deficiency may become ill at a later age.

Clinical Presentation

An excessive number of infections is the most common presenting symptom of children with SCID. However, the infections are not usually the same sorts of infections that normal children have, e.g., frequent colds. The infections of the child with SCID are usually much more serious and may even be life threatening; these may include pneumonia, meningitis or bloodstream infections.

Infections in children with SCID may be caused by the organisms that cause infections in normal children, or they may be caused by organisms which are usually not harmful in children who have normal immunity. Among the most dangerous is the chicken pox virus (varicella). Although chicken pox is annoying and causes much discomfort in healthy children, it usually is limited to the skin and mucous membranes and resolves in a matter of days. In the child with SCID, it may be fatal because it infects the lung and often the brain. Cytomegalovirus (CMV), which nearly all of us carry in our saliva glands, may cause fatal pneumonia in children with SCID. Other dangerous viruses for these children are the cold sore virus (Herpes Simplex) and the regular measles virus (rubeola). Pneumonia due to pneumocystis carinii can also be a serious problem in children with SCID.

Fungal (yeast) infections may be very difficult to treat. As an example, mouth thrush (candida) is common in most babies, and usually disappears with simple oral medication. In contrast, for the child with SCID, oral thrush persists despite all medication. The diaper area may also be involved.

Persistent diarrhea is also a very common problem in children with SCID. It may lead to severe weight loss and malnutrition. The diarrhea may be caused by the same bacteria, viruses or parasites which affect normal children. In the case of SCID, the organisms are very difficult to get rid of once they become established.

The skin may also be involved in children with SCID. The skin may become chronically infected with the same fungus (candida) that infects the mouth and causes thrush. In some cases, severe eczema can also be seen.

Diagnosis

The diagnosis is usually first suspected in children with the above clinical features. One of the easiest tests performed is to count the lymphocytes in a blood smear. There are usually over 1,200 lymphocytes (per cubic millimeter) in normal blood. SCID children usually have many fewer than this number. However, some children with SCID can have normal numbers of lymphocytes.

More complicated tests are usually necessary to make the diagnosis. The different types of lymphocytes can be identified with special stains and counted. In this way, the number of total T-lymphocytes, B-lymphocytes, helper T-lymphocytes, and killer T-lymphocytes can be counted.

Even if the patient has normal numbers of lymphocytes, they may not function normally. To test the function of lymphocytes, they are placed in test tubes and treated with various stimulants. Normal lymphocytes react when treated in this manner. In contrast, lymphocytes from patients with SCID usually do not react to the stimulus. In older children, skin tests can be used. Placing antigens from certain yeasts or bacteria into the superficial layers of the skin will cause redness and swelling in 24 to 48 hours—like a TB skin test. A positive reaction shows T-lymphocytes to be present and functioning normally.

Immunoglobulin levels are usually very low in SCID. Most commonly, all immunoglobulin classes are depressed (i.e. IgG, IgA and IgM).

The diagnosis of SCID can also be made in utero (before the baby is born). Enzyme deficiency (ADA and PNP) can be determined by amniocentesis where a small amount of fluid (which contains fetal cells) is removed from the uterine cavity. Enzyme deficiencies can be detected in any of the baby's cells. It is not necessary to test lymphocytes directly; amniotic fluid cells can be used. In other types of SCID, the diagnosis must be made from testing of the T- and B-lymphocytes. When the pregnancy is sufficiently advanced, a sample of blood can be obtained directly from the baby and testing of the lymphocytes performed. The tests which require blood from the fetus are very specialized, require great skill and experience, and present some risk to the fetus.

Inheritance

Most cases of SCID are inherited. In some families SCID is inherited as an autosomal recessive disease, while in other families the disease is inherited as a sex-linked disease. A complete explanation of how SCID is inherited is beyond the scope of this chapter and the reader should turn to the chapter on Inheritance in order to understand how autosomal recessive and sex-linked recessive diseases are inherited, the risks for having other children with the disease, and how these patterns of inheritance affect other family members. Parents should seek genetic counseling so that they are fully aware of the future risks.

It should be emphasized that there is no right or wrong decision about having more children. The decision must be made in light of the special factors involved in the family structure, the basic philosophy of the parents, their religious beliefs and background, their concept of the impact of the illness upon their lives and the lives of all the members of the family—countless factors, all of which are different for each family.

General Treatment

Children with serious chronic diseases need all the support and love that parents can provide. They must tolerate repeated hospitalizations which, in turn, are usually associated with many painful procedures. Parents need to call upon all their inner resources to learn to handle the anxiety and stress of this devastating problem. They must have well defined and useful coping mechanisms and support groups. Although the demands on the time and energies of the parents by the patient with SCID are overwhelming, if there are siblings, the parents must remember that they need to share their parents' love and care also. The parents also need to spend energy in maintaining their own relationship with each other. If the stress of the child's illness and treatment destroys the family structure, a successful therapeutic outcome for the patient is a hollow victory indeed.

The child with SCID needs to be isolated from children outside the family, especially those of school age. If there are siblings who attend school, the possibility of bringing chicken pox into the home represents the greatest danger. The parents need to alert the school authorities as to this danger, so that they can be notified when chicken pox is in the school. If the siblings have had chicken pox, there is no danger. If they have not, and if they have had a high grade exposure, they should live in another house during the incubation period. A high grade exposure is the close contact of the sibling (same reading table, eating together, playing together) with a child who breaks out in the "pox" anytime within 72 hours of that exposure. If the sibling breaks out with "pox" at home and exposes the patient, the patient should receive varicella immunoglobulin. Children who have been vaccinated with live polio vaccine may excrete live virus which could be dangerous to the SCID patient. Therefore, children who come in contact with the patient (such as siblings) should receive the killed polio vaccine.

Usually, the child with SCID should not be taken to public places (day care nurseries, church nurseries, shopping centers, etc.). Contact with relatives should be limited, especially with small children. Usually neither elaborate isolation procedures, nor the wearing of masks or gowns by the parents are indicated at home. Hand washing is essential, however.

Although no special diets are helpful, nutrition is nevertheless very important. In some instances, the child with SCID cannot absorb his food normally, which in turn can lead to poor nutrition. As a result, in some instances the child may need continuous intravenous feedings to maintain normal nutrition. Sick children generally have poor appetites, so maintaining good nutrition may not be possible in the usual fashion. (See chapter on General Care Nutrition.)

Infection with *Pneumocystis carinii*, a rare protozoan which causes pneumonia primarily in immune deficient patients, used to be a serious problem and frequent cause of death in patients with SCID. However, if these children are given prophylactic (preventing) doses of trimethoprim-sulfamethoxazole, they are protected from this infection. Therefore, all children with SCID should receive prophylaxis with trimethoprim-sulfamethoxazole until the defect in their immune system has been corrected.

LIVE VIRUS VACCINES ARE DANGEROUS. If you or your doctor suspects that your child has a serious immunodeficiency, you should not allow mumps, measles or polio vaccination until his or her immune status has been evaluated. As mentioned above, the patient's siblings should not receive live virus vaccines either. Gamma globulin (immunoglobulin) replacement therapy should also be given. Although the gamma globulin will not restore the function of the deficient T-cells, it does replace the B-cell deficiency and is therefore of some benefit.

Specific Therapy

The most successful therapy for SCID is bone marrow transplantation. Bone marrow transplantations are usually performed at medical centers which have specialized facilities. In a bone marrow transplant, bone marrow cells from a normal donor are given to the immunodeficient patient to replace the deficient cells of the patient's immune system with the normal cells of the donor's immune system. The results of hundreds of matched transplants in SCID have yielded an overall success rate of approximately 65 percent. The major factor which determines a successful outcome is the health of the patient at the time of the transplant and the presence of a normal donor with a good tissue match.

Recently, new techniques have been developed that allow bone marrow transplants from close relatives that are only a partial tissue match. Comparison studies show the results of these transplants to be nearly as good as those from completely matched donors. The details of selecting a suitable donor, the indications for a bone marrow transplantation, and the outcome of the procedure can be found in the chapter on Specific Medical Therapy.

For patients with SCID due to adenosine deaminase (ADA) deficiency, treatment with a modified form of the ADA enzyme has been used with some success. In addition, the possibility of gene therapy is nearing reality. The gene for ADA has been inserted into the T-lymphocytes of patients with ADA deficiency. These T-lymphocytes that have undergone "gene therapy" have been reinfused into the ADA deficient patients and have produced improvement in their T-lymphocyte functions.

Expectations

Severe Combined Immunodeficiency Disease is generally considered to be the most serious of the primary immunodeficiency diseases. Without a successful bone marrow transplant, the patient is at constant risk for a severe or even fatal infection. With a successful bone marrow transplantation, however, the patient's own defective immune system is replaced with a normal immune system and normal immune function is restored. The procedure is successful in approximately two thirds of patients. The first bone marrow transplantation for SCID was performed in 1968. That patient was alive and well the day this article was first published.

Chapter 10

Chronic Granulomatous Disease

Definition

Chronic Granulomatous Disease (CGD) is a genetically determined (inherited) disease characterized by an inability of the patient's phagocytic cells to kill certain microorganisms. As a result of their defect in phagocytic cell killing, these patients have an increased susceptibility to infection by certain bacteria and fungi.

The term "phagocytic cell" is a general term used to describe any white blood cell in the body that can "phagocytose" or ingest, microorganisms. In general, there are two main categories of phagocytic cells, or phagocytes:

1. polymorphonuclear leukocytes (also called neutrophils or granulocytes) and

2. mononuclear phagocytes (also called monocytes when in the blood and macrophages when in tissues).

Very complex interactions are necessary for normal function of phagocytic cells. First, the phagocyte must be able to migrate to the site of microbial invasion, whether that be under the skin, under a mucous membrane, or in an internal organ such as the lung or liver. Then the phagocyte ingests the microorganism, and brings it into the interior of the cell. After ingestion, a series of complex interactions, including metabolic and mechanical changes, are needed within the phagocyte in order for the cell to kill the bacteria or fungus.

Although phagocytic cells from patients with Chronic Granulomatous Disease can move normally and ingest microorganisms normally, they are unable to kill certain bacteria and fungi because of an abnormal metabolism within the cell. Hydrogen peroxide and other oxygen-containing compounds are produced during phagocytosis in normal phagocytes. These oxygen compounds are needed to kill certain bacteria and fungi once these microorganisms are inside the phagocytic cells. Patients with Chronic Granulomatous Disease have an inability of their phagocytic cells to process oxygen properly and create the oxygen containing compounds needed for killing. As a result, these patients lack an important mechanism of phagocytic cell killing of certain bacteria. Bacterial species such as staphylococci and serratia frequently cause infections in CGD patients because they are not killed by CGD phagocytic cells. Some bacterial species, however, such as the pneumococcus and streptococcus produce hydrogen peroxide. When these organisms are ingested by the phagocytic cells of patients with Chronic Granulomatous Disease, the microbe contributes its own hydrogen peroxide to the defective cell, the defect is circumvented, and the cells can kill these organisms. As a result, patients with Chronic Granulomatous Disease do not have an increased susceptibility to infection with these organisms. They are only susceptible to organisms, such as staphylococci, which can not produce hydrogen peroxide and other oxygen-containing compounds. Patients with Chronic Granulomatous Disease have normal antibody production, normal T-cell function, and a normal complement system; in short, the rest of their immune system is normal.

Clinical Presentation

Children with CGD are normally healthy at birth. However, CGD is a syndrome which is usually recognized during childhood. Less than 30 percent have infectious problems before three months of age. Approximately 80 percent of patients have unusually frequent or unusually severe infections before the second year of life. When infections do occur, they may be caused by staphylococci or by an unusual bacterial species.

Most infections result in the formation of granulomas, or localized, swollen collections of infected tissue. These may sometimes cause obstruction, i.e. blockage of the intestine and urinary tract, and surgical treatment may be required. In general, granulomas may require a prolonged course of intravenous antibiotic therapy before resolution is complete.

Infections may involve any organ system or tissue of the body, but usually the skin, lungs, lymph nodes, liver, or bones are involved. Infected lesions may have prolonged drainage, delayed healing and residual scarring.

Pneumonia is a recurrent problem in patients with Chronic Granulomatous Disease. In some instances, patients may develop lung abscesses. Many of the lung infections are chronic. Lymph node enlargement may be the first physical sign of CGD, and lymph glands in the neck, axilla or groin may be affected. The liver is enlarged in many young children with CGD, and liver abscesses can occur. Osteomyelitis (bone infections) frequently involve the small bones of the hands and feet. Although prolonged therapy is necessary, complete healing and return of function is the rule.

Diagnosis

The diagnosis of Chronic Granulomatous Disease is usually first suspected because of serious infections at an early age. These infections may be rather ordinary lesions with unusual bacterial species, or quite unusual lesions with ordinary bacterial species. Abscess lesions of the liver, perianal regions and small bones of hand and feet are examples of unusual lesions. Examples of unusual microbial species causing infections in CGD patients are *Serratia*, *Nocardia*, and *Aspergillus*.

The diagnosis of Chronic Granulomatous Disease is made by analyzing the metabolic function and killing capacity of the patient's phagocytic cells. Blood from CGD patients is obtained and the phagocytes are isolated. A number of tests can then be performed to test the metabolic machinery of the cell and determine if the patient's cells can metabolize oxygen correctly and produce hydrogen peroxide and other oxygen-containing compounds. Confirmation of a diagnosis of CGD is often done by measuring the capacity of the phagocytes for intracellular killing of staphylococci or other bacteria. These tests are usually done in specialized laboratories to confirm a diagnosis of CGD.

Inheritance Pattern

Chronic Granulomatous Disease is a genetic disease and therefore can be inherited or passed on in families. Although CGD most commonly occurs in males, approximately 30 percent of CGD patients are girls. There are two genetic patterns for transmission of CGD. One form of the disease is inherited in a sex-linked recessive manner; i.e. is carried on the sex chromosome or "X" chromosome (see chapter on Inheritance). Another form of the disease is inherited in an autosomal recessive fashion.

A complete discussion of the manner of inheritance of either X-Linked recessive or autosomal recessive disorders is beyond the scope of this chapter. The chapter on Inheritance covers both those patterns of inheritance in detail. It is important to understand the type of inheritance so that families can understand why a child has been affected, the risk that subsequent children may be affected, and the implications for other members of the family.

Treatment

A mainstay of therapy is the early diagnosis of infection and prompt, aggressive use of appropriate antibiotics. Empiric therapy with antibiotics aimed at the most likely offending organisms is often necessary while waiting for results of cultures. A careful search for the cause of infection is important so that sensitivity of the microorganism to antibiotics can be determined. Intravenous antibiotics are usually necessary for treating serious infections in CGD patients and clinical response may be delayed in spite of appropriate antibiotics.

Granulocyte transfusions may be helpful for some CGD patients when aggressive antibiotic and surgical therapy are failing in life-threatening infections.

Patients with CGD have such frequent infections, especially as young children, that continuous oral antibiotics (prophylaxis) is often recommended. CGD patients who receive prophylactic antibiotics may have infection-free periods and intervals between serious infections may be prolonged. The most frequently recommended agent for prophylaxis is a combination of trimethoprim-sulfamethoxazole. Patients allergic to sulfa may be given trimethoprim without sulfamethoxazole.

A recently completed international clinical trial showed that when a natural product of the immune system, gamma interferon, was given to patients with CGD they had fewer serious infections and when infections did occur their length of hospital stay was shortened. It appears that gamma interferon will significantly improve the clinical course of patients with CGD (see chapter on Therapy).

Since early treatment of infections is very important, patients are usually urged to consult their physicians about even minor infections.

Many physicians suggest that swimming should probably be confined to well-chlorinated pools since fresh water lakes and salt water swimming may expose patients to organisms which are not virulent for normal swimmers but may be infectants for CGD patients. Aspergillus is present in most samples of marijuana, so CGD patients should be discouraged from smoking "pot." Patients should also avoid dusty conditions, especially spoiled or moldy grass and hay.

Expectations

The quality of life for many CGD patients has improved remarkably with knowledge of the phagocytic cell abnormality and appreciation of the need for early, aggressive antibiotic therapy when infections occur. Recurrent hospitalizations may be required in CGD patients since multiple tests are often necessary to locate the exact site and cause of infections, and intravenous antibiotics are usually needed for treatment of serious infections.

Disease-free intervals are increased by prophylactic antibiotics and treatment with gamma interferon. Serious infections tend to occur less frequently when patients reach their teenage years. Some of the first patients identified with CGD have completed high school, attended college, and are carrying on relatively normal lives.

A Question and Answer Guide
for CGD Patients and Their Families

Source: NIH Pub. *Chronic Granulomatous Disease: A Guide for CGD Patients and Their Families.* Prepared by the NIAID. Office of Communications. National Institute of Allergy and Infectious Diseases, Division of Intramural Research.

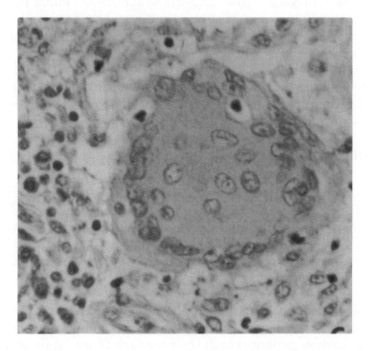

Figure 10.1. Granuloma (large gray area) in photomicrograph of lung tissue.

How is CGD diagnosed?

Recurrent infections with certain kinds of bacteria or fungi are the first clue of CGD. To confirm the diagnosis, the doctor will usually request a blood test called the nitroblue tetrazolium dye reduction test (NBT). This test indicates how well the patient's phagocytes metabolize oxygen (as in the respiratory burst described previously). If the patient has CGD, the NBT will indicate an abnormal respiratory burst. Tests of phagocyte killing of bacteria may also be performed.

Once the diagnosis is made, special X-rays, blood, and urine tests may be done to establish baseline conditions. Knowing the baseline condition can be very helpful in understanding future problems, should they occur.

What types of infections are common in CGD?

Some bacteria and fungi generate their own hydrogen peroxide, which phagocytes can use to kill the microbes themselves. Other invaders quickly destroy any hydrogen peroxide they produce so that scavenger cells cannot do their job. This latter group of microorganisms, which includes common bacteria such as *Staphylococcus aureus*, *Salmonella*, and *Pseudomonas*, and fungi such as *Aspergillus*, causes many of the troublesome infections in CGD patients.

Although these bacteria and fungi can cause infections virtually anywhere in the body, they most often target the lungs, lymph nodes, skin, liver, gastrointestinal tract, nostrils, mouth, or bones in the arms and legs.

Common signs and symptoms of these infections are diarrhea, boils (frequently in the nostrils), oozing or scaly skin and scalp rashes, canker sores, gum disease, sores near the anus, local areas of pain and tenderness, swollen lymph nodes, fever, persistent cough, and nutritional deficiencies stemming from malabsorption.

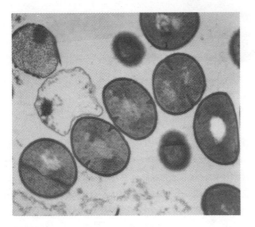

Figure 10.2. Staphylococcus aureus bacteria (photomicrograph), a common cause of CGD infections.

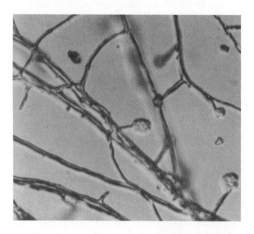

Figure 10.3. *Acremonium strictum (photomicrograph), a fungus that can cause lung infection in CGD patients, almost ever affects people with normal immune function.*

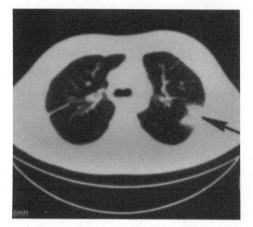

Figure 10.4. *Cross-section of lung (seen on CAT scan) showing an acremonium strictum infection (arrow) in CGD patient.*

How often do these infections occur?

CGD patients who are treated preventively with antibiotics experience an average of one serious infection every three to four years. Susceptibility to major infections varies quite a bit between patients; some CGD patients go as long as five years without any major infections, whereas others experience more frequent infections. A person whose CGD gene defect is on the X chromosome will tend to experience more infections than one whose faulty gene resides on other chromosomes.

Many patients also experience frequent minor infections. About half of all CGD patients have chronic inflammation of the gums (gingivitis), and three-quarters have frequent canker sores. Although these infections are not life-threatening, they can be annoying and uncomfortable.

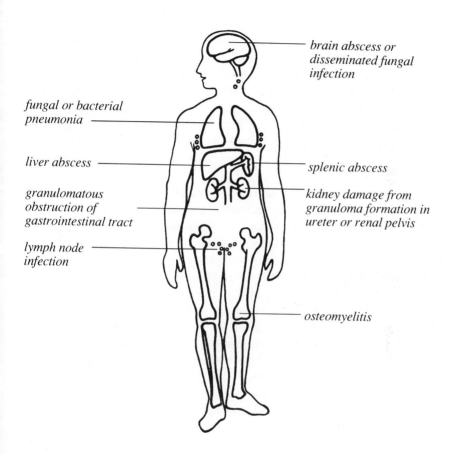

Figure 10.5. Common infection sites in CGD patients

Can CGD affect growth and development of children?

Some children with CGD have delayed growth and development. CGD children may be unusually short, with younger siblings passing them in height at an early age. However, almost all CGD children have a delayed growth spurt, occurring when other children have stopped growing. The average height of adults with CGD is the same as their parents.

What are the treatments for CGD?

Presently, the mainstay of CGD therapy is prompt and aggressive treatment of infections with appropriate antibiotics. In addition, many patients are given oral antibiotics prophylactically (as a preventive measure) to reduce the number and severity of infections.

A recently completed international study carried out at multiple medical centers indicated that interferon-gamma, a substance produced by the body's immune system, reduces the number and severity of infections in patients with CGD. These studies were especially dramatic in children less than 10 years old. These are very exciting results, and, when interferon is given with prophylactic antibiotics, the outlook is particularly promising.

It is extremely important that physicians be contacted promptly for suspected problems so that treatments can be initiated early, thereby minimizing the extent and duration of required therapy. The more serious infections are treated with antibiotics given intravenously over a period of months, which may require a prolonged hospital stay. Such long-term therapy is necessary to prevent recurrences of the infection, which can happen if the drugs are stopped after a short period of time. Steroids and other anti-inflammatory drugs are sometimes given to shrink granulomas. It is often necessary to take a tissue sample surgically (biopsy) from an infected area to determine the cause of an infection. Sometimes infected tissue must be removed or drained if the infection is not responding to antibiotic therapy. Drainage tubes placed in the chest, abdomen or other sites must sometimes remain in place for several weeks. Patients usually stay in the hospital during that time.

If antibiotics and surgery do not effectively combat serious infections, or if an infection is rapidly worsening, patients may be given transfusions of white blood cells. These transfusions contain normal phagocytes that can help curb the infection. Because white blood cell transfusions can prompt some serious side effects that worsen with each transfusion, this technique cannot be used routinely to treat infections.

Patients often experience a loss of appetite during treatment. When this happens, they may be fed intravenously to ensure proper nourishment. Sometimes intravenous fluids are administered through a tube (often called a Hickman catheter) surgically inserted in the sub-clavian or jugular vein in the neck or chest. With proper training on how to use the catheter and with help from family members, patients may be able to be fed at home and avoid a long hospital stay. The catheter can also be used at home to administer antibiotics intravenously and for obtaining blood samples for laboratory evaluation. Even when a patient is well, it is advisable to have frequent blood and urine tests, X-rays, and scans so that any abnormalities can be detected early.

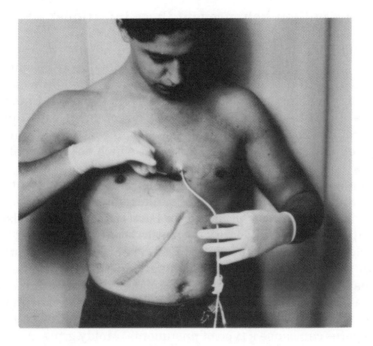

Figure 10.6. *Young CGD patient in daily cleaning of his Hickman catheter.*

Since early treatment of infections is important, patients should consult with their doctors even when experiencing minor symptoms. CGD patients should be on the lookout for the following signs of infection:

- a fever that lasts more than two days
- warm, tender, or swollen areas
- hard lumps
- sores with pus or rashes

- persistent cough or chest pain
- persistent abdominal pain
- diarrhea
- frequent or persistent headaches
- night sweats
- loss of appetite
- weight loss

How can a patient help prevent these infections?

Careful personal hygiene is important in helping to prevent minor skin and mouth infections. Although it has been recommended that CGD patients wash daily with povidine iodine scrub or hexachlorophene soaps, their skin is often very sensitive. Using harsh soaps can lead to dry skin, cracks, and breakdown with infection. Therefore, it is preferable to use a mild soap containing a high percentage of moisturizers or emollients, but which does not contain detergents or deodorants. Brushing teeth two times daily with a hydrogen peroxide and baking soda paste can limit the extent of gum disease and reduce the number of canker sores. Because dental or orthodontic procedures can introduce bacteria into the bloodstream, CGD patients should take oral antibiotics the day before and the day after undergoing such procedures. Cuts should be washed promptly with an antiseptic such as hydrogen peroxide. CGD patients should avoid using alcoholic beverages and tobacco, which can impair the immune system. In addition, they should not smoke marijuana because of the danger of inhaling mold spores the plant often harbors. These spores can cause a type of pneumonia. Moldy grass, mulch, and hay should also be avoided for the same reason.

It is important for patients to choose athletic activities that are least likely to result in scrapes and cuts, which might become infected.

To avoid a relapse of infection, it is essential for patients to take the full course of any prescribed antibiotics, even after symptoms have disappeared.

Children with CGD should receive the usual course of immunizations given to young children, including vaccines against polio, rubella, measles, and mumps. CGD patients are no more likely to develop viral infections or to have more serious viral infections than are other people.

How does CGD affect a person's quality of life?

Many people with CGD can carry on normal activities of daily life with a minimum of disruption. However, patients and their families should expect and be prepared for frequent and sometimes lengthy hospitalizations that may interfere with school or work. Many public school systems offer tutoring at home or in the hospital, which can help fill in the gaps in a child's education due to long absences from school. If a teenager with CGD is planning to go to college, he or she should choose one located near a university medical center that has physicians who are familiar with CGD.

For those patients who are unable to work steadily due to frequent illness, social security disability or welfare benefits are available.

Can CGD patients have children?

Women with CGD can become pregnant and have babies without adverse effects on their health. One potential problem for their babies, however, is that some of the drugs used to counter infections common in CGD patients can be passed from a pregnant woman to her fetus, and this may result in birth defects or miscarriage. Both women and men thinking of having children should consider the extent to which the frequency and severity of their infections would interfere with parenting responsibilities.

Genetic counseling is important for people who have CGD and want to start a family as well as for the parents of a child with CGD who are considering having another child. Blood tests together with family history can be used to assess the likelihood that a child will inherit the disease.

Prenatal tests done on amniotic fluid from the womb during the fourth month of pregnancy (amniocentesis) can determine whether the baby will have CGD.

What about the emotional strain CGD places on patients and their families?

Frequent life-threatening infections and lengthy hospital stays are stressful for both patients and their families. It is important for CGD patients and their parents to talk with a hospital social worker, who can arrange for needed therapy as well as arrange for tutoring or any other necessary community support services. Clinical social workers provide psychotherapy for patients coping with chronic illness. It is not unusual for patients and families affected by CGD to find themselves feeling afraid, angry, frustrated, or depressed. Parents of children with CGD may feel guilty about passing the disease on to their child or blame themselves for the infections their child experiences. Parents are also often torn between the needs of their child with CGD and the needs of their other children or the demands of their jobs. These competing demands can foster additional stress.

Siblings of children with CGD may become jealous of the attention given to the child who is sick. They may feel resentful and become increasingly demanding and dependent. Siblings should be encouraged to talk about their feelings and worries. Family counseling can help work through these and other problems that may arise among family members.

Patients and their families can participate in support groups for people whose lives are affected by chronic disease. Many hospitals offer support groups; if not, a hospital social worker may be able to locate such a group in the community.

Relaxation therapy can also help reduce stress. A number of relaxation techniques such as meditation, visual imagery, and therapeutic massage can relieve physical and emotional tension and promote a positive outlook. Many hospitals offer recreational therapy, such as crafts or playing musical instruments, that can make hospital stays more pleasant and help relieve boredom.

Additional resources are available to people with CGD and their families. (For further information, see the end of this chapter for organizations to contact.)

What are researchers finding about CGD?

Scientists are working to uncover the missing or defective genes and associated proteins that underlie CGD. This information can be used to develop more targeted approaches to therapy. Researchers may be able to develop drugs that either replace critical missing proteins or stimulate their production in cells. In the future, doctors may also be able to replace the defective genes in CGD patients' phagocytes with the correct ones.

How do phagocytes kill bacteria or fungi?

Normally, phagocytes envelope invading bacteria or fungi and kill them with hydrogen peroxide—key to the cell's defense mechanism.

Contact with an invading organism triggers many chemical reactions that lead to the production of hydrogen peroxide.

One of the initial reactions, conversion of glucose to water, causes release of excess electrons. Phagocytes have a special, four-protein enzyme system that picks up these excess electrons and combines them with oxygen, which was released from other chemical reactions in the cell. In the respiratory burst, the oxygen is converted to a highly energized form, called superoxide. It quickly reacts with water to form hydrogen peroxide. The hydrogen peroxide is changed by an enzyme into bleach. The bleach and the hydrogen peroxide kill the invading organisms.

Protein	% of CGD Cases	Mode of Inheritance	Group affected
1. cytochrome b, large subunit	60%	X-linked inheritance	males only
2. cytochrome b, small subunit	5%	autosomal-recessive	males and females
3. cytosol protein, 47K	30%	autosomal-recessive	males and females
4. cytosol protein, 65K	5%	autosomal-recessive	males and females

Table 10.1. Proteins Involved in Genetic Types of CGD.

What happens in CGD?

In CGD, one of the enzyme system's four proteins is either missing or defective. Therefore, the excess electrons do not combine with oxygen, no superoxide is made, and no hydrogen peroxide is produced. The phagocytes are unable to kill bacteria or fungi normally.

There are four genetically distinct types of CGD, each corresponding to an inherited abnormality of one of the four proteins (see table above). The autosomal recessive forms affect both males and females. Recent studies by NIAID scientists and others have identified a number of proteins that are missing in CGD patients. Although each protein plays a slightly different role, all are necessary for the respiratory burst, the process that is essential for phagocytes to perform their disease-fighting function. The X-linked form of CGD appears to be related to a special membrane protein, called cytochrome b558. The autosomal recessive form of the disease appears to involve defects in the cytosol, the fluid present inside the phagocyte itself. Two cytosol proteins have thus far been identified that play crucial roles in the respiratory burst.

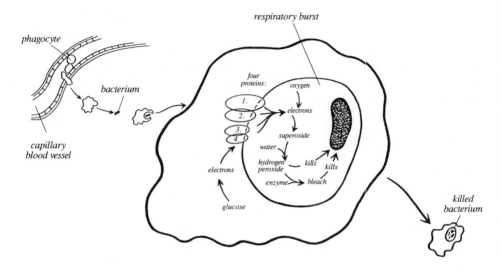

Figure 10.7.

Another experimental approach that has been tried in a few centers is bone marrow transplantation. By transfusing healthy bone marrow into a CGD patient, the specific defect of the immune system may be corrected. The major difficulties with this procedure today are the problem of rejection of the marrow by the recipient and the risk that the transplanted cells themselves may attack the donor recipient. An additional problem is the difficulty of finding suitable donors whose bone marrow is least likely to be rejected. In view of the potential complications of bone marrow transplantation, most physicians do not recommend this approach.

Recent achievements have moved scientists one step closer to their ultimate goal: to correct CGD by replacing the missing proteins or by replacing the defective genes with normal ones. NIAID scientists cloned the gene for one important protein involved in 85 percent of all autosomal recessive CGD and about one-third of all cases of CGD. In laboratory experiments, the protein made by the cloned gene restored normal function to patients' defective cells. Other investigators have identified and cloned the gene involved in X-linked CGD. It might one day be possible to replace defective CGD genes with ones that would allow phagocytes to manufacture the proteins needed to produce toxic oxygen compounds. Many questions remain about gene therapy, but both gene therapy and protein replacement therapy remain exciting prospects for the future of CGD treatment.

The rapid pace of immunologic research today brings hope that CGD and many other immune deficiency diseases will one day be conquered.

For Further Information

Many CGD patients and their families find it beneficial to keep informed about the advances made in understanding and treating CGD. The following organizations and publications may be helpful:

- The National Organization for Rare Disorders (NORD) provides newsletters, computer databases, and other information sources for a number of diseases including CGD. NORD's address is P.O. Box 8923, New Fairfield, Connecticut 06812. 1-800-999-6673

- A newsletter and publications on immune deficiency diseases are available from the Immune Deficiency Foundation, P.O. Box 586, Columbia, MD 21045.

- "The Immune System: How It Works," a booklet designed to help members of the general public understand the complexities of the immune system, can be obtained free by calling or writing the NIAID Office of Communications: 301/496-5717; Building 31, Room 7A-50. National Institutes of Health, Bethesda, MD 20892.

- Books on coping with chronic illness may be helpful and can be obtained from the public library.

Chapter 11

Ataxia-Telangiectasia

Definition

Ataxia-Telangiectasia is a primary immunodeficiency disease which affects a number of different organs in the body. It is characterized by:

1. Neurologic abnormalities resulting in an unsteady gait (Ataxia),

2. Dilated blood vessels (Telangiectasia) of the eyes and skin.

3. A variable immunodeficiency involving both cellular (T-lymphocyte) and humoral (B-lymphocytes) immune responses.

Clinical Presentation

The first presenting symptom is generally ataxia. Ataxia is a medical term used to describe an unsteady gait. It usually results from neurologic abnormalities affecting a part of the brain which controls balance. In Ataxia-Telangiectasia, it first becomes apparent when the child begins to walk, typically between 12 and 18 months of age. At this early point in time, many children are thought to have cerebral palsy or an undefined neurologic disorder and the specific diagnosis of Ataxia-Telangiectasia may not be made when symptoms first appear. Patients later develop abnormal spontaneous writhing movements of their arms and legs (choreoathetosis), jerking movements, and abnormalities in eye movements including rapidly alternating twitches of the eyes (nystagmus), difficulty in initiating voluntary eye movements (oculomotor apraxia), muscle weakness and difficulty in using the muscles needed for speech (dysarthria).

The dilated blood vessels (telangiectasia) usually become apparent after the ataxia, generally between 2 and 8 years of age. These telangiectasia usually occur first on the covering of the white portion of the eye (bulbar conjunctiva) and later on the ears, neck and extremities.

The last clinical feature which defines Ataxia-Telangiectasia, recurrent infections, is a major feature in many patients and may dominate the clinical picture. Infections most commonly involve the lungs and sinuses and are usually caused by bacteria or viruses. The infections are, at least in part, due to the variable immunodeficiency seen in Ataxia-Telangiectasia.

Patients with Ataxia-Telangiectasia may have defects in both their T-lymphocyte system and B-lymphocyte system. They may have modestly reduced lymphocyte numbers and a reduced number of peripheral blood T-lymphocytes which are defective in recognizing viral antigens. These abnormalities in T-cells are usually associated with an immature appearing thymus gland. With regard to B-lymphocytes and humoral immunity, patients produce some antibody responses against foreign antigens, such as microorganisms, but these responses are impaired, particularly anti-viral responses. These disordered antibody responses are associated with abnormal immunoglobulin levels—absent IgA in 70 percent of patients, absent IgE in 80 percent. IgG subclass deficiencies may also be found in some patients (see chapter on subclass deficiencies).

Diagnosis

The diagnosis of Ataxia-Telangiectasia is usually based on characteristic clinical findings and supported by laboratory tests. Once all of the clinical signs and symptoms of Ataxia-Telangiectasia have become obvious in an older child or young adult, the diagnosis is relatively easy. The most difficult time to diagnose Ataxia-Telangiectasia is during the period when neurologic symptoms are first apparent (early childhood) and the typical telangiectasias have not yet appeared. During this period, a history of recurrent infections and typical immunologic findings can be suggestive of the diagnosis. One of the most helpful laboratory tests used to assist in the diagnosis of Ataxia-Telangiectasia is the measurement of so-called "fetal proteins" in the blood. These are proteins which are usually produced during fetal development and may persist in some conditions (such as Ataxia-Telangiectasia) after birth. The vast majority of Ataxia-Telangiectasia patients (more than 99 percent) have elevated levels (greater than 20 ng/ml beyond 6 months of age) of serum alpha-fetoprotein. If other causes of elevations of alpha-fetoprotein can be ruled out, its elevation in the blood in association with characteristic signs and symptoms can make the diagnosis of Ataxia-Telangiectasia a virtual certainty. Patients also may have an increased frequency of spontaneous gaps and breaks in the chromosomes of their peripheral blood T-lymphocytes as well as an increased frequency of chromosomal rearrangements. Interestingly, these abnormalities involve the locations of some of the genes involved in T-cell function and immunoglobulin production.

Inheritance

Ataxia-Telangiectasia is inherited as an autosomal recessive disorder (see chapter on Inheritance). The gene responsible for the most common form of Ataxia-Telangiectasia has recently been mapped to the long arm of chromosome 11 at 11q22-23. Several other genes of immunologic interest, including those encoding part of the T-cell antigen receptor complex, are located near this location. Studies are currently underway in a number of centers to determine if X-ray sensitivity of cells cultured in test tubes can be used to detect the carrier state among asymptomatic family members of affected patients.

General Treatment

In general, treatment is largely supportive. Patients should be encouraged to participate in as many activities as possible. Children should be encouraged to attend school on a regular basis and receive support in attempting to maintain as normal a life style as possible. Physical and occupational therapists must be included in the treatment team to prevent the development of stiffness in muscles and to allow as much functional mobility as possible. A prompt diagnosis should be sought for all infections and specific therapy instituted for all suspected infections. The use of live viral vaccines should be avoided. Therapy with gamma globulin may be indicated in individuals with IgG subclass deficiencies who are having recurrent infections.

Specific Therapy

Specific therapy for Ataxia-Telangiectasia is not possible at the present time. The use of thymic transplants, thymic hormones, and bone marrow transplantation have not yet led to improvement in patients with Ataxia-Telangiectasia.

Expectations

In general, Ataxia-Telangiectasia pursues a progressive course. However, it must be stressed that the disease can be quite variable and it is difficult to predict the course in any given patient. Even within families, where the genetic defect should be the same, some children have predominantly neurologic difficulties whereas others have recurrent infections and other affected individuals may have relatively little of either for long periods of time. The course of the disease in most patients is usually characterized by progressive neurologic deterioration. Many patients are confined to a wheel chair in their teens or early twenties. Infections of the lungs (bronchitis or pneumonia) and sinuses (sinusitis) are common and may damage the lungs even if treated promptly. Malignancies or cancers are also more common in patients with Ataxia-Telangiectasia. The most common cancers affect the cells and tissues of the immune system.

It should be emphasized, however, that although the above course is the most typical, the course varies considerably from patient to patient. Some patients have survived into the fifth decade and some have been able to attend college and live independently.

Chapter 12

IgG Subclass Deficiency

Definition

Antibodies are made of proteins called immunoglobulins. There are five major types or classes of immunoglobulin (Ig): IgG, IgA, IgM, IgD and IgE. Most of the antibodies in the blood and the fluid that bathes the tissues and cells of the body are of the IgG class. The IgG class of antibodies is itself composed of four different subtypes of IgG molecules called the IgG subclasses. These are designated IgG1, IgG2, IgG3 and IgG4. Patients who suffer recurrent infections because they lack, or have very low levels of, one or two IgG subclasses, but whose other immunoglobulin levels are normal, are said to have a "selective IgG subclass deficiency"

While all the IgG subclasses are antibodies, each subclass serves somewhat different functions in protecting the body against infection. For example, the IgG1 and IgG3 subclasses are rich in antibodies against proteins such as the toxins produced by the diphtheria and tetanus bacteria, as well as antibodies against viral proteins. In contrast, antibodies against the polysaccharide (complex sugar) coating (capsule) of certain disease-producing bacteria (e.g. the *pneumococcus* and *Haemophilus influenzae*) are predominantly of the IgG2 type. Some of the IgG subclasses can cross the placenta very well and enter the unborn infant's bloodstream, while others do not. Antibodies of certain IgG subclasses interact readily with the complement system, while others interact poorly if at all with the complement proteins Thus, an inability to produce antibodies of a specific subclass may render the individual susceptible to certain kinds of infections.

The IgG circulating in the bloodstream is 60-70 percent IgG1, 20-30 percent IgG2, 5-8 percent IgG3 and 1-3 percent IgG4. The amount of the various IgG subclasses varies with age as well as with certain genetic factors. IgG1 and IgG3 reach normal adult levels by 5-7 years of age while IgG2 and IgG4 levels rise more slowly, reaching adult levels at about 10 years of age. In young children, the ability to make antibodies to the polysaccharide coatings of bacteria, antibodies which are most commonly of the IgG2 subclass, develops more slowly than the ability to make antibodies to proteins. Some individuals have genes which cause the IgG2 levels to be somewhat reduced, but this does not appear to make them unusually susceptible to infection. All these factors must be taken into account before an individual is considered to be abnormal either by virtue of having a low IgG subclass level or an inability to make a specific type of antibody.

Clinical Presentation

Recurrent ear infections, sinusitis, bronchitis and pneumonia are the most frequently observed illnesses in patients with IgG subclass deficiencies. Both males and females may be affected. Some patients will show an increased frequency of infection beginning in their second year of life; however, in other patients the onset of infections may occur later. Often a child with IgG subclass deficiency will first come to the physician's attention because of recurrent ear infections. Somewhat later recurrent or chronic sinusitis, bronchitis and/or pneumonia may make their appearance. In general, the infections suffered by patients with selective IgG subclass deficiencies are not as severe as those suffered by patients who have marked deficiencies of IgG, IgA and IgM (for example X-Linked Agammaglobulinemia and Common Variable Immunodeficiency). Occasionally, subclass deficient patients have suffered recurrent episodes of meningitis or bacterial infections of the bloodstream (e.g. sepsis).

Selective IgG1 subclass deficiency is very rare. IgG2 subclass deficiency is the most frequent subclass deficiency in children, while IgG3 subclass deficiency is the most common deficiency seen in adults. IgG4 deficiency most often occurs in association with IgG2 deficiency. The significance of selective IgG4 deficiency is unclear at this time.

Diagnosis

IgG subclass deficiency may be suspected in children and adults who have a history of recurrent infections of the ears, sinuses, bronchi and lungs. An individual is considered to have a selective IgG subclass deficiency if one or more of the IgG subclass levels in their blood is below the normal range for age and the levels of other immunoglobulins (i.e. IgG, IgA and IgM) are normal or near normal. An individual may have very low levels or absence of one or more IgG subclasses and yet the total amount of IgG in their blood may be normal or near normal. Therefore, to make the diagnosis of selective IgG subclass deficiency, quantitation of IgG subclasses is required along with measurement of serum IgG, IgA, and IgM. IgG subclass deficiencies often accompany IgA deficiency (see Chapter on IgA deficiency). Combined deficiencies of IgA with IgG2 and IgG4 deficiency are frequently observed. IgG2 and IgG4 deficiency as well as IgA and IgE deficiency also occur in association with Ataxia-Telangiectasia (see chapter on Ataxia-Telangiectasia).

Many patients with selective IgG2 subclass deficiency or IgA and IgG2 deficiency are unable to produce protective levels of antibody when immunized with vaccines against *Streptococcus pneumoniae* (the *pneumococcus*) or *Haemophilus influenzae* bacteria. Patients with IgG subclass deficiencies usually make normal amounts of antibodies to protein vaccines such as the diphtheria and tetanus toxoids in the routine DPT immunizations.

Patients with IgG subclass deficiencies have normal numbers of B- and T-lymphocytes, and their T-lymphocytes function normally when tested by delayed hypersensitivity skin tests or by lymphocyte stimulation tests in the laboratory.

Inheritance

No clear cut pattern of inheritance has been observed in the IgG subclass deficiencies. Occasionally two individuals with IgG subclass deficiency may be found in the same family. In some families IgG subclass deficiencies have been found to be associated with IgA deficiency, Common Variable Immunodeficiency and/or complement component deficiency.

Natural History

The natural history of patients with selective IgG subclass deficiency is not completely understood. It has been apparent that selective IgG subclass deficiencies occur more often in children than in adults and that the type of subclass deficiency in children (i.e. predominantly IgG2) differs from that most commonly seen in adults (i.e. IgG3). These findings suggested that at least some children may "outgrow" their subclass deficiencies. In fact, recent studies have shown that many, but not all, children who were subclass deficient during early childhood (i.e. under the age of 5 years) develop normal subclass levels as well as the ability to make antibodies to polysaccharide vaccines as they get older. However, IgG subclass deficiencies may persist in some children as well as in adults and in some instances a selective IgG subclass deficiency may evolve into Common Variable Immunodeficiency (see chapter on Common Variable Immunodeficiency). At present it is not possible to determine which patients will have the transient type of subclass deficiency and in which patients the subclass deficiency may be permanent or the forerunner of a more serious immunodeficiency. For these reasons, periodic reevaluation of immunoglobulin and IgG subclass levels are necessary.

Treatment

Patients with IgG subclass deficiency frequently suffer recurrent or chronic infections of the ears, sinuses, bronchi and lungs. Treatment of these infections usually requires antibiotics. One goal of treatment is to prevent permanent damage to the ears and lungs which might result in hearing loss or chronic lung disease. Another goal is to maintain patients as symptom-free as possible so that they may pursue their activities of daily living such as school or work. Sometimes antibiotics may be used for prevention (i.e. prophylaxis) of infections in patients who are unusually susceptible to ear or sinus infections. Some IgG subclass deficient patients also have reactive airways disease and may experience episodes of wheezing and shortness of breath particularly when they have a sinus infection or other respiratory tract infections. These patients may require treatment with drugs called bronchodilators which relieve the constriction of the muscles of the bronchi, which is the cause of wheezing and shortness of breath. If patients have developed chronic lung disease and bronchiectasis, physical therapy and daily postural drainage may be necessary.

For immunodeficiency diseases, in which patients are unable to produce adequate levels of the major immunoglobulin classes (i.e. IgG, IgA and IgM) and fail to make antibodies against proteins as well as polysaccharide antigens (X-Linked Agammaglobulinemia and Common Variable Immunodeficiency), immunoglobulin (gammaglobulin) replacement therapy is clearly needed. Immunoglobulin replacement therapy can be done by giving either injections of gamma globulins into a muscle or by giving gamma globulins intravenously. Since larger amounts of gamma globulins can be given intravenously than by intramuscular injection, the intravenous method of treatment is most often used (see Chapter on Specific Medical Therapy). The use of gamma globulin replacement therapy in patients with IgG subclass deficiencies is not as clear cut as for X-Linked Agammaglobulinemia and Common Variable Immunodeficiency patients. Patients with IgG subclass deficiency have a more limited antibody and immunoglobulin deficiency than patients with X-Linked Agammaglobulinemia and Common Variable Immunodeficiency. In those patients in which infections and symptoms can be controlled with antibiotics, gamma globulin replacement therapy may not be necessary. However, in those patients in which infections cannot be readily controlled with antibiotics, gamma globulin replacement therapy should be considered. Since many young children appear to outgrow their IgG subclass deficiency as they get older, it is important to reevaluate the patient to determine if the subclass deficiency is still present. If the subclass deficiency has resolved, gamma globulin replacement therapy may be discontinued and the patient observed. If the deficiency has persisted, gamma globulin therapy may be re-instituted. In teenagers and adults, disappearance of the subclass deficiency is less likely.

Expectations

The outlook for patients with IgG subclass deficiency is generally good. Many children appear to outgrow their deficiency as they get older. For those patients in whom the deficiency persists, the use of antibiotics and gamma globulin replacement therapy can usually prevent serious infections and the development of impaired lung function, hearing loss or injury to other organ systems.

Chapter 13

The Wiskott-Aldrich Syndrome

Definition

The Wiskott-Aldrich Syndrome (WAS) is a primary immunodeficiency disease which is inherited in an X-Linked recessive fashion and therefore affects only males. It has a generally consistent pattern of clinical problems including:

1. Recurrent infections from defects in T-lymphocytes and B-lymphocytes of the immune system.

2. Abnormal bleeding caused by a deficiency in blood platelets.

3. Eczema of the skin.

The immune deficiency in this disorder affects both the T-lymphocyte and B-lymphocyte systems and therefore is classified as a "combined immunodeficiency." However, unlike children with other combined immunodeficiencies, such as Severe Combined Immunodeficiency (SCID), the defects in the T- and B-lymphocyte systems in the WAS are each partial defects. This results in the affected boys having problems with certain types of micro-organisms while being able to defend against other types of micro-organisms almost normally.

Affected children are able to make some protective antibodies to certain organisms such as tetanus but are incapable of producing antibodies to other bacteria like *Hemophilus influenzae* or the *pneumococcus*. The immune system normally eliminates these organisms by producing antibodies against the outer capsule portion of the bacteria (the capsular polysaccharide antigens). It is now known that a principal defect in the WAS B-lymphocyte system is an inability to make protective antibodies to any polysaccharide antigen. Therefore, infections with these types of bacteria can not be fought off normally by boys with the WAS, and they may develop frequent and/or recurrent ear infections (otitis), lung infections (pneumonia), or even meningitis.

The T-lymphocyte system also has partial defects. T-lymphocytes are usually present in near normal numbers, but they function abnormally. This defect may result in the boys experiencing infections with "opportunistic organisms" such as yeast, *pneumocystis carinii*, or one of the herpes viruses. These infections may not be a problem unless the patient also requires treatment with immunosuppressive drugs (like corticosteroids). In this case great caution must be exercised to prevent serious infections from developing.

Platelets are tiny blood cells that function to help prevent and stop bleeding. In the WAS the platelet count in the blood is usually markedly reduced. The platelet count only averages from 15,000-35,000 compared with a normal of 200,000-400,000. Because of this low platelet count (called thrombocytopenia), patients with the WAS may bleed into their skin, their mucous membranes or internal organs either spontaneously or after relatively minor trauma. In addition to having very few platelets, the platelets they do have are much smaller in size than normal platelets. In fact, the small platelet size is the best single test to confirm the diagnosis of WAS in a boy with thrombocytopenia. The WAS is the only known disease known to have tiny platelets.

Eczema is a scaling, itchy skin rash that is found in almost all boys with the WAS. It may be very mild in some and severe in others.

Clinical Presentation

Boys with the WAS usually present with symptoms related to their:

- thrombocytopenia (low platelets),
- an increased susceptibility to infection related to their immunodeficiency, and/or
- eczema.

They may have symptoms relating to all three of these (i.e. thrombocytopenia, infection and eczema) or just one of them initially.

One of the most common clinical presentations is thrombocytopenia and a tendency to bleed. Affected boys may be noticed to have purple spots on their skin soon after birth, but this is often attributed to bruising from the birth process. The bleeding may be small and resemble pinheads in size (petechiae) or may be larger and resemble bruises (purpura). They may also have bloody bowel movements, bleeding gums, and prolonged nose bleeds. Serious hemorrhage into the brain is also a danger to these boys and before the era of modern treatment, caused the deaths of about one-third of the boys with this syndrome.

Their increased susceptibility to infection may take many forms. They may have recurrent episodes of otitis media (middle ear infections), bacterial or viral pneumonias, blood infections (bacteremia and sepsis), and/or meningitis.

Finally, their eczematous skin rash may also be a prominent clinical symptom. In infants it may be seen as "cradle cap" or as a severe diaper rash. In older boys it usually occurs in the skin creases around the front of the elbow, around the wrists and neck, and behind the knees. It can be very frustrating because the itching is intense and the boys will scratch themselves until they bleed. They often scratch their skin even while asleep.

One of the problems that is recognized to be quite common in older boys and men with the WAS is a high incidence of "autoimmune-like" symptoms. The name "autoimmune" describes conditions that appear to be the result of the immune system reacting against part of the patient's own body. In the WAS a variety of different symptoms occur including, for example, episodes of high fever without infection. New skin rashes unrelated to eczema may appear, often associated with painful swollen joints at the ankle, knee, hip and elsewhere. The boys may also develop painful, hot and discolored places on their legs which do not involve the joints but are nevertheless so severe that they prevent them from walking. Sometimes the thrombocytopenia becomes worse because a new autoimmune platelet disorder adds to the problem they already have with low platelets. Occasionally inflammation of arteries (vasculitis) in the skin, heart, brain or elsewhere can develop which causes a wide range of confusing symptoms. This autoimmune disorder can occur at any age and episodes may last only a few days or may occur in waves which recur over a period of many years.

Diagnosis

Frequently the WAS is incorrectly diagnosed at first, being confused with other, more common, causes of thrombocytopenia. The diagnosis of WAS is more easily established when a clear family history is present. Since it is an inherited disease transmitted as an X-Linked recessive trait, these boys frequently have brothers or maternal uncles (their mother's brother) with the same disease. About 60 percent of cases will have such a positive family history. As mentioned above, the best single test to confirm the diagnosis is a careful determination of the platelet size in these boys. The most common platelet disease in children, Idiopathic Thrombocytopenia Purpura (ITP), is associated with platelets that are larger than normal while WAS platelets are about only half the normal size. In infants, platelet size may be the only reliable test to confirm the diagnosis. In children over the age of 2, a variety of immunologic abnormalities can also be used to help with the diagnosis. Skin tests used to test T-lymphocyte function usually show a negative response and tests of T-cell function performed in test tubes may also be normal. Certain types of serum antibodies are characteristically low or absent in boys with the WAS. They have low levels of antibodies to blood group antigens (the isohemagglutinins) and fail to produce antibody when given a vaccine to pneumococcal or *Hemophilus Influenzae* polysaccharides. Their lymphocytes may also have an abnormal appearance when examined under the scanning electron microscope and they may have an abnormality in a cell surface glycoprotein (sialophorin). In addition, patients with this disease often have tests indicating abnormal function of their monocytes and granulocytes.

Inheritance

As described earlier, the WAS is inherited as an X-Linked recessive trait so that only boys are affected with the disease. See the chapter on Inheritance for more complete information on how X-Linked recessive disorders are passed on from generation to generation. Often the question of having additional children is raised when a family is identified as carrying the WAS gene. Statistically, each male child has a 50 percent chance of having the WAS. The decision about having future children is a highly personal one dependent upon many factors including the basic philosophical and religious beliefs of the parents, their concept of the impact of a child's illness on their lives and the lives of other members of the family, and a number of other factors which are different for each family.

Treatment

As soon as the diagnosis of the WAS is clearly established, one of several treatment options should be initiated. First, if the boy has normal siblings, the family should be tissue typed to determine whether there are any HLA-identical siblings (good tissue matches) who could serve as a donor for a bone marrow transplant. The results with HLA-identical sibling donor bone marrow transplantation in the WAS are better than any other disease treated by this procedure with an overall success (cure) rate of over 85 percent. This is probably the treatment of choice for a boy with the WAS. If there is no identical sibling donor, bone marrow transplantation using an unrelated HLA matched donor or a partially matched family member as a donor could be considered. The results with these transplants have been much less successful (less than 30 percent cure) and other treatments should probably be tried, at least initially.

Hemorrhage can be life threatening in boys with the WAS. The most serious bleeding problem is the development of hemorrhage into the brain (intracerebral hemorrhage). Historically, this complication has occurred in nearly one half of the boys at some time during their lives. Since intracerebral hemorrhage is often fatal, major efforts to prevent it from occurring are an essential part of the treatment plan for this disease.

Since hemorrhage is such a major problem in the WAS, treatment to eliminate this complication is essential. Surgical removal of a lymphoid organ in the abdomen called the spleen (splenectomy) results in correction of the thrombocytopenia in over 90 percent of the cases. The spleen normally functions as a type of bloodstream filter. In the WAS the spleen mistakenly filters the platelets from the blood and destroys them. The operation is relatively simple and has been used successfully in WAS patients who were not candidates to receive bone marrow transplantation. To help prevent infections in WAS boys after the spleen has been removed, daily antibiotics and/or regular infusions of intravenous gammaglobulin are given.

This combination of splenectomy and antibiotics/gammaglobulin has been very effective in controlling many of the problems of the WAS. Boys are able to ride bicycles, participate in contact sports, and do most of the other activities that they were unable to do when their platelet counts were very low. This combination treatment has also been responsible for lessening the incidence of bacterial infections in these boys and has permitted a greatly improved quality of life for most patients. It is not necessary to isolate the affected boys from contact with other children to protect them from possible infections. Their immune defect is not as severe as that found in children with SCID, where isolation is advisable. In fact, contact with other children is encouraged so that boys with the WAS can develop socially. Splenectomy at an early age is often recommended because a fatal brain hemorrhage may occur as the result of simple head trauma, as may occur when an infant is learning to walk. Until a splenectomy can be performed, it is advisable to restrict the activity of affected boys to prevent rough-house types of physical activity that could result in head trauma.

As in the case with children with other primary immunodeficiency diseases, boys with the WAS must not be given live virus vaccines since there is the remote possibility that the vaccine strains of the virus may cause disease in these children because of their defective immune systems.

In addition to controlling infection with antibiotics and intravenous gammaglobulin, and performing a splenectomy to correct the thrombocytopenia, skin care is another problem needing attention in most boys with WAS. Eczema is usually controlled by following a few simple guidelines. Avoid excessive bathing since frequent baths actually dry the skin and make the eczema worse. Use bath oil during the bath and a moisturizing cream after bathing (such as Eucerine) and twice daily to areas of dry skin/eczema. Steroid creams applied sparingly to areas of particular inflammation can be very helpful, but their overuse should be avoided. Although no special diets are helpful, complete and balanced nutrition is important. Occasionally specific foods (eggs, wheat, etc.) are identified which seem to worsen the eczema and these should be avoided, but as a general rule no such offending foods are identified.

Symptoms relating to auto-immune diseases may present a difficult treatment dilemma because it may become necessary to use drugs which suppress the boy's immune system even though this system is weak already. Nonsteroidal anti-inflammatory drugs such as indomethacin may be helpful in controlling the autoimmune symptoms and the use of corticosteroids.

Any child with a serious chronic illness needs all the support and love that parents can provide. They must tolerate repeated hospitalizations which, in turn, may be associated with painful procedures. Parents need to call upon all their inner resources to learn to handle the anxiety and stress associated with having a child with this serious disease and need to develop mechanisms to help them cope and outside sources for emotional support. The demands on the time and energies of the parents of a child with the WAS can be overwhelming, and if there are normal unaffected siblings, the parents must remember that these children need to share their parents' love and care as well. The parents also need to spend energy in maintaining their own relationship with each other. If the stress of the child's illness and treatment destroys the family structure, a successful therapeutic outcome for the patient will be a hollow victory indeed.

Expectations

The Wiskott-Aldrich Syndrome was formerly one of the most severe of the immunodeficiency diseases with survival beyond childhood very unlikely. Although it remains a serious disorder with some deaths occurring in childhood, many affected males are now living productive lives into their third and fourth decades, even without having been treated by bone marrow transplantation. Some of these young men have become fathers themselves and, despite the problems posed by a chronic medical condition, have been successful in becoming productive and responsible adults capable of living full lives.

Chapter 14

The DiGeorge Anomaly

Definition

The DiGeorge Anomaly is a primary immune deficiency disease which is caused by abnormal development of certain cells and tissues of the head and neck during growth and differentiation of the fetus. Tissues which are dependent upon a single group of embryonic cells for their normal fetal development are called "fields." Although the tissues and organs that ultimately develop from a "field" may appear to be unrelated in the fully formed child, they are related in that they have developed from the same embryonic or fetal tissues or "field."

The field that is affected in the DiGeorge Anomaly controls the development of the face, parts of the brain, the thymus, the parathyroid glands, the heart and the aorta. The original control of the development of this field is found in a group of cells which originate in the face of the developing embryo. In order for the components of the field to develop properly, these cells must migrate out from the face during fetal development to the areas of the developing heart, thymus and parathyroid glands. If this normal development of the field does not occur, then normal facial, thymus, parathyroid and heart development may not occur. The anomalies seen in the DiGeorge Anomaly are the consequence of abnormal development of this field.

It is possible that some organs develop normally while others do not. Therefore, patients with DiGeorge Anomaly do not all show the same organ involvement. Also, a given organ may be mildly to severely involved. Infants and children with the DiGeorge Anomaly therefore may have abnormalities in any or all of these organs. Patients with the DiGeorge Anomaly may have any or all of the following:

- **Facial appearance**. Affected children may have an upward bowing of their mouth, an underdeveloped chin, eyes that slant somewhat downward, and defective upper portions of their ear lobes. These facial characteristics vary greatly from child to child and may not be very prominent in many affected children.

- **Parathyroid gland abnormalities.** Affected children may have underdeveloped parathyroid glands (hypoparathyroidism). These are small glands found in the neck near the thyroid gland (hence the name "parathyroid"). They function to control the normal metabolism and blood levels of calcium. Therefore, children with the DiGeorge Anomaly may have trouble maintaining their normal levels of calcium and this in turn may cause them to have seizures (convulsions). In some cases, the parathyroid abnormality is relatively mild or not present at all. The parathyroid defect may become less severe with time.

- **Cardiac defects.** Affected children may also have a variety of heart defects. For the most part, these anomalies involve the aorta and the part of the heart from which the aorta develops. As with the other organs affected in the DiGeorge Anomaly, the heart defects vary from child to child and in some children may be very mild or absent.

- **Thymus gland abnormalities.** Affected infants and children also may have abnormalities of their thymus. The thymus gland is normally located in the upper area of the front of the chest. However, the thymus begins its development high in the neck during the first three months in utero. As the thymus gets bigger and matures, it drops down into the chest to its ultimate site underneath the breast bone and over the heart. The thymus controls the development and maturation of one kind of lymphocyte, the T-lymphocyte ("T" for "Thymus"). T-lymphocytes are important for resistance to certain viral and fungal infection and also help B-lymphocytes to develop into plasma cells and produce immunoglobulins or antibodies (see chapter on Understanding the Immune System). Thus, patients with the DiGeorge Anomaly may have defects in their T-lymphocyte function and as a result, an increased susceptibility to viral, fungal and bacterial infections. As with the other defects in the DiGeorge Anomaly, the T-lymphocyte defect is extremely variable from patient to patient; in fact, modest deficiencies may disappear with time.

Diagnosis

The diagnosis of the DiGeorge Anomaly is usually made on the basis of signs and symptoms that are present at birth or develop soon after birth. Affected children may show signs of low calcium as a result of their hypoparathyroidism. This may show up as a low blood calcium on a routine blood test or the infant may be "jittery" or have seizures (convulsions). Affected children may also show signs and symptoms of a heart defect. They may have a heart murmur that shows up on a routine physical exam, they may show clinical signs of heart failure, or they may have low oxygen content of their arterial blood and appear "blue" or cyanotic. Finally, affected children may show signs of infection because of the underdevelopment of their thymus gland and low T-lymphocyte function. Some children present at birth or while they are still in the nursery, while others may not show signs or symptoms until they are a few weeks or months older.

In some children, all of the different organs and tissues are affected; that is, they have the characteristic facial characteristics, they have low blood calcium from their hypoparathyroidism, they have heart defects and they have a deficiency in their T-lymphocyte number and function. A T-lymphocyte count can predict whether the immune defect is likely to resolve spontaneously. In other children all of the different organs and tissues may not be affected and those organs and tissues that are affected may be affected to different degrees. Thus, there is a great deal of variation in the DiGeorge Anomaly from child to child. Not only do the children differ in which of the organs and tissues are affected but they also differ from each other in terms of how severely a given organ or tissue is affected.

Therapy

Therapy of the DiGeorge Anomaly is aimed at correcting the defects relating to each of the organs or tissues that are affected and, therefore, depends on the nature of the defect and how severe it is. The treatment of the low calcium and hypoparathyroidism may involve calcium supplementation and replacement of the missing parathyroid hormone. The cardiac defect may require medications to improve the function of the heart or may require corrective surgery in some cases. If surgery is required, the exact nature of the surgery will depend on the nature of the heart defect. Surgery can be performed before any immune defects are corrected. However, all precautions usually taken with immunodeficient children need to be observed.

As mentioned above, the immunologic defect in T-lymphocyte function varies from child to child and therefore the need for therapy of their T-lymphocyte defect varies from child to child. Many children with the DiGeorge Anomaly have perfectly normal T-lymphocyte function and therefore require no therapy for an immunodeficiency. Many children initially have mild or modest defects in T-lymphocyte function and their T-lymphocyte function improves significantly as they grow older. The spontaneous improvement and increase in T-lymphocyte immunity can be attributed to growth of a tiny but normal thymus gland. A feature of these small glands is that they do not make the normal descent from the neck into the chest during early fetal development. In the normal child, the thymus begins high in the neck during the first three months of development in utero. As the thymus grows bigger and bigger, it drops down to its ultimate site underneath the breast bone in the chest. In most cases of the DiGeorge Anomaly, the tiny thymus remains high in the neck, but ultimately grows enough to provide adequate T-lymphocyte function. In the remaining children (approximately 25 percent), the thymus is either completely absent or never grows enough to develop adequate numbers of T-lymphocytes. The severity of the defect is basically dependent upon how much thymus tissue the child develops. The degree of associated B-cell deficiency depends upon the number of helper T-cells which the thymus can generate.

As can be seen from the preceding paragraph, not all children with the DiGeorge Anomaly require therapy for their immunodeficiency. In those children who do require therapy for their immunodeficiency, some form of transplantation of normal immune system tissue may be of help. The immune defect in the DiGeorge Anomaly involves the thymus and T-lymphocytes. Therefore, thymus transplants have been used in children with the DiGeorge Anomaly. In fact, fetal thymuses were successfully transplanted for the DiGeorge Anomaly as early as

1968. The overall success rate is difficult to determine accurately, because of different techniques which are employed and also because it is unclear whether or not some of the children who received transplant would have improved spontaneously. Recently, bone marrow transplants from matched sibling donors (see chapter on Therapy) have been performed with successful outcomes. Also, newer methods of thymus transplantation have shown improved long term results.

Expectations

The outlook for a child with the DiGeorge Anomaly depends in large part on the degree to which the child is affected. The severity of the heart disease is usually the most important determining factor. As mentioned above, 75 percent of the children have no immune deficit or only a transient problem with their immune system. If the immunodeficiency is persistent, correction is necessary.

Part Three

Autoimmune Diseases and Disorders

Chapter 15

Autoimmune Diseases

Integral to our well-being is the ability of the immune system to distinguish that which is self from that which is nonself or foreign. More simply put, our immune system will not attack our own tissues. When this discrimination process fails, the body begins to manufacture antibodies to its own constituents. These "autoantibodies" cause what are termed "autoimmune" diseases (Table 15.1), including familiar conditions such as rheumatoid arthritis (RA), systemic lupus erythematosus (SLE), and insulin-dependent diabetes mellitus (IDDM or type 1).

Although the precise mechanism of autoimmunity is not understood, scientists think that early in our development, we possess cells that are capable of recognizing and attacking our own tissue. However, nature has provided a system for eliminating or inactivating these cells under normal circumstances. The events that regulate this negative selection are unknown, as are the reasons why it fails to occur. Nevertheless, this mechanism suggests an inherent or genetic cause for autoimmune disease. Other evidence indicates that autoimmune syndromes can result from chronic infection. For example, one of the clinical manifestations of the tick-borne disease Lyme borreliosis is a condition remarkably similar to rheumatoid arthritis.

By understanding the events that direct self-recognition on a genetic and cellular level, scientists will be able to develop more precise therapeutic strategies for controlling autoimmune diseases, rather than merely treating their symptoms.

NIH Pub No. 91-2414.

Table 15.1. Antibodies and antigens in Lupus and other diseases.

Clinical Designation	Antigen Molecular Identity	Autoantibody Frequency (%) Lupus	Other Diseases
Native DNA	Double-strand DNA	40	
Denatured DNA	Single-strand DNA	70	80 (DLE)[a]
Histones	H1, H2A, H2B, H3, H4	70	> 95 (DLE)
Sm	Proteins 29(B'), 28(B), 16(D), 13(E) kD complexed with U1, U2, U4-U6 snRNAs	30	
Nuclear RNP	Proteins 70, 33(A), 22(C) kD complexed with U1 snRNA	32	> 95 (MCTD)[a]
SS-A/Ro	Proteins 60, 52 kD complexed with Y1, Y3-Y5 RNAs	35	60 (SS)[a]
SS-B/La	Protein 48 kD complexed with nascent RNA pol III transcripts	15	40 (SS)
Ku	Proteins 86, 66 kD; DNA-binding proteins	10	
Ki	Protein 29.5 kD	14	
PCNA/Cyclin	Protein 36 kD; auxiliary protein of DNA polymerase δ	3	
Ribosomal RNP	Proteins 38, 16, 13 kD associated with ribosomes	10	

[a] *DLE=Drug-induced lupus erythematosus; MCTD=mixed connective tissue disease; SS=Sjögren's syndrome.*

Overview

Among the many important scientific observations made during the past decade have been the crystallographic analysis of the MHC (major histocompatibility complex) class I antigen HLA (human leukocyte antigen)-A2, and the elucidation of the antigen-specific receptor on T lymphocytes. During the 1980s, scientists promulgated the argument that autoimmune diseases are diseases of the T cell repertoire in which lymphocytes bearing autoreactive receptors either are not eliminated or are activated inappropriately with resultant tissue damage. Current studies of autoimmunity now center on the T inducer cell as the major participant in autoimmune responses. The cascade of the immune response is guided by this T inducer cell. This approach is a marked change from concepts of the 1950s and 1960s, which cited aberrant responses of either T cells or B cells as the underlying focus of autoimmunity.

Significant advances have been made in understanding how the repertoire of T cell receptors for antigen is shaped. Evidence indicates that the initial event in the selection of the T cell receptor repertoire is a positive selection event that occurs intrathymically. This initial positive selection is followed by at least three different forms of negative selection. The first of these negative selections appears to occur as an intrathymic event. It can be demonstrated by the presence of a certain subset of T cell receptors that is deleted prior to the cell's exit from the thymus. The antigens that drive this negative selection are not yet understood.

Another level of T cell receptor inactivation seems to be a peripherally induced state of anergy. This state has been observed following the insertion of MHC products as transgenes in ectopic sites that seemingly exclude presentation within the thymus. Scientists have not yet understood the mechanisms that underlie the anergic state, the consequences of this anergy, and the nature of activation signals that can override this anergy.

Other important studies have demonstrated an association between particular MHC gene products and autoimmune diseases. For example, patients who develop seropositive RA have an HLA-DR4 gene product that confers susceptibility to the development of the disease. Patients with type I diabetes have an HLA-DQ product that allows development of IDDM. Initial studies suggested that ectopic expression of MHC products might result in the development of autoimmunity. However, recent evidence indicates that ectopic expression of MHC class II gene products alone does not lead to autoimmunity.

Scientists have not determined definitively whether autoimmune diseases are the result of infectious agents. One striking finding in the 1980s was the observation that persistent infection with the spirochete *Borrelia burgdorferi* led to the development of certain features of autoimmunity. Lyme arthritis is an example of a disease resulting from chronic infection that is identical to seronegative RA in many respects.

Another major finding of the past decade was the observation that products of certain infectious agents, such as staphylococcal enterotoxins, serve as "super antigens." These super antigens can activate large numbers of T cells that bear germ-line-encoded T cell receptors, despite the fine antigen specificity of these cells. Although these studies are in their infancy, they may lead to important insights with respect to the etiologic events that allow aberrant T cell activation with potential autoimmune consequences.

Finally, immunologists continue to work on specific and quasi-specific forms of immunotherapy that will inactivate T cells within the repertoire that participate in the induction of autoimmunity. These new models of immunotherapy have many targets of opportunity, and several forms have proven successful in animal models of autoimmune disease.

Characterization of the Events That Initiate and Perpetuate Antiself Responses (Autoimmunity)

The major unresolved issue in autoimmunity continues to be why the body develops an immune response to its own tissues. To answer this question, scientists are considering recent observations concerning the mechanisms of deletion or inactivation of self-reactive cells; the role of infectious agents in triggering or perpetuating an autoimmune response; and the role of certain genes, such as MHC and T cell receptor genes, in conferring susceptibility to autoimmune disease.

Research Opportunities

- Characterize the self antigens that are the targets of autoimmunity.

- Define the role of infectious agents in the induction and perpetuation of autoimmunity.

- Characterize the mechanisms whereby certain genes confer susceptibility to the development of autoimmune disease.

- Define further the mechanisms of self tolerance whose breakdown leads to autoimmune sequelae.

Development of Specific Immunosuppressive Therapies

New strategies to suppress the autoimmune process have been suggested by recent advances in our understanding of the events involved in the initiation of immune responses to foreign antigens. These strategies are designed to inhibit the immune response to self-antigens by influencing early initiating events rather than late-stage events. This approach will allow the development of interventions that are relatively selective for specific antigens involved in the autoimmune process, as opposed to therapies that produce a global suppression of immunity.

Scientists need to develop innovative new strategies that target specific elements of the autoimmune process. These targets include gene products, such as MHC and T cell receptor genes, that are associated with autoimmune disease; activated lymphocytes whose inappropriate recognition of self-antigens leads to autoimmune sequelae; purposeful tolerization against the self-antigens that are targets of autoimmune responses; and infectious agents that are involved in the induction and perpetuation of autoimmune disease.

Research Opportunities

- Develop new and specific immuno-therapies for autoimmune diseases.

- Develop early clinical application of therapies that have been successful in preclinical models.

Use of Animal Models in Studies of Autoimmune Disease

The use of animal models will enhance our understanding of the mechanisms that lead to autoimmunity as well as aid the development of new treatment strategies for autoimmune diseases. Effective

153

animal models include both naturally occurring models of disease, such as the non-obese diabetic mouse, and models such as transgenic mice that are created through molecular biological techniques. Specialized knowledge, equipment, and facilities are needed to create, characterize, standardize, produce, and distribute these animals. As a result, scientists studying autoimmune diseases have not had optimal access to these invaluable animal models. A centralized facility is needed, therefore, to serve as a resource for scientists studying animal models of autoimmunity.

Research Opportunity

- Initiate a resource facility for maintaining, producing, and distributing animal models of autoimmunity.

Bibliography

Aca-Orbea, H.; Steinman, L.; McDevitt, H.O. T cell receptors in murine autoimmune diseases. *Annual Review of Immunology* 7: 311-405, 1989.

Bjorkman, P.J.; Saper, M.A.; Samraoui, B.; Bennett, W.S.; Strominger, J.L.; Wiley, D.C. Structure of the human class I histocompatibility antigen HLA A2. *Nature* 329: 506512, 1987.

Kronenberg, M.; Siu, G.; Hood, L.E.; Shastri, N. The molecular genetics of the T cell antigen receptor and GT cell antigen recognition. *Annual Review of Immunology* 4: 529-591, 1986.

Wraith, D.C.; McDevitt, H.O.; Steinman, L.; Aca-Orbea, H. T cell recognition as the target for immune intervention in autoimmune disease. *Cell* 57: 709-715, 1989.

Chapter 16

Organ-Specific Immune-Mediated Diseases

In autoimmune disease, the body's immune system inappropriately identifies some of the body's own tissue as foreign and attacks it. Many of the resultant diseases are familiar conditions such as type I (insulin-dependent) diabetes, multiple sclerosis, and systemic lupus erythematosus (SLE). Less familiar diseases include autoimmune diseases of the skin (pemphigus), the eye (uveitis), the colon (Crohn's disease), and the thyroid gland (Graves' disease). Virtually every tissue and organ system is susceptible to attack from immune dysregulation, and the accompanying suffering and expense are immense.

Scientists have not yet determined what controls these unfortunate events. Incidence of autoimmune disease in families is strong evidence that genetic factors are involved. However, conflicting data have emerged from studies of twins in which only one of the pair has an autoimmune disease. This finding would suggest that environmental factors influence and cause confusion of our immune system. In some of these diseases, progress is being made in understanding the genetic correlations as well as the precise targets of the immune system. For instance, the pancreatic cells are the target in insulin-dependent diabetes, and a chemical receptor is the target in myasthenia gravis. However, scientists still need to learn why the immune system goes awry and how to predict and prevent the ensuing diseases.

NIH Pub No. 91-2414.

Overview

The past decade has been characterized by remarkable advances in the techniques for studying immune disorders as well as in the understanding of basic immunology. These advances include the generation and utilization of monoclonal antibodies, discovery of the T cell receptor, characterization of a series of lymphokines, the ability to sequence and clone genes rapidly and ultimately produce peptides in vitro, and the development of animal models with selected disorders that permit the direct manipulation of certain genes. During the 1980s, scientists also identified an increasing number of organ-specific autoimmune disorders and now are addressing a series of questions concerning this large group of human diseases (Table 16.1). Answers to these questions will have a significant impact on the treatment of autoimmune disorders.

Current knowledge has enabled scientists to recognize the immunologic basis of a diverse range of disorders, including type I diabetes (IDDM), pemphigus, myasthenia gravis, and uveitis. To define specific immunopathogenic mechanisms within the general framework of autoimmunity, scientists are investigating each of these diseases for answers to a series of identical questions. These questions can be categorized as either basic or clinical:

Basic

- What genes determine susceptibility to disease?
- What triggers the development of autoimmunity?
- What are the target molecules?
- What are the effector molecules?
- What are the effector mechanisms?

Clinical

- Can one predict who will develop the disorder?
- Can one predict the timing of overt disease and its clinical course?
- Can one prevent the disorder?
- Can one cure the disorder or prevent the development of morbidity and mortality?
- Can one develop disease-specific therapies?

The likelihood of obtaining definitive answers to particular questions varies across the spectrum of organ-specific autoimmune diseases. The rate of progress toward answering these questions for a given disease is determined by several factors. For example, answers concerning IDDM will be expedited by the frequency with which this disorder occurs and the existence of spontaneous animal models with the genetics of the disease. Other factors include the nature of the effector molecules for the disorder and the identified inciting factors, such as drug-induced hemolytic anemias. The answers derived for one disease will have considerable bearing on research addressing the other diseases. The rapidly accelerating pace of obtaining answers to these questions is reinforcing the hope that safe, preventive, curative, or palliative therapies soon will be developed for this series of illnesses.

In addition to classical autoimmune disorders and recently recognized autoimmune disorders such as IDDM, there almost certainly are many conditions that have not yet been recognized as organ-specific autoimmune diseases. For other disorders, the magnitude of the role of autoimmunity is not yet clear. In the coming decade, scientists are likely to make major advances in recognizing the contribution of autoimmunity to various common disorders.

Several themes are common to organ-specific autoimmune disorders. These themes include a very strong genetic component in disease susceptibility. However, a less than 100 percent concordance for disease in identical twins suggests that, in some disorders, autoimmunity is triggered by environmental factors or random events such as somatic mutations. Specific susceptibility alleles apparently are necessary for most disorders but are not sufficient for the subsequent development of disease. In addition, one or more susceptibility genes are located within the major histocompatibility complex. Susceptibility to organ specific autoimmune diseases is inherited through multiple genes. In some cases, each genetic locus is necessary but not sufficient for overt disease. The non-obese diabetic mouse model of IDDM is an example of this type of inherited susceptibility.

Multiple environmental events can trigger the development of autoimmunity or affect the probability of subsequent disease. A diverse range of events can affect the development of different disorders. For example, ingesting the wheat protein gliadin can trigger celiac disease or dermatitis herpetiformis; receiving the drug penicillamine can actuate myasthenia gravis or pemphigus; having congenital rubella can trigger thyroiditis or type I diabetes; and receiving a blood transfusion can incite post-transfusion purpura.

When the effector molecule for a disease is an antibody, a prominent neonatal form of the disorder is associated with specific auto-antibodies. For example, congenital heart block, hyperthyroidism, myasthenia gravis, and pemphigus are associated with antibodies that react with the Rh antigen, thyroid-stimulating hormone, acetylcholine receptor, and epithelial cell surface molecules, respectively. For each autoimmune disorder, a series of normal molecules of the target cell can become targets of autoimmunity. The potential to direct molecular synthesis of given molecules to ectopic organs should rapidly enhance the ability of scientists to discern the primacy of a given target molecule for most organ-specific autoimmune diseases.

The scope of the human suffering and expense caused by organ-specific autoimmune diseases is immense. Because this type of autoimmunity is more common in older individuals, the impact is certain to grow as populations age. The recognition of additional disorders with autoimmune bases will increase this impact further. By solving the fundamental riddles and developing effective antigen-specific therapies for specific autoimmune diseases, scientists hope to devise a treatment that can be generalized to all related disorders.

Therapy of Organ-Specific Immune Disorders

Scientists have only recently identified the actual or putative autoimmune bases for organ-specific autoimmune diseases such as type I diabetes and multiple sclerosis. Although these disorders have significant morbidity and mortality, researchers have not yet determined if intervention at an appropriate stage with existing immunotherapeutics will beneficially alter the course of disease. Furthermore, therapy with immunosuppressive agents for these and other previously defined organ-specific autoimmune diseases is associated with considerable morbidity and mortality. Therefore, new agents and modalities of drug delivery need to be developed and evaluated. With a more thorough understanding of the genetics and pathogenesis of organ-specific autoimmune diseases, scientists should be able to develop safer, more specific, and more effective therapies for these disorders.

Research Opportunity

- Develop innovative clinical trials that use currently available agents as well as newly emerging immunotherapies to prevent or treat organ specific auto immune diseases.

Table 16.1. Organ-specific diseases.

Disease	Gene	Trigger	Target	Pathogenesis	Therapy
Graves'	HLA	ND[a]	TSH receptor >?"ganglioside"	Ab[b]	Thyroid ablation
Graves' ophthalmopathy	ND	ND	ND	ND	Immuno-suppression
Thyroiditis	HLA	Subset iodine	Thyroglobulin thyroid peroxidase	?T cell/Ab	Thyroxine replacement
Addison's	HLA	ND	ND	?T cell	Hormone replacement
Hypoparathyroidism	ND	ND	ND	?T cell	Vitamin D, calcium
Hypophysitis	ND	ND	ND	ND	Secondary hormone replacement
Ovarian/testicular failure	ND	ND	ND	ND	Androgen or estrogen replacement; no Rx for infertility
Type I diabetes	HLA ?other	Rarely, congenital rubella	Insulin islet ganglioside 64 kD antigen	?T cell	Palliative insulin treatment

[a] ND = not determined.
[b] Ab = antibody.

159

Characterization of the Role of Disease-Associated Genes and Environmental Factors

Over the past decade, scientists have made remarkable progress in understanding how genes in the HLA (human leukocyte antigen) region of the sixth chromosome contribute to a wide variety of organ-specific autoimmune disorders. Studies of these genes have been particularly extensive for pemphigus, celiac disease, Graves' disease, uveitis, and IDDM.

Techniques finally are available at the molecular genetic level to identify the genes associated with certain autoimmune diseases and to define their role in these disorders. For example, researchers now can create transgenic animals with specific disease susceptibility genes and can directly study the interaction between these genes and potential target molecules. Using these techniques, scientists have learned that a specific protein, gliadin, interacts with specific HLA and appears to activate the intestinal destruction associated with celiac disease. In a mouse model of IDDM, investigators prevented disease by introducing a normal HLA gene into the animal.

Other studies, particularly those using animal models of auto-immunity, have demonstrated that non-HLA genes also can be critical for the development of autoimmunity. However, even the chromosomal localization of most of these genes is unknown.

Research Opportunities

- Define MHC (major histocompatibility complex) and non-MHC genes that create susceptibility to organ specific autoimmune diseases.
- Identify additional environmental agents that are associated with autoimmune diseases.
- Define the mechanism whereby environmental agents and other known factors trigger autoimmunity and interact with genetic susceptibility to activate diseases.

Characterization of the Target Molecules of Organ-Specific Autoimmune Diseases

In many diseases, antibodies or immune cells are able to destroy or interfere with the normal function of specific organs. For example, both myasthenia gravis and Graves' disease are caused by a reaction between antibodies and specific cell surface receptors. In pemphigus, antibodies cause the separation of epidermal cells, leading to the formation of life-threatening blisters. In these and other diseases that are mediated by antibodies, infants of affected mothers receive maternal antibodies and thus often are born with transient disease. Although the major target molecules for some disorders are unknown, initial molecular identification has been accomplished for the majority of diseases. More extensive knowledge of the molecules that are targeted by the immune system will enable scientists to develop more specific and rational therapies for organ-specific autoimmune diseases.

Research Opportunity

- Characterize the molecules within specific organ systems that are targets of the autoimmune process and develop antigen-specific immunotherapies based on these findings.

Bibliography

Caspi, C.C. Basic mechanisms in immune-mediated uveitic disease. In: Immunology of Eye Diseases, *Immunology in Medicine Series*, Vol. 13, edited by S. Lightman. Dordrecht. The Netherlands: Kluwerr Academic Publishers, p. 61, 1989.

Castano, L.; Eisenbarth, G.S. Type I diabetes: a chronic autoimmune disease of man, mouse, and rat. *Annual Review of Immunology* 8: 1990 (in press).

Elson, C.O. The immunology of inflammatory bowel disease. In: *Inflammatory Bowel Disease* (3rd ed.), edited by J.B. Kirsner, R.G. Shorter. Philadelphia: Lea & Febiger, p. 97, 1988.

Gammon, W.R.; Heise, E.R.; Burke, W.A.; Fine, J.D.; Woodley, D.T.; Brihggaman, R.A. Increased frequency of HLA-DR2 in patients with autoantibodies to epidermolysis bullosa acquisita antigen: evidence that the expression of autoimmunity to Type VII collagen is HLA class II allele-associated. *Journal of Investigative Dermatology* 91: 228-232, 1988.

Jordon, R.E.; Sawana, S.; Fritz, K.A. Immunopathologic mechanisms in pemphigus and bullous pemphigoid. *Journal of Investigative Dermatology* 85: 72s-78s, 1985.

Kawashima, H.; Fujino, Y.; Mochizuki, M. Effects of a new immunosuppressive agent, FK506, on experimental autoimmune uveoretinitis in rats. *Investigative Ophthalmology and Visual Science* 29: 1265-1271, 1989.

Krueger, G.G.; Stingl, G. Immunology/inflammation of the skin: A 50-year perspective. *Journal of Investigative Dermatology* 92: 32s-51s, 1989.

Linton, A.L.; Clark, W.F.; Driedger, A.A. Acute interstitial nephritis due to drugs. *Annals of Internal Medicine* 93: 735, 1980.

Neilson, E.G. Pathogenesis and treatment of interstitial nephritis. *Kidney International* 35: 1257-1271, 1989.

Rodgers, V.D.; Kagnoff, M.F. Acquired immunodeficiency syndrome and disease of the gastrointestinal tract. In: *Immunology and Allergy Clinics of North America: Gut and Intestinal Immunology* (vol. 8, no. 3) edited by M. Kagnoff. Philadelphia: W.B. Saunders Co., p. 451, 1988.

Chapter 17

Arthritis, Rheumatic Diseases, and Related Disorders

Arthritis and related musculoskeletal disorders can affect people of all ages. However, the prevalence of many of these diseases tends to increase with age. Several of them occur predominantly in women; others are more common in men.

The term "arthritis," which literally means joint inflammation, refers to a family of over 100 rheumatic diseases that attack the joints and connective tissues. Each rheumatic disease has different symptoms and patterns and can vary greatly from person to person, and each requires different treatments.

Rheumatic and musculoskeletal diseases and disorders are the most frequently reported causes of impairment affecting adults, the leading cause of mobility limitation, and the second leading cause of activity restriction in the United States. More than 37 million Americans are afflicted by one or more of the rheumatic diseases. In addition, more than 25 million Americans have osteoporosis, and countless millions have other musculoskeletal disorders. These diseases have an enormous impact on the U.S. population; they cost tens of billions of dollars each year in medical care and lost productivity. Because the U.S. population is aging, the public health importance of arthritis and musculoskeletal diseases such as osteoarthritis and osteoporosis will continue to grow in the years to come.

NIH Pub No. 93-3413. National Institutes of Health, National Institute of Arthritis and Musculoskeletal and Skin Diseases. *For more detailed information on arthritis and rheumatic disorders see Omnigraphics' <u>Arthritis Sourcebook</u>.*

Research is beginning to uncover fundamental causes of many rheumatic and musculoskeletal diseases. The application of molecular biology techniques, coupled with advances in our understanding of genetics and the immune system, is providing insight into immunologic abnormalities, genetic factors, inflammatory responses and their mediators, infectious agents, and metabolic and hormonal derangements that are involved in these diseases. Ultimately, this knowledge should enable design of highly specific preventive agents and treatments.

The Many Guises of Arthritis

The most common forms of arthritis are osteoarthritis, rheumatoid arthritis, and gout. Osteoarthritis is the most prevalent, and its prevalence increases with age. It involves the breakdown of tissue that allows the joints to move smoothly. Some 16 million Americans are afflicted with it, according to the National Institute of Arthritis and Musculoskeletal and Skin Diseases.

Osteoarthritis. The common symptoms of osteoarthritis are pain and stiffness. Pain is usually felt when certain joints are used, especially finger joints and those that bear the body's weight—namely knees, hips and spine. Disability most often occurs in these weight-bearing joints.

Rheumatoid arthritis. Rheumatoid arthritis generally starts between the ages of 20 and 45 and affects almost three times as many women as men. Rheumatoid arthritis involves many joints, but most commonly the small joints of the hand. Inflammation and thickening of tissue around the joints may cause destruction of the bones, deformity, and eventually disability. In some cases the disease may be mild; in others it can be crippling. While the cause is unknown, some scientists believe rheumatoid arthritis may be sparked by a virus and linked to a disruption of the body's defense, or immune system.

Gout. Gout is the easiest form of arthritis to diagnose and treat, and it is the best understood. It most commonly affects the joints of the feet, particularly the big toe, although other joints may be involved. Most cases of gout occur in men. Gout gets its start when too much of a certain body chemical, uric acid, is deposited in the tissues. Crystals of uric acid form in the joints, causing inflammation and severe pain. Attacks of gout may follow minor injury, excessive eating or drinking, overexercise, or surgery, or may occur for no apparent reason.

Juvenile rheumatic arthritis. Arthritis in children can take many forms. The most common is juvenile rheumatoid arthritis. It affects primarily those under 8, causes growth disturbances, and can produce high fever and skin rash. It can be controlled with proper treatment.

Psoriatic arthritis. Psoriatic arthritis affects about 10 percent of the people who have psoriasis, a common but sometimes severe skin disease.

Systemic lupus erythematosus. Systemic lupus erythematosus, an uncommon form of arthritis, affects the skin, joints, and internal organs. Like rheumatoid arthritis, women suffer more often than men from this variation of the disease, and it usually crops up between the ages of 20 and 40.

Ankylosing spondylitis. Ankylosing spondylitis, also known as **rheumatoid spondylitis** or **Marie-Strumpell disease**, affects mostly males in late adolescence or young adulthood. Back pain, stiffness, and loss of spinal mobility are the main symptoms.

Bursitis. Bursitis is inflammation of a bursa, a small sac containing fluid that lies between a tendon and the bone over which the tendon moves. Popular names for bursitis are "tennis elbow" and "housemaid's knee."

Fibrositis. Fibrositis involves pain, stiffness or soreness of the fibrous tissue, especially in the coverings of the muscles. It does not affect joints directly.

Scleroderma. A disease of the body's connective tissue with accompanying symptoms of arthritis in the joints is called scleroderma. This disease causes thickening and hardening of the skin and sometimes inflammatory and other changes in internal organs, including the esophagus, intestinal tract, heart, lungs, and kidneys. Scleroderma strikes more women than men and can occur at any age, although it most often starts in the 40s and 50s.

Research Explores New Therapies for Rheumatoid Arthritis

More than 2 million Americans, the majority of them women, are affected by rheumatoid arthritis, a chronic inflammatory disease of unknown cause. The primary target of this crippling disorder is the joint lining or synovial membrane, which becomes inflamed and invades and damages nearby bone and cartilage. This results in pain, stiffness, loss of movement, and eventually complete destruction of the joint. Rheumatoid arthritis usually affects multiple joints and can also cause inflammation of the blood vessels and the outer lining of the heart and lungs.

Both genetic and non-genetic factors have been implicated in the development of rheumatoid arthritis. The application of new techniques in molecular biology and genetics is enabling continued progress in our understanding of immunogenetic markers for susceptibility to rheumatoid arthritis and other rheumatic diseases These findings are making it possible to determine, with increasing sensitivity, those people who are genetically predisposed to developing rheumatoid arthritis and certain other rheumatic diseases.

Current concepts of infection and of autoimmune disease (diseases in which the body is attacked by its own immune system, as is the case in rheumatoid arthritis and some other rheumatic diseases) are increasingly overlapping. Rheumatoid arthritis has been widely suspected to be caused by an infectious agent, and while this has not been proven, bacteria have been linked to many "reactive" types of arthritis.

NIAMS intramural scientists induced a rheumatoid arthritis-like inflammatory disease in an inbred strain of rat by injecting them with the cell walls of streptococcal bacteria. This research group has obtained evidence that the susceptibility of these rats to inflammatory disease is due to a defect in the complex neural and hormonal system that controls the body's response to inflammatory stimuli such as infectious agents. The possibility that similar defects play a role in rheumatoid arthritis in humans is being explored.

As in the case of osteoarthritis, molecular biology studies in patients with rheumatoid arthritis have provided evidence that collagen-destroying enzymes are involved in the mechanism of disease. In fact, these destructive enzymes seem to play a more prominent role in rheumatoid arthritis than in osteoarthritis. Several NIAMS-supported research groups have obtained evidence that the production of these enzymes, and of a factor that can inhibit these enzymes, is localized specifically to cells in the synovial lining. Thus, future therapies for rheumatoid arthritis may include agents that can block production or actions of these destructive enzymes in the synovium.

At present, treatment for rheumatoid arthritis consists primarily of drugs that control the symptoms of the disease. An exciting new area of basic and clinical research involves the development of various "biologics" for treating rheumatoid arthritis. These agents, which include various antibodies and specific inhibitors of inflammatory factors, are designed specifically to target various components of the immune system that mediate the inflammation and destruction of the joints that occur in rheumatoid arthritis. Thus, these new approaches are aimed at preventing symptoms, rather than treating them once they occur. A number of potential biologic therapies for rheumatoid arthritis are being tested in controlled clinical trials in humans, and some newer therapies are being tested in animal models.

NIAMS is also conducting a clinical trial to assess the efficacy of minocycline in the treatment of rheumatoid arthritis. In one study, 219 patients were enrolled in the 48-week trial. A report on the results of this study was scheduled for release in 1994.

Clinical Trial Evaluates Treatment of Arthritis In Children

An estimated 200,000 children in the United States have some form of arthritis. Research is providing evidence that specific genetic markers, similar to those associated with rheumatoid arthritis in adults, are associated with increased susceptibility to juvenile rheumatoid arthritis (JRA). Specific genetic variants of T-cell receptors, key components of the immune response, may also play a role in some forms of juvenile arthritis.

While about one-third of all patients with juvenile arthritis can be treated effectively with nonsteroidal anti-inflammatory drugs, the remainder are resistant to these drugs and are candidates for additional therapy. A carefully controlled clinical trial performed by the Pediatric Rheumatology Collaborative Study Group and their collaborators in Russia, and funded by NIAMS and the Arthritis Foundation, showed that low doses of methotrexate given once a week by mouth are effective in the treatment of resistant JRA. Methotrexate is a drug that had been shown previously to be effective in treating rheumatoid arthritis in adults. The methotrexate regimen used in the children was shown to be safe, with few side effects, over the 6-month treatment period. The results justify the use of methotrexate as the second-line agent for treating resistant cases of JRA.

Scleroderma Disease Mechanisms Being Explored

Systemic sclerosis, or scleroderma, is a potentially life-threatening connective tissue and small blood vessel disorder that affects about four times more women than men. Individuals with this disease develop thickening of the skin and damage to internal organs such as the kidneys, lungs, and heart as a result of excessive accumulation of the structural protein collagen. Scleroderma is also a disease of the immune system. Antinuclear autoantibodies have been found in up to 90 percent of scleroderma patients.

Scleroderma usually begins with Raynaud's disease, a relatively common disorder characterized by blanching and cooling of the fingers and toes due to abnormal changes in small blood vessels, which affect the circulation. Researchers at the University of Connecticut in Farmington studied patients with Raynaud's disease to determine the relationship between autoantibodies and long-term clinical outcome. They found that the presence of two antinuclear antibodies in Raynaud's patients was associated with the subsequent development of scleroderma or other connective tissue disease. Tests for these antibodies should provide a sensitive method to detect those Raynaud's patients who are at risk for scleroderma.

Molecular studies of skin or isolated skin cells from scleroderma patients are yielding numerous insights into the disease mechanisms. The role of certain growth factors in mediating the abnormal production of collagen that leads to hardening of the skin in scleroderma is being elucidated. Adhesion molecules, the glue-like molecules that cause inflammatory white blood cells to adhere to their target tissues, are also being implicated in the development of scleroderma. Once the details of these processes are worked out, it should be possible to develop specific treatments for scleroderma that target and block these processes at the molecular level.

National Institute of Allergy and Infectious Diseases

The National Institute of Allergy and Infectious Diseases (NIAID) funds research aimed at elucidating the pathogenesis and etiology of rheumatoid arthritis. Scientists are trying to identify the causative agents of rheumatoid arthritis. They are also studying the genes that are involved in the predisposition to and development of arthritis, the mechanisms of autoantibody production and the biochemistry and physiology of molecules that induce inflammation and tissue damage.

An in vitro system was established by NIAID-supported researchers in which suspensions of lymphocytes (white blood calls important for immune defense) and synovial cells from the joints of patients with rheumatoid arthritis were cultured, producing an outgrowth of tissue. This outgrowth closely resembled the inflammatory material on the lining layer of synovial cells inside a joint, the hallmark of human rheumatoid arthritis. Scientists found that the continuous growth of this tissue depended on the presence of cytokines, T cells, and a portion of a particular kind of bacterium.

This system, a novel technologic advance, is a valuable tool with which to study the interaction between the immune system and the fibroblasts (cells that produce connective tissue) in the joint. It could also prove very useful in assessing the pharmacologic effects of new drugs and biologicals designed to stop or reverse inflammatory tissue damage.

National Institute of Child Health and Human Development

For women of reproductive age, autoimmune diseases are among the more common disorders. As a rule, estrogens exacerbate autoimmune diseases, while androgenic substances (male sex hormones) suppress them. The role of progestogens in the course of diseases of immune origin has not been satisfactorily determined.

For women of late reproductive age, rheumatoid arthritis is reported to occur less frequently among women who have used contraceptive steroids. The role of sex hormones in this disease has been inferred from the fact that many more woman than men have rheumatoid arthritis and from the observation that pregnancy often improves the symptomatology of rheumatoid arthritis.

The National Institute of Child Health and Human Development (NICHD) just completed a large case-controlled study to identify whether current or past use of oral contraceptives containing estrogens or progestogens reduced the risk of rheumatoid arthritis. The investigators recruited 349 people with rheumatoid arthritis and 1,357 control subjects.

Rheumatoid arthritis risk declined with longer duration of oral-contraceptive use and with increasing estrogen dose. Little association was observed with cumulative progestogen dose, estrogenic of progestogenic potency of currently used preparations, timing of oral contraceptive use, or past use in women over 45. Current or past use appears to reduce the risk of rheumatoid arthritis in women under 45 by about 30 percent.

Further data analysis will help clarify mechanisms by which contraceptive hormones protect women from rheumatoid arthritis. The further analysis will focus on the relation between rheumatoid arthritis and postmenopausal hormone use, past pregnancy and childbearing history, and personal characteristics known to influence endogenous hormone levels such as smoking, weight, and age of menarche.

For more information about arthritis, write to:

National Institute of Arthritis and Musculoskeletal and Skin Diseases
Building 31, Room 4C05
Bethesda, MD 20892

Chapter 18

Coping with Connective Tissue Diseases

"I woke up one morning and noticed that my hands and feet were swollen. I said to myself, 'what is this?'" says Carol Grogul, a 29 year-old administrative assistant in a New York City investment company.

She went to work and didn't think much more about it. But over the course of the next few weeks, Grogul began to experience severe pain in her knees and hips.

"One minute I was fine, the next minute the pain was so bad I couldn't move," she recalls.

When her fingers started curling into a claw shape, she became frightened. After seeking help from several doctors to no avail, Grogul was referred to a rheumatologist. The diagnosis: scleroderma (thickening of the skin), also called systemic sclerosis, which is one of a family of disorders known collectively as connective tissue diseases (CTDs). Within a matter of weeks, she was to feel the full brunt of scleroderma's distressing symptoms.

"Now the skin on my face is so tight I can hardly open my mouth. I have no muscle energy at all. I walk with a cane, like an old woman, and I'm losing my hair," she says.

These severe symptoms followed a bout with kidney failure, also the result of scleroderma. "This disease may not kill you, but you will suffer," she says. "I never have a day when I feel really good, but I just have to keep going."

Seven years ago, when Tina Kline of Clyde, N.C., was pregnant with her second child, she noticed rashes on her knuckles, nose, eyes, and

FDA Consumer November 1992.

chest. She assumed was experiencing a reaction to picking strawberries. She also felt completely exhausted, which she attributed to her pregnancy.

"A few days later, my arms would not go over my head. I couldn't get dressed or undressed. My legs were so weak, I had to crawl up the stairs," she recalls.

Tests taken in the emergency department of her local hospital were inconclusive, so Kline was referred to various specialists for additional tests. Ultimately, a rheumatologist made the diagnosis: polymyositis/dermatomyositis (PM/DM), another CTD with potentially devastating consequences.

Today, at age 36, Kline, who founded a PM/DM support group, is in remission from the disease. But she suffers from bone deterioration, a side effect of the prednisone (a corticosteroid medication) prescribed to lessen her symptoms.

After six weeks, during which she took 60 milligrams of oral prednisone daily, the joints in her legs began to deteriorate. She was hospitalized and given 150 milligrams daily of the immunosuppressive drug azathioprine (Imuran) to combat the deterioration. However, she continued taking prednisone to treat PM/DM. The disease had also caused her lungs to become infected.

Over the next few years, in a rare instance of widespread joint deterioration, Kline said that her hip and shoulder joints "collapsed," even though prednisone was tapered to lower levels. She has since had her hips and shoulders surgically replaced, and "my knees are next," she says. "There are days when I feel angry and frustrated, sick of having to deal with the disease nonstop, day in and day out," Kline admits. "But I've learned to be grateful for what I can do, for whatever physical independence I have."

Today, Tina Kline, founder of a support group for people with polymyositis/dermatomyosits, looks like almost any healthy 30-something woman as she stands at her kitchen counter slicing vegetables. The PM/DM that first attacked her seven years ago during a pregnancy is in remission. But during her fight with the disease she was confined to a wheelchair, her hips and shoulder joints collapsed, she developed a back hump and distended stomach, and she lost hair and gained 50 pounds.

Immune System at Fault

In scleroderma, PM/DM, and systemic lupus erythematosus (SLE), the immune system goes awry. (See "Living with Lupus.")

172

"The body ceases to recognize 'self as self,' and mounts an attack against itself," explains Joseph Markenson, M.D., associate professor of clinical medicine at Cornell University Medical College in New York City. In such an "autoimmune reaction" the body produces antibodies—substances normally secreted by certain white blood cells to combat disease-causing viruses, bacteria, and other microorganisms—against its own cells and tissues. This triggers an array of symptoms, from joint pain to rashes to internal organ damage.

These CTDs have been in the news lately because of claims by some women and physicians that silicone leakage from breast implants and collagen injected into the skin to reduce acne scars and wrinkling cause CTDs. Although scientific evidence linking these products with CTDs is not conclusive, the media attention has sparked much curiosity about these disorders.

The fact is, the vast majority of the millions of Americans who suffer from a CTD—many of whom are women in their 20s, 30s and 40s—have no clue why the disease has struck them. This includes an estimated 2 million Americans with rheumatoid arthritis (see "Arthritis: Modern Treatment for that Old Pain in the Joints" in the July-August 1991 *FDA Consumer*), a CTD that thus far has not been associated with silicone implants or collagen injections. It also includes an estimated 500,000 Americans with SLE or another variant of lupus; 300,000 with scleroderma; and an unknown number who suffer from PM/DM. Many people who have a CTD develop "overlap" syndromes, which means they have symptoms of more than one CTD simultaneously.

CTDs are potentially life-threatening, and even mild cases can significantly impair quality of life. Disabling symptoms interfere with the ability to work or take care of a family. There is also an emotional toll when other people's unfounded fears lead them to treat a person with a CTD as an outcast.

"I know a woman with lupus who lost her job; people in her office wouldn't go near her or let her sit on their chairs," says Ronni Shulman, a 38-year-old public relations consultant from Westchester, N.Y., who has had scleroderma for 10 years. "I've noticed women hold on to their children when I walk by." Yet these disorders aren't contagious or infectious. No one can "catch" them from someone else.

What Causes CTDs?

The causes of CTDs are unknown, although scientists are investigating factors that may play a role in triggering the disorders. Suspected culprits are defective genes, overproduction of hormones, and faulty clearing from the body of antibodies and the substances with which they react.

"There appears to be a combination of some environmental agents acting on certain genetic backgrounds in these diseases," says Fred Miller, M.D., Ph.D., medical officer in FDA's Center for Biological Evaluation and Research, molecular immunology laboratory. He notes that occupational exposure to silica dust and polyvinyl chlorides have been associated with scleroderma. Drug-induced lupus, a variant of SLE, can be traced to the use of drugs such as hydralazine (a high blood pressure medication), procainamide (a treatment for irregular heartbeats), and isoniazid (a tuberculosis drug). When a patient stops the suspected drug, lupus symptoms may clear up. But why some people become ill after exposure to these agents remains unclear.

The idea that an environmental agent can trigger a CTD in susceptible people has led to conjecture about a possible link between silicone, collagen injections, and CTDs. Yet the data offered to support a connection are "very sparse and weak," says FDA's Miller.

Because FDA feels further study of silicone breast implants is warranted, the agency has restricted the use of these implants to women undergoing breast reconstruction following mastectomy and a limited number of women choosing the devices for augmentation (see "Silicone Breast Implants Available Under Tight Controls" in the June 1992 *FDA Consumer*).

Many physicians are urging caution with collagen injections. "It [the procedure] worries me a lot," says Judith Anderson, M.D., a hematologist and associate professor of internal medicine in the Division of Hematology/Oncology, Wayne State University School of Medicine. She points out that there is no standardization of the type of collagen used for injection. Most physicians use collagen products made from bovine (cow) collagen. Such products are likely to be properly purified and free of contaminants because they are prepared in large quantities for commercial use.

However, "unethical practitioners" may use collagen from cadavers, which may not be subject to the same high standards of quality control, Anderson says. Cadaver collagen may be contaminated with white cells that can cause an autoimmune reaction in a person who receives collagen injections. There is also potential for viral contamination of cadaver collagen. "If I were a young woman with a cleft chin or wrinkles, I would think 100 times before having collagen injections," she says.

Although patients are given a preliminary injection to test for allergic reaction before undergoing treatment, "that doesn't mean you won't develop problems several years down the road," adds Sara Kramer, M.D., a rheumatologist and instructor of clinical medicine at New York University Medical Center. "My feeling is, if you don't need the procedure for medical reasons, you're better off not having it done."

FDA holds that evidence is insufficient to show that collagen injections cause CTDs in people without a history of these diseases. Even so, this does not mean there is no risk of developing CTDs from these injections. The agency has mandated that collagen products' labels carry a warning about the possible association between collagen injections and PM/DM. People considering undergoing the procedure should ask their physicians for the patient information brochure, which lists the possible adverse effects of the products, and discuss these risks with their doctors.

Diagnosing CTDs

One reason it's so difficult to determine if silicone, collagen injections, or anything else triggers CTDs is that the illnesses themselves are not easily diagnosed. No single test can definitively determine whether a person has a CTD, and symptoms are very often vague, mimicking those of other diseases. As Shulman says about scleroderma, "It's like the snowflake of diseases—no two cases are alike."

A CTD is usually diagnosed by the patient's symptoms, medical history, and the results of a number of tests that assess the status of the immune system and tissues in the body.

- **Blood Tests:** Several blood tests are used to help determine whether a patient has a CTD and, if so, what type. A physician may first order a complete blood count and other standard blood tests. Depending on results, the doctor may also order an antinuclear antibody test (ANA). This is a nonspecific test that determines if a patient has auto-antibodies that react with parts of the cell nuclei. However, results may be positive for conditions other than a CTD, such as infectious diseases or endocrine disease.

  Disease-specific antibody tests may also be done. These tests indicate the presence of antibodies for specific CTDs. For example, the anti-DNA and anti-Sm antibody tests are specific to

SLE. There are also specific antibody tests for scleroderma and PM/DM. However, many people with CTDs have negative antibody tests. These tests can help confirm a diagnosis in a patient with symptoms or a family history, but can't be used alone to make diagnoses.

- **Electromyography:** This test assesses the electrical activity in muscles and is used in the diagnosis of PM/DM.

- **Biopsy:** The removal of a small piece of tissue for inspection under a microscope can be a useful diagnostic tool. A biopsy of muscle tissue can help diagnose PM/ DM. A biopsy of kidney tissue can give evidence that SLE has affected that organ.

Symptom Management

Just as the causes of CTDs are unknown, so are the cures. All CTDs are chronic, but people may have long periods of remission when they are symptom-free. For this reason, treatment focuses on symptom "management."

Since few people with CTDs suffer from all symptoms characteristic of a specific disorder, the treatment plan for each patient must be individualized. Because the drugs used to treat severe symptoms can have very serious side effects—such as the bone deterioration Kline developed from taking corticosteroids—physicians continuously weigh the benefits of treating symptoms against the risks of adverse drug effects (see "Distinguishing CTDs" below).

Looking Ahead

Studies are under way in medical centers around the country to test investigational therapies for CTDs. These include the use of certain orphan drugs and combinations of new immunosuppressive drugs, biologic agents (antibodies produced in a laboratory), plasmapheresis (removal of plasma from blood cells, and reinfusion), and photophoresis (use of a drug activated by ultraviolet light).

"The upside to all the media attention focused on CTDs lately is increased awareness among physicians and the public about the toll these diseases take on people's lives," says hematologist Anderson. She and others hope this will spur greater interest in exploring the causes that underlie these disorders and result in better ways to manage and even cure connective tissue diseases.

Clinical Trials

Patients interested in participating in clinical trials of investigational therapies for CTDs should talk with their physicians or contact the following organizations:

National Organization for Rare Disorders (NORD)
P.O. Box 8923
New Fairfield, CT 06812-1783
(203) 746-6518

Scleroderma Society
1182 Teaneck Road
Teaneck, NJ 07666
(201) 837-9826

The National Support Group for Dermatomyositis
RD 3, Box 80
Clyde, NC 28721
(704) 627-9908

Lupus Foundation of America, Inc.
4 Research Place, Suite 180
Rockville, MD 20850-3226
(301) 670-9292 or (800) 558-0121

Arthritis Foundation
1314 Spring St., N.W.
Atlanta, GA 30309
(404) 872-7100

The National Arthritis and Musculoskeletal and Skin Diseases Information Clearinghouse
Box AMS
Bethesda, MD 20892
(301) 495-4484

Distinguishing CTDs

CTDs have some symptoms in common and others that are specific to each disorder. Here's a look at the most common symptoms of scleroderma, PM/DM and SLE and how they are treated.

- **Scleroderma:** The most common early symptom of scleroderma is Raynaud's phenomenon (but not everyone who has Raynaud's phenomenon develops scleroderma). In Raynaud's phenomenon, the blood vessels of the hands and feet constrict in response to cold exposure, and the affected skin turns white, blue, then red. Vasodilators, drugs that relax and dilate blood vessels, are used to treat this condition.

  Swelling of the hands or feet is managed with diuretics (drugs that help eliminate excess water from the body) or nonsteroidal anti-inflammatory drugs (NSAIDs).

  There are no proven treatments as yet to treat or alter the course of fibrosis, the skin thickening that gives scleroderma its name. Experimental therapies, such as the use of penicillamine, a drug that interferes with collagen production, are being explored.

  Skin sores must be cleansed to prevent bacterial infection, usually caused by staphylococcus bacteria. If infection occurs, it may be treated initially by soaking the affected area in warm water and applying an antiseptic such as hydrogen peroxide or Betadine (povidone-iodine solution). If infection continues, a broad-spectrum antibiotic such as erythromycin may be prescribed.

  ACE inhibitors (a type of blood pressure medication) are frequently prescribed to treat kidney involvement and prevent kidney failure. A variety of experimental therapies are being used to treat involvement of other organs.

  A wide range of over-the-counter and prescription medicines are used to treat less severe symptoms, such as dry, itchy skin and digestion problems.

  Physical therapy may help early in the process to prevent joint contracture. Range of motion exercises can also help protect joints and keep them limber.

- **Polymyositis/Dermatomyositis(PM/DM):** Muscle weakness—particularly in the shoulders, arms and legs—is the hallmark of polymyositis. When the muscle weakness is preceded or accompanied by a red rash on the nose, cheeks, knees, or knuckles and a purple coloring on the eyelids, the disorder is called dermatomyositis. The two are usually grouped together as PM/DM.

Corticosteroids are the mainstay of treatment, says rheumatologist Kramer. In severe cases, immunosuppressive drugs such as methotrexate or cyclophosphamide may be prescribed. Physical therapy can help prevent muscles from shrinking as they heal.

- **Systemic Lupus Erythematosus (SLE):** Milder symptoms of SLE, such as joint pain, rashes, and mild pleurisy (inflammation of the lung lining) often respond to NSAIDs. Corticosteroids are used to treat more severe symptoms, such as kidney disease, and milder symptoms that don't respond to NSAIDs.

Antimalarial drugs may be prescribed to reduce joint swelling, pain and rash, including the patchy, crusty red skin patches associated with this disorder. Immunosuppressive drugs may be used to treat patients with very severe symptoms, such as advanced kidney disease or central nervous system disease.

SLE patients are advised to avoid the sun, which can precipitate or aggravate a flare-up of the disease. Daily sunblock use is recommended, even for those patients who don't spend much time in the sun.

—by Marilynn Larkin

Marilynn Larkin is a medical writer in New York City.

Chapter 19

Insulin-Dependent Diabetes Mellitis

Diabetes is the sixth leading cause of death by disease in the United States today and a factor in more than 300,000 deaths a year. A chronic and physically disabling disease, diabetes can cause damage to virtually every part of the body. In addition to physical hardship, diabetes heaps financial burden on those it afflicts. People with the disorder spend three times as much on medical care as the average American. The disease costs the United States an estimated $20 to $40 billion annually in lost worker productivity, health care costs, disability payments, and premature deaths.

Diabetes interferes with the body's ability to metabolize glucose (sugar) for energy. It is estimated that between 13 and 14 million Americans have diabetes; approximately 700,000 new cases are diagnosed every year. Adults over 55 and certain minorities including blacks, Hispanics, Native Americans and Native Hawaiians are most vulnerable to the disorder. Experts say that half of those who have the disease do not know it and consequently are not receiving medical care.

By far the most devastating aspect of diabetes is the long-term complications it can cause. The longer someone has the disease the greater the risk of eye disease and blindness, heart disease, strokes nerve damage, leg and foot amputations, and kidney failure. People with diabetes are more prone to digestive disorders and gum and skin infections, and babies born to mothers with diabetes are at increased

NIH Pub No. 94-3422.

risk for birth defects. Those with diabetes also experience a greater number of medical emergencies and hospitalizations than the average person. Untreated, abnormally high or low blood glucose levels can cause unconsciousness, coma and even death.

Diabetes Interferes With Glucose Metabolism

The end product of carbohydrate metabolism, glucose is found in the blood of all animals and is the body's chief source of energy. When the amount of glucose in blood rises, as it does after a meal is digested, beta cells in the pancreas release the hormone insulin. Insulin enables the body to use the amount of glucose it needs for fuel and then store the rest. Diabetes occurs when the body produces little or no insulin or when the body does not respond to the insulin that is produced (insulin resistance). When this happens, glucose builds to dangerously high levels in the blood, damaging areas of the body it is meant to nourish. At the same time, the overflow is excreted in urine, robbing the body of energy it needs to survive. Scientists now know that diabetes is not a single disease as was once believed, but rather a complex group of disorders. Its primary forms are insulin-dependent diabetes mellitus (IDDM) and non-insulin-dependent diabetes mellitus (NIDDM).

The focus of this chapter is IDDM, an autoimmune disease. For more information on this and other forms of diabetes, see Omnigraphics' *Diabetes Sourcebook*.

Insulin-Dependent Diabetes Strikes the Young

Approximately 750,000 Americans have insulin-dependent diabetes, also known as Type I diabetes. It usually strikes individuals under 30 although it can occur at any age. An autoimmune disease, IDDM occurs when the immune system—that protects the body from foreign invaders such as viruses and bacteria—instead mistakes the insulin-secreting beta cells in the pancreas for foreign bodies and destroys them. Scientists do not yet understand why this happens, but they believe both genetic and viral factors are involved. By the time the symptoms of diabetes occur, most of the body's ability to produce insulin is gone. Those with IDDM must have daily insulin injections to survive.

Discovery of Diabetes Genes Key to Predicting, Preventing IDDM

Studies of the incidence of IDDM in pairs of identical twins and in families confirm the disease's genetic component. Recently, NIDDK-supported scientists identified several genes that may play a role in a person's predisposition to IDDM. The discovery of these and other diabetes-susceptibility genes may lead to the development of screening tests for diabetes and methods of preventing or delaying onset of the disease in those at risk.

In research that holds great promise, investigators for the National Institute of Diabetes and Digestive and Kidney Diseases (NIDDK) are examining the relationship between the development of IDDM and specific genes in one area of the mammalian genome, the major histocompatibility complex (MHC). The MHC helps shape an organism's immune response to the environment, and scientists believe that inheriting certain genes in this complex increases one's risk of developing IDDM. This year, NIDDK-supported investigators at Massachusetts General Hospital and the Joslin Diabetes Center in Boston found, for the first time, a defect in the immune systems of IDDM rodent models and humans predisposed to IDDM. The immune defect involves genes of the MHC. Scientist discovered that among nonobese diabetic (NOD) mice—a strain of mice prone to development of diabetes—those with a decreased expression of MHC class I proteins were more susceptible to IDDM. (MHC class I antigens are present on all body cells and signal the cell as "self.")

In related research supported by NIDDK, investigators have identified additional susceptibility genes on chromosome 1. The products of these genes control the movement of lymphocytes or immune system cells into the pancreatic islets where the insulin-producing beta cells are located.

Also using a rodent model, NIDDK-supported scientists have implicated at least three other genes in the development of IDDM. Several other groups of investigators supported by NIDDK are examining a specific alteration in DNA in the region of the insulin gene that may be associated with IDDM.

These advances demonstrate that an altered gene product seems linked to the development of IDDM. Now that scientists have discovered several diabetes-related genes, they can begin studying each gene's role in the disease process.

Work Continues on IDDM Screening Tests

In research related to the genetics of IDDM, scientists are closer to developing a blood test to screen individuals for certain diabetes-related antibodies. An important advance was reported last year when researchers at the University of Washington in Seattle discovered, cloned, and sequenced the gene for the antigen GAD-2, a protein found in human beta cells. Antibodies to GAD-2 appear up to seven years before onset of IDDM and are found in 80 percent of patients at the time of diagnosis. This year the same researchers discovered and mapped the chromosomal location of several genes for the antigens that trigger antibodies against beta cells. They also sequenced—determined the sequence of molecular bases that make up a gene—carboxypeptidase-H, a component of beta cells that appears to be associated with the development of IDDM. Some scientists believe that identifying these beta cell autoantigens eventually will help prove whether viral infections can initiate IDDM by presenting the immune system with molecules so similar to GAD-2 that beta cells become the target.

In the hope of devising methods to predict and measure a person's risk of developing the disorder, scientists are studying close relatives of IDDM patients. NIDDK-supported researchers have discovered that relatives who have a particular type of islet cell antibody (ICA) have a markedly lower risk of developing diabetes. On the other hand, the scientists found that among relatives who have a positive result on the standard ICA test, which does not distinguish between different ICAs, an abnormal reading on a test that measures beta cell function, called the intravenous glucose tolerance test (IVGTT), predicts onset of diabetes within 1.5 years. Results of a populations-based study indicate that measuring ICA, anti-insulin antibodies (AIA) and GAD antibodies, and conducting the IVGTT, may help identify high risk individuals.

Research Implicates Role of Cow's Milk in IDDM Susceptibility

A finding by Finnish and Canadian researchers supports a long-held theory that proteins in cow's milk, like certain viruses, may mimic a beta cell antigen. Study results suggest that patients with IDDM have an immune response to cow's milk and have developed anti-bodies to albumin (a protein found in milk) that are capable of reacting with a particular beta cell protein. Such antibodies could participate in the development of islet dysfunction. Similar research conducted by NIDDK-supported scientists suggest that breast-feeding of infants may provide a protective influence against the risk of IDDM later in life. However, NIDDK-supported scientists at the University of Florida in Gainesville caution that it is premature to eliminate cow's milk from the diets of growing infants and children considered to be at risk for IDDM, until additional studies confirm recent findings.

Early Insulin Treatment Could Slow IDDM Onset

Once methods are established for developing diabetes, intervention therapies can be designed to prevent onset of the disease. Research has shown that oral administration of insulin delays onset and reduces incidence of diabetes in nonobese diabetic mice. Preliminary results in humans suggest that injections of insulin may delay onset or prevent IDDM. Further research should show whether oral administration of insulin may be useful in preventing IDDM in susceptible individuals.

Transplantation Research Promises a Treatment

There is no cure for diabetes. Treatment involves the daily administration of insulin, either by injection or infusion, in combination with a diet and exercise program. Scientists believe that islet transplantation could eliminate a patient's need for insulin injections. Pancreas and islet transplants have reversed insulin dependence in selected patients who have had a kidney transplant and therefore already are taking immunosuppressive drugs to prevent graft rejection. However, the toxicity of these immunosuppressive drugs prohibits the use of islet cell transplants in most patients. A standing goal of NIDDK-supported scientists is to achieve islet cell transplantation without the use of immunosuppressive drugs.

Implantation of islets in a site where they are not recognized as foreign, is a technique being studied at the University of Pennsylvania. There NIDDK grantees have discovered that the thymus, the organ in which certain immune system cells mature, is an ideal location. In ongoing research in animal models, the scientists injected islets into the thymus glands of 18 diabetes-prone newborn rodents and gave placebo injections to 14 other diabetes-prone newborns. Seven of the 14 rodents that received the placebo developed diabetes, but none of the 18 that received the islet injection developed the disorder. In addition, biopsies showed that the 18 rodents who received the islets had normal pancreases. According to the study's principal investigator, who recently reported similar results in adult rodents, implanting islets into the thymus glands of people at risk for developing diabetes may be a way of "reeducating" their immune systems to prevent the disease.

Other NIDDK-supported researchers are seeking to protect islet transplants by developing barriers to autoimmune destruction. For the first time, NIDDK grantees at Washington University in St. Louis have corrected diabetes in mice by implanting islets, encapsulated in porous tubes, just beneath the skin. Because the tubes are selectively permeable, they protect the transplanted islets from being rejected. Holes in the sides of the tube are large enough to permit oxygen and nutrients to enter and insulin produced by the cells to flow out into the bloodstream. Yet the holes are small enough to keep the attacking immune system cells out. The investigators plan to test the technique in dogs and monkeys and if these results are successful, human trials could begin in two years.

An islet transplant study conducted by NIDDK grantees at the University of Minnesota provides the clearest evidence yet that transplantation of as few as 265,000 islets, a fraction of what is normally used in transplantation, can result in the release of insulin and glucagon (another hormone involved in glucose metabolism) at appropriate times. Islet transplantation can provide prolonged periods of insulin independence for those who are dependent on insulin injections. The subjects in the study were people whose pancreases had to be removed, but who then had their own islets implanted in the liver. As a result, no immunosuppression was needed. The scientists reported that the body's rejection of islets, rather than insufficient numbers of islets, is probably the reason for unsuccessful islet transplantation.

While research in islet transplantation holds great promise, harvesting islets from human cadavers and animals is expensive and labor-intensive. Therefore, a group of NIDDK-supported scientists are approaching transplantation from a different perspective. Investigators at the University of Texas Southwestern Medical Center at Dallas have created the first genetically engineered beta cells. The cells were made by adding the genes for human insulin and glucose transporter protein, Glut-2, to an insulin-secreting cell line. This research represents the first time genetic engineering has been used to produce a cell line that releases insulin in response to changes in glucose concentration. The scientists have not tested the cells in animals or humans yet because they still need to design a barrier method to protect the cells from attack.

Chapter 20

What Is Guillain-Barré Syndrome?

Guillain-Barré (ghee-yan bah-ray) syndrome is a disorder in which the body's immune system attacks part of the nervous system. The first symptoms of this disorder include varying degrees of weakness or tingling sensations in the legs. In many instances the weakness and abnormal sensations spread to the arms and upper body. These symptoms can increase in intensity until the muscles cannot be used at all and the patient is almost totally paralyzed. In these cases the disorder is life threatening—potentially interfering with blood pressure, heart rate, and breathing—and is considered a medical emergency. The patient is often put on a respirator to assist with breathing and is watched closely for problems such as an abnormal heart beat, infections, blood clots, and high or low blood pressure. Most patients, however, recover from even the most severe cases of Guillain-Barré syndrome, although some continue to have minor problems.

Guillain-Barré syndrome can affect anybody. It can strike at any age and both sexes are equally prone to the disorder. The syndrome is rare, however, afflicting only about one person in 100,000. Usually Guillain-Barré occurs a few days or weeks after the patient has had symptoms of a respiratory or gastrointestinal viral infection. Occasionally pregnancy, surgery, or vaccinations will trigger the syndrome. The disorder can develop over the course of hours or days, or it may take up to 3 to 4 weeks. Most people reach the stage of greatest weakness within the first 2 weeks after symptoms appear, and by the third week of the illness 90 percent of all patients are at their weakest.

NIH Pub No. 92-2902.

What Causes Guillain-Barré Syndrome?

No one yet knows why Guillain-Barré strikes some people and not others. Nor does anyone know exactly what sets the disease in motion. What scientists do know is that the body's immune system begins to attack the body itself, causing what is known as an autoimmune disease. Usually the cells of the immune system attack only foreign material and invading organisms. In Guillain-Barré syndrome, however, the immune system starts to destroy the myelin sheath that surrounds the axons of many nerve cells, or even the axons themselves (axons are long, thin extensions of the nerve cells; they carry nerve signals). The myelin sheath surrounding the axon speeds up the transmission of nerve signals and allows the transmission of signals over long distances.

In diseases in which the nerve cells' myelin sheaths are injured or degraded, the nerves cannot transmit signals efficiently. That is why the muscles begin to lose their ability to respond to the brain's commands, commands that must be carried through the nerve network. The brain also receives fewer sensory signals from the rest of the body, resulting in an inability to feel textures, heat, pain, and other sensations. Alternately, the brain may receive inappropriate signals that result in tingling, "crawling-skin," or painful sensations. Because the signals to and from the arms and legs must travel the longest distances they are most vulnerable to interruption. Therefore, muscle weakness and tingling sensations usually first appear in the hands and feet.

When Guillain-Barré is preceded by a viral infection, it is possible that the virus has changed the nature of cells in the nervous system so that the immune system treats them as foreign cells. It is also possible that the virus makes the immune system itself less discriminating about what cells it attacks. Scientists are investigating these possibilities and others to find why the immune system goes awry in Guillain-Barré syndrome and other autoimmune diseases. The cause and course of Guillain-Barré syndrome is an active area of neurological investigation, incorporating the cooperative efforts of neurological scientists, immunologists, and virologists.

How Is Guillain-Barré Syndrome Diagnosed?

Guillain-Barré is called a syndrome rather than a disease because it is not clear that a specific disease-causing agent is involved. A syndrome is a medical condition characterized by a collection of symptoms (what the patient feels) and signs (what a doctor can observe or measure). Because the signs and symptoms of the syndrome can be quite varied, doctors may find it difficult to diagnose Guillain-Barré in its earliest stages. Several disorders have symptoms similar to those found in Guillain-Barré, so doctors examine and question patients carefully before making a diagnosis. Collectively, the signs and symptoms form a certain pattern that helps doctors differentiate Guillain-Barré from other disorders. For example, physicians will note whether the symptoms appear on both sides of the body (most common in Guillain-Barré) and the quickness with which the symptoms appear (in other disorders muscle weakness may progress over months rather than days or weeks). In Guillain Barré, reflexes such as knee jerks are usually lost. Because the signals traveling along the nerve are slower, a nerve conduction velocity (NCV) test can give a doctor clues to aid the diagnosis. In Guillain-Barré patients, the cerebrospinal fluid that bathes the spinal cord and brain contains more protein than usual. Therefore a physician may decide to perform a spinal tap, a procedure in which the doctor inserts a needle into the patient's lower back to draw cerebrospinal fluid from the spinal column. Laboratory scientists, working with clinical neurologists, are conducting research that may help provide physicians with more precise and reliable diagnostic tests for this disorder.

How Is Guillain-Barré Treated?

There is no known cure for Guillain-Barré syndrome. However, there are therapies that lessen the severity of the illness in most patients, and there are a number of ways to treat the complications of the disease.

Currently, plasmapheresis and high-dose immunoglobulin therapy are used in the more serious cases of Guillain-Barré syndrome. Plasmapheresis is a method by which whole blood is removed from the body and processed so that the red and white blood cells are separated from the plasma, or liquid portion of the blood. The blood cells are then returned to the patient without the plasma, which the body quickly replaces. Scientists still don't know exactly why plasmapheresis works, but the technique seems to reduce the severity and duration of the Guillain Barré episode. This may be because the plasma portion of the blood contains elements that the immune system needs to function. When these elements are removed along with the plasma, the immune system is not able to attack the nervous system as effectively.

In high-dose immunoglobulin therapy, doctors give intravenous injections of the proteins that the immune system uses to attack invading organisms. Investigators have found that these immunoglobulins, when given to Guillain-Barré patients, can lessen the immune attack on the nervous system. Investigators don't know why this is, but some suggest that the immunoglobulins may overwhelm the immune system and keep it from attacking the nerve cells and their myelin sheaths. The use of steroid hormones has also been tried as a way to reduce the severity of Guillain-Barré, but controlled clinical trials have not demonstrated that this treatment is effective.

Much of the treatment for this syndrome consists of keeping the patient's body functioning during recovery of the nervous system. This can sometimes require placing the patient on a respirator, a heart monitor, or other machines that assist body function. The need for this sophisticated machinery is one reason why Guillain-Barré syndrome patients are usually treated in hospitals, often in an intensive care ward. In the hospital, doctors can also look for and treat the many problems that can afflict any paralyzed patient complications such as pneumonia or bed sores.

Often, even before recovery begins, care-givers may be instructed to manually move the patient's limbs to help keep the muscles flexible and strong. Later, as the patient begins to recover limb control, physical therapy begins. Carefully planned clinical trials of new and experimental therapies are the key to improving the treatment of patients with Guillain-Barré syndrome. Such clinical trials begin with the research of basic and clinical scientists who, working with clinicians, identify new approaches to treating patients with the disease.

What Is the Long-Term Outlook for Those with Guillain-Barré Syndrome?

Guillain-Barré syndrome can be a devastating disorder because of its sudden and unexpected onset. In addition, recovery is not necessarily quick. As noted previously, patients usually reach the point of greatest weakness or paralysis days or weeks after the first symptoms occur. Symptoms then stabilize at this level for a period of days, weeks, or, sometimes, months. The recovery period may be as little as a few weeks or as long as a few years. About 30 percent of those with Guillain-Barré still feel a residual weakness after 3 years. About

3 to 5 percent may suffer a relapse of muscle weakness and tingling sensations many years after the initial attack.

Guillain-Barré syndrome patients face not only physical difficulties, but emotionally painful periods as well. It is often extremely difficult for patients to adjust to sudden paralysis and dependence on others for help with routine daily activities. Patients sometimes need psychological counseling to help them adapt.

What Research Is Being Done?

Scientists are concentrating on finding new treatments and refining existing ones. Scientists are also looking at the workings of the immune system to find which cells are responsible for beginning and carrying out the attack on the nervous system. The fact that so many cases of Guillain-Barré begin after a viral infection suggests that certain characteristics of these viruses may activate the immune system inappropriately. Investigators are searching for those characteristics. As noted previously, neurological scientists, immunologists, virologists, and pharmacologists are all working collaboratively to learn how to prevent this disorder and to make better therapies available when it strikes.

Where Can I Go for More Information?

The National Institute of Neurological Disorders and Stroke conducts and supports a wide range of research on neurological disorders, including Guillain-Barré syndrome. For more information on this or other neurological disorders, or on the Institute and its research programs, contact:

Office of Scientific and Health Reports Neurological Institute
P.O. Box 5801
Bethesda, MD 20824
(301) 496-5751 (800) 352-9424

The organization listed below provides printed information and assistance to Guillain-Barré patients and other interested parties.

Guillain-Barré Syndrome Foundation International
P.O. Box 262
Wynnewood, PA 19096
(215) 667-0131

Chapter 21

Immune Thrombocytopenic Purpura

What Is It?

Immune Thrombocytopenic Purpura (ITP) is a disorder of the blood. Immune refers to the immune system's involvement in this disorder. Antibodies, part of the body's immunologic defense against infection, attach to blood platelets, cells that help stop bleeding, and cause their destruction. Thrombocytopenia refers to decrease in blood platelets. Purpura refers to the purplish-looking areas of the skin and mucous membranes (such as the lining of the mouth) where bleeding has occurred as a result of decreased platelets.

Some cases of ITP are caused by drugs, and others are associated with infection, pregnancy, or immune disorders such as systemic lupus erythematosus. About half of all cases are classified as "idiopathic," meaning the cause is unknown.

What are the symptoms of ITP?

The main symptom is bleeding which can include bruising ("ecchymosis") and tiny red dots on the skin or mucous membranes ("petechiae"). In some instances bleeding from the nose, gums, digestive or urinary tracts may also occur. Rarely, bleeding within the brain occurs.

NIH Pub No. 93-2114.

How Is ITP Diagnosed?

The physician will take a medical history and perform a thorough physical examination. A careful review of medications the patient is taking is important because some drugs can be associated with thrombocytopenia. A complete blood count will be done. A low platelet count will establish thrombocytopenia as the cause of purpura. Often the next procedure is a bone marrow examination to verify that there are adequate platelet-forming cells (megakaryocytes) in the marrow and to rule out other diseases such as metastatic cancer (cancer that has spread to the bone marrow) and leukemia (cancer of the blood cells themselves). Another blood sample may be drawn to check for other conditions sometimes associated with thrombocytopenia such as lupus and infection.

Acute and Chronic Forms of Thrombocytopenic Purpura

Acute (temporary) thrombocytopenic purpura is most commonly seen in young children. Boys and girls are equally affected. Symptoms often, but do not necessarily, follow a viral infection. About 85 percent of children recover within one year and the problem doesn't return.

Thrombocytopenic purpura is considered chronic when it has lasted more that six months. The onset of illness may be at any age. Adults more often have the chronic disorder and females are affected two to three times more than males. The onset of illness may be at any age.

How Is ITP Treated?

If the doctor thinks a drug is the cause of the thrombocytopenia, standard treatment involves discontinuing the drug's use. Infection, if present, is treated vigorously since control of the infection may result in a return of the platelet count to normal.

The treatment of idiopathic thrombocytopenic purpura is determined by the severity of the symptoms. In some cases, no therapy is needed. In most cases, drugs that alter the immune system's attack on the platelets are prescribed. These include corticosteroids (i.e., prednisone) and/or intravenous infusions of immune globulin. Another treatment that usually results in an increased number of platelets is removal of the spleen, the organ that destroys antibody-coated platelets. Other drugs such as vincristine, azathioprine (Imuran), Danazol, cyclophosphamide, and cyclosporine are prescribed for patients only in the severe cases where other treatments have not shown benefit since these drugs have potentially harmful side effects. Except in certain situations (e.g., internal bleeding and preparation for surgery), platelet transfusions usually are not beneficial and, therefore, are seldom performed. Because all therapies can have risks, it is important that overtreatment (treatment based solely on platelet counts and not on symptoms) be avoided. In some instances lifestyle adjustments may be helpful for prevention of bleeding due to injury. These would include use of protective gear such as helmets and avoidance of contact sports in symptomatic patients or when platelet counts are less than 50,000. Otherwise, patients usually can carry on normal activities, but final decisions about activity should be made in consultation with the patient's hematologist.

Where Can I Obtain Further Information on ITP?

Blood specialists (hematologists) are experts in the diagnosis and treatment of these disorders. These doctors practice in most mid- and large-sized cities. A majority of medical centers have hematology divisions in their medicine or pediatrics departments, and patients who need evaluation, treatment, or information can often be referred there.

Clinical studies on ITP are being conducted at the National Institute of Diabetes and Digestive and Kidney Diseases (NIDDK), one of the National Institutes of Health (NIH). For information about these studies, doctors can contact Dr. N. Raphael Shulman, Clinical Hematology Branch, NIDDK, NIH, Building 10, Room 8C101, Bethesda, Maryland 20892.

Additional information can also be obtained from the National Organization for Rare Disorders at P.O. Box 8923, New Fairfield, Connecticut 06812; telephone (203) 746-6518.

Chapter 22

Systemic Lupus Erythematosus: The Disease with a Thousand Faces

Definition

Lupus is a chronic, autoimmune disease which causes inflammation of various parts of the body, especially the skin, joints, blood and kidneys. The body's immune system normally makes proteins called antibodies to protect the body against viruses, bacteria and other foreign materials. These foreign materials are called antigens. In an autoimmune disorder such as lupus, the immune system loses its ability to tell the difference between foreign substances (antigens) and its own cells and tissues. The immune system then makes antibodies directed against "self." These antibodies, called "auto-antibodies," react with the "self" antigens to form immune complexes. The immune complexes build up in the tissues and can cause inflammation, injury to tissues, and pain.

More people have lupus than AIDS, cerebral palsy, multiple sclerosis, sickle-cell anemia and cystic fibrosis combined. LFA market research data show that between 1,400,000 and 2,000,000 people reported to have been diagnosed with lupus. (Study conducted by Bruskin/Goldring Research, 1994.) For most people, lupus is a mild disease affecting only a few organs. For others, it may cause serious and even life-threatening problems. Thousands of Americans die each year from lupus-related complications.

What is Lupus; Lupus and Infections and Immunizations; Pregnancy and Lupus; Lupus in Men; Laboratory Tests Used in the Diagnosis of Lupus; Living Well with Lupus. © Lupus Foundation of America, Inc. Reprinted with permission.

Types of Lupus

There are three types of lupus: discoid, systemic, and drug-induced. Discoid lupus is always limited to the skin. It is identified by a rash that may appear on the face, neck and scalp. Discoid lupus is diagnosed by examining a biopsy of the rash. In discoid lupus the biopsy will show abnormalities that are not found in skin without the rash. Discoid lupus does not generally involve the body's internal organs. Therefore, the ANA test, a blood test used to detect systemic lupus, may be negative in patients with discoid lupus. However, in a large number of patients with discoid lupus, the ANA test is positive, but at a low level or "titer."

In approximately 10 percent of the people with lupus, discoid lupus can evolve into the systemic form of the disease, which can affect almost any organ or system of the body. This cannot be predicted or prevented. Treatment of discoid lupus will not prevent its progression to the systemic form. Individuals who progress to the systemic form probably had systemic lupus at the outset, with the discoid rash as their main symptom.

Systemic lupus is usually more severe than discoid lupus, and can affect almost any organ or system of the body. For some people, only the skin and joints will be involved. In others, the joints, lungs, kidneys, blood or other organs and/or tissues may be affected. Generally, no two people with systemic lupus will have identical symptoms. Systemic lupus may include periods in which few, if any, symptoms are evident (remission) and other times when the disease becomes more active (flare). Most often when people mention "lupus," they are referring to the systemic form of the disease.

Drug-induced lupus occurs after the use of certain prescribed drugs. The symptoms of drug-induced lupus are similar to those of systemic lupus. The drugs most commonly connected with drug-induced lupus are hydralazine (used to treat high blood pressure or hypertension) and procainamide (used to treat irregular heart rhythms). However, not everyone who takes these drugs will develop drug-induced lupus. Only about 4 percent of the people who take these drugs will develop the antibodies suggestive of lupus. Of those 4 percent, only an extremely small number will develop overt drug-induced lupus. The symptoms usually fade when the medications are discontinued.

Although drug-induced lupus and discoid lupus share features of systemic lupus, the rest of this chapter primarily discusses systemic lupus.

Cause

The cause(s) of lupus is unknown, but environmental and genetic factors are involved. While scientists believe there is a genetic predisposition to the disease, it is known that environmental factors also play a critical role in triggering lupus. Some of the environmental factors that may trigger the disease are: infections, antibiotics (especially those in the sulfa and penicillin groups), ultraviolet light, extreme stress, and certain drugs.

Although lupus is known to occur within families, there is no known gene or genes which are thought to cause the illness. Only 10 percent of lupus patients will have a close relative (parent or sibling) who already has or may develop lupus. Statistics show that only about 5 percent of the children born to individuals with lupus will develop the illness.

Lupus is often called a "woman's disease" despite the fact that many men are affected. Lupus can occur at any age, and in either sex, although it occurs 10-15 times more frequently among adult females than among adult males. The symptoms of the disease are the same in men and women. People of African, American Indian, and Asian origin are thought to develop the disease more frequently than Caucasian women, but the studies that led to this result are small and need corroboration.

Hormonal factors may explain why lupus occurs more frequently in females than in males. The increase of disease symptoms before menstrual periods and/or during pregnancy support the belief that hormones, particularly estrogen, may be involved. However, the exact hormonal reason for the greater prevalence of lupus in women, and the cyclic increase in symptoms, is unknown.

Pregnancy and Lupus

Since lupus primarily affects young women, pregnancy often becomes a crucial question. Years ago, all medical texts said that lupus patients could not have children, and if they become pregnant, they should have therapeutic abortions. Clearly, these early conclusions are wrong. Currently, 50 percent of all lupus pregnancies are completely normal, and 25 percent deliver normal babies prematurely. Fetal loss, due to spontaneous abortion (miscarriage) or death of the baby accounts for the remaining 25 percent. While not all of the problems of pregnancy with Lupus have been solved, pregnancies are possible, and normal children are the rule.

While it is certainly possible for lupus patients to have children, pregnancy may not be easy. It is important to note that although many lupus pregnancies will be completely normal, all lupus pregnancies should be considered "high risk." "High risk" is a term commonly used by obstetricians to indicate that solvable problems may occur and must be anticipated. Pregnant lupus patients should be managed by obstetricians who are thoroughly familiar with high risk pregnancies and work in close concert with the woman's primary physician. Delivery should be planned at a hospital that has access to a unit specializing in the care of premature newborns. SLE mothers should not attempt home delivery, or be overly committed to "natural" childbirth, since treatable complications during delivery are frequent. However, under close observation, the risk to the mother's health is lessened, and healthy babies can be born.

Will Pregnancy Flare My Lupus?

Although older medical texts suggest that SLE flares are common in pregnancy, recent studies indicate that flares are uncommon and are usually easily treated. In fact, 6-15 percent of lupus patients will actually experience an improvement in lupus symptoms during pregnancy. Flares most often occur during the first or second trimester, or during the two months immediately after delivery. Most of the flares tend to be mild. The most common symptoms of these flares are arthritis, rashes and fatigue. Approximately 33 percent of lupus patients will have a decrease in platelet count during pregnancy, and about 20 percent will have an increase in or new occurrence of protein in the urine.

Women who conceive after 5-6 months of remission are less likely to experience a lupus flare than those who get pregnant while their lupus is active. Lupus nephritis before conception also increases the chance of experiencing a lupus flare during pregnancy.

It is important to distinguish the symptoms of a lupus flare from the normal body changes that occur during pregnancy. For example, because the ligaments that hold the joints together normally soften in pregnancy, fluid may accumulate in the joints, especially in the knees, and cause swelling. Although this may suggest an increase in inflammation due to lupus, it may simply be the swelling that occurs during a normal pregnancy. Similarly, lupus rashes may appear to worsen during pregnancy, but this is usually due to an increased blood flow to the skin that is common in pregnancy (the "blush" of a pregnant woman). Many women also experience new hair growth during pregnancy, followed by a dramatic loss of hair after delivery. Although hair loss is certainly a symptom of active SLE, this again is most likely a result of the changes that occur during a normal pregnancy.

When Is the Best Time to Get Pregnant?

The answer is simple: when you are at your healthiest. Women in remission have much less trouble than do women with active disease. Their babies do much better, and everyone worries less.

Good health rules are essential: rest well, take medications as prescribed, visit your doctor(s) regularly, don't smoke, don't drink, and certainly don't use "recreational" drugs.

Why Are Frequent Doctor Visits So Important in a Lupus Pregnancy?

Frequent doctor visits are important in any high risk pregnancy because many conditions which may occur can be prevented or treated more easily, if found early.

About 20 percent of lupus patients will have a sudden increase in blood pressure, protein in the urine, or both during pregnancy. This is called toxemia of pregnancy (or preeclampsia, or pregnancy-induced hypertension). It is a serious condition, and will require immediate treatment and usually immediate delivery. Toxemia is more common in older women, in black women, in women with twins, in women with kidney disease, in women with high blood pressure, and in women who smoke. Serum complement and blood platelet count may be abnormal in these cases. Since complement levels and blood platelet counts are also abnormal during SLE flares, it may be difficult for the doctor to be certain that a flare is not causing these symptoms. If toxemia is promptly treated the woman should be in no danger, but there is a high risk that the baby will die if it is not rapidly delivered. If toxemia is ignored, both the woman and her baby are in danger.

As pregnancy progresses it is often wise for the doctor to check the baby's growth with sonograms (which are harmless). The doctor should also regularly check the baby's heart beat. Abnormalities in either the baby's growth or heart beat may be the first signs of trouble that can be treated.

Can I Take Medications During Pregnancy?

It is always unwise to take unnecessary medications during pregnancy. However, necessary medications should not be discontinued. Most medications commonly taken by SLE patients are safe to use during pregnancy. Prednisone, Prednisolone, and probably methylprednisolone (Medrol) do not get through the placenta and are safe for the baby. Specifically, dexamethasone (Decodrol, Hexadrol) and betamethasone (Celestone) do reach the baby and are used **ONLY** when it is necessary to treat the baby as well. For example, these medications might be used to help the baby's lungs mature more rapidly if the baby will be premature. Aspirin is safe (but see the FDA warning below); it is often used to protect against a complication known as toxemia of pregnancy. Preliminary reports suggest that azathioprine (Imuran) and hydroxychloroquine (Plaquenil) do not harm babies but the final word is not yet in on these. Cyclophosphamide (Cytoxan) is definitely harmful if taken during the first three months of pregnancy.

Editor's note: The September, 1990 issue of the *FDA Consumer* draws attention to the FDA's warning to pregnant women not to take aspirin during the last three months of pregancy without a physician's consent. As of September 1991, all oral and rectal nonprescription aspirin and drugs containing aspirin must carry this warning. The article notes that aspirin can impede fetal circulation and uterine contractions, causing damage to the fetus and complicating delivery. This warning is similar to one issued earlier for nonprescription medication containing ibuprofen. The FDA decided to issue the warning based on recommendations from its Advisory Review Panel on OTC (over-the-counter) Internal Analgesic and Antirheumatic Drug Products which is composed of non-government experts.

What about "Prophylactic" (Preventative) Treatment with Prednisone?

A few doctors feel that all pregnant women with lupus should take small doses of Prednisone to prevent early abortion. However, there are no confirmed data that this is necessary. Similarly, some physicians feel steroids should be given or increased after the baby is born to prevent "post partum flare." Again, there is no evidence that this is necessary in most cases either. For patients recently on steroids, however, "stress" steroid is usually given during labor to supplement what the mother can't make herself.

What Are Anti-phospholipid Antibodies and Why Are They Important?

About 33 percent of lupus patients have antibodies that interfere with the function of the placenta. These antibodies are called anti-phospholipid antibodies, the lupus anticoagulant or anti-cardiolipin antibodies. These antibodies may cause blood clots, including blood clots in the placenta, that prevent the placenta from growing and functioning normally. This usually occurs during the second trimester. Since the placenta is the passageway for nourishment from the mother to the baby, the baby's growth slows. The baby can be delivered at this time and will be normal if it is big enough.

Treatment for lupus patients who have these antibodies is still being tested. Aspirin, Prednisone, Heparin and plasmapheresis have all been suggested as possible therapies. However even with the use of such medications, these antibodies may still lead to miscarriage.

Will My Baby Be Normal?

Prematurity is the greatest danger to the baby. About 50 percent of lupus pregnancies end before 9 months, usually because of the complications previously discussed. Babies born after 30 weeks or over 3 pounds usually do well. Premature babies may have difficulty breathing, may develop jaundice, and may become anemic. In modern neonatal units, these problems can be easily treated. Babies weighing more than three pounds at birth grow normally. Even babies as small as 1 pound, 4 ounces have survived and have been healthy in every way, but the outcome is uncertain for babies of this size. There are no congenital abnormalities that occur only to babies of lupus patients (except as described below), and no unusual frequency of mental retardation.

Will My Baby Have Lupus?

About 33 percent of lupus patients have an antibody known as anti-Ro or anti-SSA antibody. About 10 percent of women with Anti-Ro antibodies, or about 3 percent of all lupus women, will have a baby with a syndrome known as neonatal lupus. Neonatal lupus is not SLE. Neonatal lupus consists of a transient rash, transient blood count abnormalities, and a special type of heart beat abnormality. If the heart best abnormality occurs, which is very rare, it is treatable, but it is permanent. Neonatal lupus is the only type of congenital abnormality found in children of mothers with lupus. For babies with neonatal lupus who do not have the heart problem, there is no trace of the disease by 3-6 months of age, and it does not recur. Even babies with the heart beat abnormality problem grow normally. If a mother has had one child with neonatal lupus, there is about a 25 percent chance of having another child with the same problem.

Will I Have to Have a Caesarian Section?

Very premature babies, babies showing signs of stress, babies of mothers with low platelets, and babies of mothers who are very ill are almost always delivered by Caesarian section. This is often both the safest and fastest method of delivery in these cases. Usually the decision about type of delivery is not made in advance because the specific circumstances at the time of delivery are the determining factors.

Can I Breast-feed?

Although breast feeding is possible for lupus patients, breast milk may not come if the baby is born very prematurely because very premature babies are not strong enough to suckle, and thus, cannot draw the milk. However, milk can be pumped from the breast to feed a premature baby if the baby is not strong enough to suckle and the mother wishes to do this. Plaquenil and the cytotoxic drugs (Cytoxan, Imuran) are passed through the milk to the baby. Some medications, such as Prednisone, may prevent milk from being produced. If you are taking any medication it is best not to breast feed; but if your doctor approves, you may.

Who Will Care for the Baby?

Prospective parents often do not ask what will happen after the baby is born if the mother is ill and unable to care for the child. Since it is likely that a lupus patient will have future periods of illness, it is wise to think of this possibility in advance and to have plans for alternate child-care (spouse, grandparent, etc.) if needed.

Symptoms

Although lupus can affect any part of the body, most people experience symptoms in only a few organs. Table 22.1 lists the most common symptoms of people with lupus.

ymptom	Percentage
chy joints (arthralgia)	95%
ever over 100 degrees F (38 degrees C)	90%
rolonged or extreme fatigue	81%
rthritis (swollen joints)	90%
kin Rashes	74%
nemia	71%
idney Involvement	50%
ain in the chest on deep breathing (pleurisy)	45%
utterfly-shaped rash across the cheeks and nose	42%
un or light sensitivity (photosensitivity)	30%
air loss	27%
aynaud's phenomenon (fingers turning white nd/or blue in the cold)	17%
eizures	15%
outh or nose ulcers	12%

Table 22.1. Table of Symptoms.

Diagnosis

Because many lupus symptoms mimic other illnesses, are sometimes vague and may come and go, lupus can be difficult to diagnose. Diagnosis is usually made by a careful review of a person's entire medical history coupled with an analysis of the results obtained in routine laboratory tests and some specialized tests related to immune status. Currently, there is no single laboratory test that can determine whether a person has lupus or not. To assist the physician in the diagnosis of lupus the American Rheumatism Association issued a list of 11 symptoms or signs that help distinguish lupus from other diseases. A person should have four or more of these symptoms to suspect lupus. The symptoms do not all have to occur at the same time.

The Eleven Criteria Used for the Diagnosis of Lupus Erythematosus

Malar Rash. Rash over the cheeks.

Discoid Rash. Red raised patches.

Photosensitivity. Reaction to sunlight, resulting in the development of or increase in skin rash.

Oral Ulcers. Ulcers in the nose or mouth, usually painless.

Arthritis. Non-erosive arthritis involving two or more peripheral joints (arthritis in which the bones around the joints do not become destroyed).

Serositis. Pleuritis or pericarditis.

Renal Disorder. Excessive protein in the urine (greater than 0.5 gm/day or 3+ on test sticks) and/or cellular casts (abnormal elements the urine derived from red and/or white cells and/or kidney tubule cells).

Neurologic Disorder. Seizures (convulsions) and/or psychosis in the absence of drugs or metabolic disturbances which are known to cause such affects.

Hematologic Disorder. Hemolytic anemia or leukopenia (white blood count below 4,000 cells per cubic millimeter) or lymphopenia (less than 1,500 lymphocytes per cubic millimeter) or thrombocytopenia (less than 100,000 platelets per cubic millimeter). The leukopenia and lymphopenia must be detected on two or more occasions. The thrombocytopenia must be detected in the absence of drugs known to induce it.

Immunologic Disorder. Positive LE prep test, positive anti-DNA test, positive anti-Sm test or false positive syphilis test (VDRL).

Antinuclear Antibody. Positive test for antinuclear antibodies (ANA) in the absence of drugs known to induce it.

Adapted from: Tan, E.M., et. al. The 1982 Revised Criteria For the Classification of SLE. *Arth Rheum* 25: 1271-1277.

Flares (What Triggers Lupus?)

What triggers an attack of lupus in a susceptible person? Scientists have noted common features in many lupus patients. In some, exposure to the sun causes sudden development of a rash and then possibly other symptoms. In others an infection, perhaps a cold or a more serious infection, does not get better, and then complications arise. These complications may be the first signs of lupus. In still other cases, a drug taken for some illness produces the signaling symptoms. In some women, the first symptoms and signs develop during pregnancy. In others, they appear soon after delivery. Many people cannot remember or identify any specific factor. Obviously, many seemingly unrelated factors can trigger the onset of the disease.

Treatment

For the vast majority of people with lupus, effective treatment can minimize symptoms, reduce inflammation, and maintain normal bodily functions.

Preventive measures can reduce the risk of flares. For photosensitive patients, avoidance of (excessive) sun exposure and/or the regular application of sun screens will usually prevent rashes. Regular exercise helps prevent muscle weakness and fatigue. Immunization protects against specific infections. Support groups, counseling, talking to family members, friends, and physicians can help alleviate the effects of stress. Needless to say, negative habits are hazardous to people with lupus. These include smoking, excessive consumption of alcohol, too much or too little of prescribed medication, or postponing regular medical checkups.

Treatment approaches are based on the specific needs and symptoms of each person. Because the characteristics and course of lupus may vary significantly among people, it is important to emphasize that a thorough medical evaluation and ongoing medical supervision are essential to ensure proper diagnosis and treatment.

Medications are often prescribed for people with lupus, depending on which organ(s) are involved, and the severity of involvement. Effective patient-physician discussions regarding the selection of medication, its possible side effects, and any changes in doses are vital. Commonly prescribed medications include:

Nonsteroidal Anti-inflammatory Drugs (NSAIDs): These medications are prescribed for a variety of rheumatic diseases, including lupus. The compounds include acetylsalicylic acid (e.g., aspirin), ibuprofen (Motrin), naproxen (Naprosyn), indomethacin (indocin), sulindac (Clinoril), tolmetin (Tolectin), and a large number of others. These drugs are usually recommended for muscle and joint pain, and arthritis. Aspirin may cause stomach upsets for some people. This effect can be minimized by taking them with meals, milk, or antacids. The other NSAIDs work in the same way as aspirin, but tend to be less irritating to the stomach than aspirin, and often require fewer pills per day to have the same effect as aspirin.

Acetaminophen: Acetaminophen (e.g., Tylenol) is a mild analgesic that can often be used for pain. It has the advantage of less stomach irritation than aspirin, but it is not nearly as effective at suppressing inflammation as aspirin.

Corticosteroids: Corticosteroids (steroids) are hormones that have anti-inflammatory and immunoregulatory properties. They are normally produced in small quantities by the adrenal gland. This hormone controls a variety of metabolic functions in the body. Synthetically produced corticosteroids are used to reduce inflammation and suppress activity of the immune system. The most commonly prescribed drug of this type is Prednisone. Because steroids have a variety of side effects, the dose has to be regulated to maximize the beneficial anti-immune/anti-inflammatory effects and minimize the negative side effects. Side effects occur more frequently when steroids are taken over long periods of time at high doses (for example, 60 milligrams of Prednisone taken daily for periods of more than one month). Such side effects include weight gain, a round face, acne, easy bruising, "thinning" of the bones (osteoporosis), high blood pressure, cataracts, onset of diabetes, increased risk of infection and stomach ulcers.

Anti-malarials: Chloroquine (Aralen) or hydroxychloroquine (Plaquenil), commonly used in the treatment of malaria, may also be very useful in some individuals with lupus. They are most often prescribed for skin and joint symptoms of lupus. It may take months before these drugs demonstrate a beneficial effect. Side effects are rare, and consist of occasional diarrhea or rashes. Some anti-malarial drugs, such as quinine and chloroquine, can affect the eyes. Therefore, it is important to see an eye doctor (ophthalmologist) regularly. The manufacturer suggests an eye exam before starting the drug and one exam every six months thereafter. However your physician might suggest a yearly exam as sufficient.

Cytotoxic Drugs: Azathioprine (Imuran) and cyclophosphamide (Cytoxan) are in a group of agents known as cytotoxic or immunosuppressive drugs. These drugs act in a similar manner to the corticosteroid drugs in that they suppress inflammation and tend to suppress the immune system. The side effects of these drugs include anemia, low white blood cell count, and increased risk of infection. Their use may also predispose an individual to developing cancer.

People with lupus should learn to recognize early symptoms of disease activity. In that way they can help the physician know when a change in therapy is needed. Regular monitoring of the disease by laboratory tests can be valuable because noticeable symptoms may occur only after the disease has significantly flared. Changes in blood test results may indicate the disease is becoming active even before the patient develops symptoms of a flare. Generally, it seems that the earlier such flares are detected, the more easily they can be controlled. Also, early treatment may decrease the chance of permanent tissue or organ damage and reduce the time one must remain on high doses of drugs.

Nutrition and Diet

Although much is still not known about the nutritional factors in many kinds of disease, no one questions the necessity of a well-balanced diet. Fad diets, advocating an excess or an exclusion of certain types of foods, are much more likely to be detrimental than beneficial in any disease, including lupus. Scientists have shown that both antibodies and other cells of the immune system may be adversely affected by nutritional deficiencies or imbalances. Thus, significant deviations from a balanced diet may have profound effects on a network as complex as the immune system.

There have been suggestions about various foods and the treatment of lupus. One example is fish oil. However, these diets have been used only in animals with limited success and should not become the mainstay of a person's diet.

Prognosis

The idea that lupus is generally a fatal disease is one of the gravest misconceptions about this illness. In fact, the prognosis of lupus is much better than ever before. Today, with early diagnosis and current methods of therapy, 80-90 percent of people with lupus can look forward to a normal lifespan if they follow the instructions of their physician, take their medication(s) as prescribed, and know when to seek help for unexpected side-effects of a medication or a new manifestation of their lupus. Although some people with lupus have severe recurrent attacks and are frequently hospitalized, most people with lupus rarely require hospitalization. There are many lupus patients who never have to be hospitalized, especially if they are careful and follow their physician's instructions.

New research brings unexpected findings each year. The progress made in treatment and diagnosis during the last decade has been greater than that made over the past 100 years. It is therefore a sensible idea to maintain control of a disease that tomorrow may be curable.

The Lupus Foundation of America

The Lupus Foundation of America (LFA) was incorporated as a nonprofit health agency in 1977. The purpose of the LFA is to assist local chapters in their efforts to provide supportive services to individuals living with lupus, to educate the public about lupus, and to support research into the cause and cure of lupus. Last year over 200,000 people received service from the LFA and its chapters.

Since its establishment the Lupus Foundation has remained a grassroots, volunteer-driven organization. Volunteers, through an extensive network of over 500 constituent chapters, branches, support groups and International Associated groups, provide the majority of services which link the Lupus Foundation to thousands of lupus patients and their families. Last year LFA volunteers contributed over 375,000 hours of service at the local and national levels.

The Lupus Foundation of America is the largest lupus group in the world with nearly 46,000 members in 98 chapters throughout the U.S. Thousands of others are associated with the LFA through the 73 International Associated Groups in 37 countries worldwide. The LFA and its chapters contributed more than $1,000,000 for lupus research in the past two years.

The LFA sets standards and provides direction and general support to its chapters, leading the efforts to operate a patient-oriented, nonprofit, voluntary health agency in an ethical and professional manner. The LFA has developed specific services and programs to provide chapters with assistance in meeting patients' needs and organizational goals. These include chapter support, volunteer leadership training, research, patient education programs, public awareness activities, professional education, advocacy, and resource development.

For more information about various aspects of lupus, contact the Lupus Foundation of America.

Lupus Foundation of America, Inc.
4 Research Place, Suite 180
Rockville, MD 20850-3226
301-670-9292
800-558-0121

Infections and Immunizations

Better techniques for diagnosis, evaluation and disease management combined with more judicious use of medications have significantly improved the prognosis for lupus patients over the past two decades. Thirty five years ago, only 40 percent of the people living with lupus were expected to live more than three years following diagnosis. With early diagnosis and current methods of therapy, 80–90 percent of lupus patients now live for more than 10 years after their diagnosis and many can look forward to a normal lifespan.

Prior to the medical advances made in lupus diagnosis and treatment, most patient deaths were the result of renal failure or central nervous system involvement. Today, as many patients with lupus will die from infection as from active systemic disease. This is an important reason for developing an increased awareness about lupus and its relationship to infections and immunizations.

Lupus patients are more susceptible to infection than most people for two reasons:

- Lupus directly affects a person's immune system, reducing his or her ability to prevent and fight infection.

- Many of the drugs used to treat lupus suppress the function of the immune system, leaving the patient more prone to infection.

Direct Effects of Lupus on the Immune System

Lupus patients have abnormalities in their immune systems that predispose them to develop infections.

Effects of Medications Used In the Treatment of Lupus

Cortisone-like drugs (Prednisone) and cytotoxic drugs such as azathioprine (Imuran) and cyclophosphamide (Cytoxan) increase a person's susceptibility to infections because they suppress both normal and abnormal immune function. However, the control of lupus activity is usually more important than the danger posed by a possible infection due to the use of immunosuppressive medications.

The risk of infection parallels the dose and the duration of treatment with steroids. A daily dose of 20 mg. of Prednisone is enough to impose a significant risk. Administration of steroids every other day ("alternate day" treatment) decreases the risk and incidence of infections.

Lupus patients are more susceptible to infection even if they do not take corticosteroids. Lupus experts such as Dr. Marian Ropes sparingly used steroids in treating her patients in the 1940s and 1950s. Yet, Dr. Ropes published data showing that the majority of her patients developed serious infections during their disease course—even on low dose steroids.

Types of Infection in SLE

Infections that occur in people with lupus fall into two categories. The first category includes infections caused by organisms which can induce infection in persons with lupus and in the general population as well. This category includes organisms such as streptococcus (which causes strep throat) and staphylococcus (which causes staph infections).

The second category consists of "opportunistic" infections. Opportunistic infections are caused by organisms capable of inducing disease only when one's immune system is weakened. Most of the opportunistic infections are fungal, parasitic or protozoan.

The most common infections that lupus patients contract involve the respiratory tract, skin and urinary tract and do not usually require hospitalization. Fortunately, only a few lupus patients will need aggressive hospital treatment for infections. However, infections in lupus patients tend to last longer and require a longer course of treatment with antibiotics than infections in people who do not have lupus. Lupus patients are at an unusually high risk for contracting salmonella, herpes zoster and candida (yeast) infections.

Clinical Evaluation of Possible Infection

Active lupus and infection may share many symptoms. Further, infection can induce a lupus flare or be difficult to distinguish from a lupus flare. For example, fever and decreased energy are nonspecific symptoms that may be associated with both lupus flares or infections. More specific symptoms, like sore throat or pain on taking a deep breath, may also occur with either a flare of lupus or with infection. Therefore, it is important for a person with lupus to contact his or her physician whenever symptoms are suggestive of either a disease flare or an infection, so that a medical history and physical examination can be performed.

Laboratory tests including white blood cell counts may help a physician to distinguish an infection from a lupus flare. A low white blood cell count usually suggests active lupus (although certain viruses can also give a low white count) while a high count suggests infection. The physician may also wish to get a throat, urine, blood or stool culture and a complete blood count (CBC) or chest X-ray. Some physicians find a C-reactive protein (CRP) blood test to be helpful in differentiating active lupus from infection, but this is controversial.

Fevers may be due to an infection, a drug reaction or active lupus.

Any lupus patient with a fever should be thoroughly evaluated, especially if the patient is also taking aspirin, nonsteroidal medications (e.g., Advil, Naprosyn) or steroids which lower body temperature.

If necessary, patients with suspected life-threatening infections of unknown source may need to be hospitalized. Here, the patient may be observed, cultures taken and tests such as gallium scanning, bone marrow biopsy, lymph node biopsy or bronchoscopy can be performed to help make a rapid diagnosis.

Treatment and Prevention of Infection

The treatment of infections in lupus patients is basically the same as for other patients. Even those taking high doses of immunosuppressive medications for their lupus may respond well to antibiotics. The use of sulfa drugs in the treatment of infections should be avoided whenever possible, because they can increase photosensitivity. To prevent possible infections, patients at high risk of infection often benefit from taking antibiotics before dental treatment or surgical procedures. In general, individuals with lupus should avoid exposure to people with colds or other infections.

Prevention of Infection: Immunization

The risk of certain types of infection can be decreased with immunization (vaccinations).

Nearly all individuals with lupus have been vaccinated against a variety of diseases with little difficulty. However it is possible that immunization with vaccines that use live viruses will result in a lupus flare. Nevertheless, polio, measles and tetanus vaccines, which all use live viruses have been given to hundreds of thousands of lupus patients with no adverse reactions. Passive immunization (i.e., vaccinating the patient with a killed virus), poses no problems in lupus patients. Gammaglobulin is an example of a vaccine which uses a nonspecific antibody instead of a live virus.

It should be noted that lupus patients may have adverse reactions to two types of immunizations. First, some lupus patients who receive allergy shots (immunotherapy) will experience a lupus flare following this treatment. For this reason, in 1989 the World Health Organization recommended that patients with autoimmune diseases should not receive certain types of allergy shots. Allergy shots (immunotherapy) might cause the patient to make more anti-DNA and other lupus-related antibodies in addition to making antibodies against the agent causing the allergy. Lupus patients are advised to consult their rheumatologist before receiving any type of allergy immunotherapy.

Some lupus patients may also experience difficulties after receiving tetanus or flu vaccines. It seems that flu vaccines do not work as well if the patient has lupus, antibody levels against the flu virus achieve only half the desired level for half as long in those with lupus. Additionally, up to 20 percent of patients with lupus may feel sick or achy for a few days following a flu vaccination. This is twice as many people as in the general population, where only 10 percent of individuals will suffer such adverse effects following a flu shot. Because of these potential problems, lupus patients should consult their physician before receiving any vaccine.

Lupus in Men

Who Gets Lupus?

Systemic lupus erythematosus (SLE) is often called a "woman's disease" because it occurs 10-15 times more frequently among adult females than among adult males. However, lupus can occur in either sex, and at any age.

The higher occurrence of the disease in women might depend partially on the age at which it occurs. Before puberty, approximately one young male is affected for every three females, whereas in the adult years, approximately 10 females are affected for every male. After the menopause (that is, after the mean age of 55), there are approximately 8 females for every male affected. These differences in sexual preference apply only to systemic lupus erythematosus and not to discoid lupus, which is lupus of the skin. Discoid lupus affects more men than does SLE.

More men than women develop drug-induced lupus, because most of the medications that produce drug-induced lupus are used more frequently in men than in women. The two most common drugs that produce drug-induced lupus are procainamide, which is used to treat various types of heart abnormalities; and hydralazine, which is used to control high blood pressure. Since more males than females suffer heart attacks which may result in irregular heartbeats afterwards, procainamide is used more often by males. Similarly, hydralazine is used more often by men than by women, for reasons that are not clear.

The Clinical Course

The symptoms of SLE are identical in men and women at the time of initial presentation of the disease. However, some researchers suspect that the later manifestations of SLE may differ between the sexes. Several studies conclude that there is more severe renal, neurologic, and vascular disease in men with SLE than in women. Such findings, however, have not been confirmed, and more research is needed in this area. At this time, there is no substantial evidence to document a significant difference between the severity of SLE in men and women. The clinical course of the disease is the same in both sexes.

Hormones

For years investigators had been looking at hormonal differences between males and females which might explain the higher prevalence of lupus in women. Studies have considered estrogens (female hormones) and androgens (male hormones). Some data indicates that there is a difference in the way estrogen is metabolized (chemically changed) in normal individuals, versus the way it is metabolized in individuals with lupus. Although there is no significant difference in the way estrogen is metabolized by men and women with lupus, there is a difference in the way that androgens are metabolized by male and female lupus patients. Therefore, while there does not appear to be a significant increase in estrogen in men with lupus, there is a suggestion that women with lupus metabolize androgens at a faster rate than women without lupus.

There is also evidence that lower testosterone levels (a male hormone) in both young and old men may predispose these men to autoimmune-like diseases. Drugs which lower testosterone levels in men are associated with rheumatic symptoms but have not been specifically associated with the onset of SLE.

Sexual Factors

There are significant differences in the way men might react to the diagnosis of SLE. They might have the misconception that lupus is a "woman's disease" and therefore that a man with SLE is less masculine than a mon who does not have SLE. This is simply not true. Men with lupus are fertile, sexually active and potent, and have normal reproductive histories. Many are also very hirsute (hairy). None of these characteristics would be apparent if males with SLE were any different hormonally than males who do not have lupus. Thus, as far as sexual factors are concerned, males with lupus are not different than males without lupus.

Coping

The emotional stresses for men with lupus are the same as those experienced by women with SLE. In some ways, it may be even more difficult for men to cope with having lupus because of the cultural and societal expectations of men. For example, the same incapacitating feelings that women with SLE feel may be more apparent in males because they may no longer be able to perform or progress in their work environment, or they may not even be able to continue to work in order to support a family. They may have difficulty in performing duties which involve physical labor. The inability to work and earn a living, because of disability due to illness, may result in significant emotional and mental stress for the male. This may not be the case in all instances for the female with lupus. The roles and expectations of males and females in society are changing, but these changes take a long time. The above stresses, coupled with the fact that lupus is commonly referred to as a "woman's illness," only makes it more difficult for males to cope with this chronic disease.

There are cosmetic changes that are of some concern to men with lupus. Symptoms such as rashes, hair loss, and weight gain are usually not as incapacitating for men as they are for women. On the other hand, men may be more concerned than women with a change or loss of job, a decrease in job performance, a significant loss of independence and problems with self-esteem, and false feelings about a "loss of masculinity."

There is a significant lack of written and published material geared to men with lupus, or men who suffer from any chronic disease, for that matter. In addition, lupus support groups are comprised mostly of women, and as a result, men with lupus feel ostracized or deprived of what few normal counseling mechanisms exist. The Lupus Foundation of America is attempting to change this approach in its support groups.

Laboratory Tests uses in the Diagnosis of Lupus

Because many symptoms of systemic lupus erythematosus (SLE) mimic those of other illnesses, lupus can be a difficult disease to diagnose. Diagnosis is usually made by a careful review of three factors:

- the patient's entire medical history;

- the patient's current symptoms; and

- an analysis of the results obtained in routine laboratory tests and some specialized tests related to immune status.

To make a diagnosis of SLE, an individual must show clinical evidence of a multi-system disease (i.e. has shown abnormalities in several different organ systems). The following are typical manifestations which might lead to suspicion of SLE:

- **Skin:** butterfly rash; ulcers in the mouth; hair loss.

- **Joints:** pain; redness and swelling.

- **Kidney:** abnormal urinanalysis suggesting kidney disease.

- **Lining membranes:** pleurisy; pericarditis and/or peritonitis (taken together this type of inflammation is known as polyserositis).

- **Blood:** hemolytic anemia (the red cells are destroyed by autoantibodies); leukopenia (low white blood cell count); thrombocytopenia (low platelets).

- **Lungs:** infiltrates that are transient.

- **Nervous system:** convulsions; psychosis; nerve abnormalities that cause strange sensations or alter muscular control or strength.

If an individual has several of these symptoms, the physician will then usually order a series of tests to examine the functioning of the individual's immune system. In general, physicians look for evidence of autoantibodies.

Although there is no one test that can definitely say whether a person has lupus or not, there are many laboratory tests which aid the physician in making a lupus diagnosis.

Commonly used tests in the diagnosis of SLE are:

- **The anti-nuclear antibody test (ANA):** a test to determine if autoantibodies to cell nuclei are present in the blood.

- **The anti-DNA antibody test:** to determine if the patient has antibodies to the genetic material in the cell.

- **The anti-Sm antibody test:** to determine if there are antibodies to Sm, which is a protein found in the cell nucleus.

- Tests to detect the presence of **immune complexes** in the blood.

- Tests to examine the total level of **serum complement**—a group of proteins which can occur in immune reactions—and tests to assess the specific level of C3 and C4, two proteins of this group.

- **LE cell prep:** An examination of the blood looking for a certain kind of cell which has ingested the swollen antibody-coated nucleus of another cell. This test is used less frequently than the ANA test, because the ANA is more sensitive for SLE than the LE cell prep.

The first laboratory test ever devised was the LE (lupus erythematosus) cell test. The LE cell prep is positive in about 40-50 percent of patients with systemic lupus. Unfortunately, the test can also be positive in up to 20 percent of patients with rheumatoid arthritis, in some patients with other rheumatic conditions like Sjogren's syndrome or scleroderma, in patients with liver disease, and in persons taking certain drugs (such as procainamide, hydralazine, and others).

The immunofluorescent anti-nuclear antibody (ANA, or FANA) test is more sensitive for lupus than the LE cell prep test. The ANA test is positive in almost all patients with Systemic lupus, and is the best diagnostic test currently available for identifying systemic lupus. A negative ANA test is strong evidence against lupus as the cause of a person's illness, although there are very infrequent instances where SLE is present without detectable anti-nuclear antibodies. However, a positive ANA test, by itself, is not proof of lupus since the test may also be positive in:

1. Individuals with other connective tissue diseases;

2. Patients being treated with certain drugs, including procainamide, hydralazine, isoniazid, and chlorpromazine;

3. Individuals with conditions other than lupus, such as: scleroderma, Sjogren's syndrome, rheumatoid arthritis, thyroid disease, liver disease, infectious mononucleosis, and other chronic infectious diseases such as hepatitis, lepromatous leprosy, subacute bacterial endocarditis, and malaria.

The test can even be weakly positive in about 20 percent of healthy individuals. While a few of these healthy people may eventually develop lupus symptoms, the majority will never develop any signs of lupus or related conditions. The chances of a person having a positive ANA test increases as he or she ages.

ANA reports include a titer (number) and a pattern. The titer tells us how many times the technician had to dilute plasma from the patient's blood to get a sample free of the anti-nuclear antibodies. Thus, a titer of 1:640 shows a greater concentration of anti-nuclear antibodies than a titer of 1:320 or 1:160.

The apparent great difference between various titers can be misleading. Since each dilution involves doubling the amount of test fluid, it is not surprising that titers increase rather rapidly. In actuality, the difference between a 1:160 titer and a 1:320 titer is only a single dilution. This does not necessarily represent a major difference in disease activity. ANA titers go up and down during the course of the disease, and a high or low titer does not necessarily mean the disease is more or less active. Therefore, it is not always possible to determine the severity of the disease from the ANA titer.

A titer above 1:80 is usually considered positive. However, some laboratories may interpret different titer levels as positive, so one cannot compare titers from different laboratories.

The pattern of the ANA test can sometimes be helpful in determining which autoimmune disease is present and which treatment program is appropriate. The homogeneous (smooth) pattern is found in a variety of connective tissue diseases as well as in patients taking particular drugs such as certain anti-arrhythmics, anti-convulsants or antihypertensives. This pattern is also the pattern that is most commonly seen in healthy individuals who have positive ANA tests. The speckled pattern is found in SLE and other connective tissue diseases, while the peripheral (or rim) pattern is found almost exclusively in SLE. The nucleolar (a pattern with a few large spots) pattern is found primarily in patients who have scleroderma.

Because the ANA is positive in so many conditions, the results of the ANA test have to be interpreted in light of the patient's medical history, as well as his or her clinical symptoms. Thus, a positive ANA alone is NEVER enough to diagnose lupus. On the other hand, a negative ANA argues against lupus but does not rule out the disease completely.

The ANA can be looked at as a screening test. If it is positive in a person who is not feeling well and who has other symptoms or signs of lupus, the physician will probably want to conduct further tests for lupus. If the ANA is positive in a person who is feeling well and in whom there are no other signs of lupus, it should be ignored. If there is any doubt, a consultation with a rheumatologist may clarify the situation.

In those individuals with a positive ANA, additional tests for certain particular antibodies that may better establish a diagnosis of SLE can be done. The knowledge of which particular antibody is responsible for the positive ANA test can sometimes be helpful in determining which autoimmune disease is present. For instance, antibodies to DNA (the protein that makes up the body's genetic code) are found primarily in SLE. Antibodies to histones (DNA packaging proteins) are usually found in patients with drug-induced lupus. However, these antibodies may also be found in SLE. Antibodies to the Sm antigen are found almost exclusively in lupus, and often help to confirm the diagnosis of SLE. Antibodies to RNP (ribonucleoprotein) are found in a variety of connective tissue diseases. When present in very high levels, RNP antibodies are suggestive of mixed connective tissue disease, a condition with symptoms like those of SLE, polymyositis, and scleroderma.

Antibodies to Ro/SS-A are found in patients with either lupus or Sjogren's syndrome and are almost always found in babies who are born with neonatal lupus. Antibodies to PM-Scl are associated with certain cases of polymyositis and antibodies to Jo-1 are associated with polymyositis. Antibodies to Scl-70 are found in people with a generalized form of scleroderma, while antibodies to the centromere (a structure involved in cell division) are found in patients with a limited form of scleroderma which tends to have a chronic course.

Laboratory tests which measure complement levels in the blood may also be helpful to the physician in making a diagnosis of SLE. Complement is a blood protein that destroys bacteria and also mediates inflammation. Complement proteins are identified by the letter "C and a number. The most common complement tests are C3, C4, and CH50. If the total blood complement level is low, or the C3 or C4 complement values are low and the patient also has a positive ANA, some weight is added to the diagnosis of lupus. Low C3 and C4 complement levels in individuals with a positive ANA may signify the presence of lupus kidney disease.

Sometimes examination of a tissue sample (biopsy) can be helpful in making a diagnosis. The biopsy is one of the best ways to evaluate an organ or tissue. The procedure involves removal of a small sliver of tissue, which is then examined under a microscope. The doctor can use the biopsy to identify the amount of inflammation and damage to the tissue. Further tests can be performed on the specimen in order to determine whether the problem is due to lupus or is caused by some other factor such as infection or medication. Almost any tissue can be biopsied, the most common sites biopsied in lupus are the skin and kidney. The results of the biopsy, like any other laboratory test should be examined in combination with the clinical history.

The interpretation of all these tests, and their relationship to symptoms, can be difficult. When someone has many symptoms and signs of lupus and has positive tests for lupus, physicians have little problem with making a correct diagnosis and initiating treatment. However, a more common problem occurs when an individual presents with vague, seemingly unrelated symptoms of achy joints, fever, fatigue, or pains.

Powerful new diagnostic tools have been developed which are useful in the diagnosis of SLE. Like other such tests in medicine, they are useful only in the hands of skilled physicians who understand their strengths and limitations. Fortunately, with growing awareness of lupus, an increasing number of physicians will consider the possibility of lupus in the diagnosis.

Living With Lupus

What Is Wellness?

How can a person with a chronic illness live well? For many people with lupus, living well means adopting a wellness philosophy. Wellness is an approach to living and the first step in achieving wellness is understanding what it means to be "well." A wellness lifestyle requires attention to the body, the mind and the spirit. It requires thoughtful planning and carefully adjusting your daily routines. Living well with lupus is a struggle at times, but is achievable and well worth the effort.

Wellness means making a decision to be the best you can be and then taking responsibility for doing what helps or hinders your life. This requires you to understand and accept that everything you do to your body, think with your mind and believe with your heart has an impact on your state of health. Health is affected by your state of wellness, but wellness is about more than health. People who are ill, disabled and even those in their final days of living can experience wellness. Wellness is choosing options and making commitments which enhance life. To live well with the challenges of lupus requires coping with the impact that a chronic illness has on the body, the mind and the spirit. These three areas are inseparable; improvement in one leads to improvement in the others.

Wellness doesn't just happen, it must be worked on every day. It must be carefully planned with a positive outlook and a realistic evaluation of your potential. Living well with lupus requires a balanced plan. Maintaining balance includes:

- identifying what you want to do in each area,
- setting goals and
- making a contract with yourself.

In essence, you make a commitment to start living and enjoying a wellness lifestyle. This commitment puts you in control instead of being controlled by an illness.

The Wellness Mind

People with lupus are not responsible for developing the disease, but they are responsible for the way they react to it. Attitudes, feelings and thoughts have an impact on health. The wellness-oriented mind is one that chooses to see the world in a positive light. To live well with lupus, focus on your abilities rather than your disabilities. Whether you choose to view yourself as active and responsible for you life or as a victim of disease is a personal choice.

Planning includes thinking through your daily and weekly commitments and then looking for energy-saving short cuts. Visualize what needs to be done and decide if you are physically up to it. Be flexible, if you don't have the strength to do it today, it may wait. Or tackle the task piece-meal; do what you can now and save the rest for later. If you push yourself when you do not have the physical energy to complete a task, you may pay for this with more fatigue. A positive attitude coupled with a well thought-out plan of action will increase the likelihood of success.

Your attitudes, thoughts and feelings are truly your own and you are free to change them as you develop a wellness mind set. If you find you are afraid, bored, confused, distressed or depressed in your life, there is nothing that says you have to keep those thoughts and feelings or be controlled by them. You can choose to change. You can make the decision to adopt a new attitude, and then take steps to make the change happen. Life is a choice and it is yours to make.

The Wellness Body

To operate efficiently the human body requires fitness, nutrition, and stress management. Fitness is important because it can prevent unwanted problems such as obesity, muscle weakness, low energy or fatigue. It also can cause desirable effects such as increased stamina, vitality and confidence. The joint pain, fatigue and muscle weakness frequently found in people with lupus can lead to physical inactivity and reduced fitness. Rest is an important component in managing fatigue. It may be necessary to increase the length or number of rest periods in times of a lupus flare. As important as rest is, it is necessary to seek a balance between sufficient and excessive rest. Excessive rest is harmful to the joints, muscles, bones and overall fitness. A lack of fitness may be indicated by: unexpected weight gain, sore muscles after routine or increased use, or a loss of strength or endurance.

Studies show fitness can be improved in people with chronic systemic diseases without undesirable side effects. Your doctor or a physical therapist can recommend an individualized home exercise program. The keys to achieving your ideal level of fitness are:

- to find an activity that interests you
- to make a commitment (and put it in writing) to your exercise plan
- to recognize ways you might try to talk yourself out of sticking to your plan
- to list the payoffs you expect from fitness
- to chart your progress. You can take pride in taking control and being as strong and fit as possible with lupus.

Nutrition provides the necessary fuel for the body to carry on its normal functions. Your body requires a balance of nutrients. Fad diets are to be avoided because they are nutritionally unsound. Eating well and wisely are essential to achieving fitness and living well. There are no specific dietary guidelines for people with lupus other than to observe a balanced diet that includes the appropriate amounts of food from each food group. Several studies on the effects of diet on disease have identified three dietary recommendations for general health:

1. Eat a balanced diet

2. Include a variety of foods from all food groups; eat foods that are: low in fat, high in fiber, and less refined

3. Eat and exercise to maintain ideal body composition.

Corticosteroids often increase the appetite and unless you are careful, unwanted weight gain can occur. Realizing that overeating is inconsistent with a wellness lifestyle is a step toward controlling weight and practicing wellness.

If you want to lose weight, focus on two things: increasing your exercise and decreasing your fat intake. Exercise increases the amount of lean muscle mass and increases the body's capacity to burn up fat. How do you know if you are eating too much fat? Record everything you eat for one day. Consult a dietician or nutrition book to determine your fat and caloric intake. Fat calories should make up no more than 30 percent of the total calories. Set realistic goals for how you will improve your diet. Be patient; changes in diet take time (weeks) before results are seen. Be wary of reports that make outrageous claims for easy weight loss. Reports from genuine scientific research that use controlled studies and find the same results in more than one laboratory, are probably authentic. When it comes to wellness, there are no quick fixes. The most important actions you can take to maintain physical wellness include eating properly, exercising and maintaining your weight at a proper level.

Stress management can be achieved by using various self-help techniques. Lupus affects many aspects of living: family and intimate relationships, vocational status, finances, self-esteem, mood, morale and one's sense of personal control. Managing the stress that occurs in these areas can be a struggle and at times, it can be overwhelming. Scientific studies show that people who are actively involved and believe they have some control in life situations are more healthy than people who are passive and believe they are helpless victims.

Participation in a support group can provide social and emotional help. Support groups can also help individuals develop or improve their coping skills which alleviate some stresses of chronic illness. Support group participation bolsters self-esteem, morale and self-reliance. Working to improve patient-doctor communications is a way to help one gain a sense of control and reduce stress. This can be accomplished by the following:

- prepare for doctor visits by making a list of questions and a brief outline of current problems
- keep a medical diary
- take medications with you
- ask how and why a medication needs to be taken

- if a medication causes a problem, notify your doctor
- make it a goal to understand your doctor's advice. You and your doctor are equally responsible for maintaining clear communication about your health and wellness.

The Wellness Spirit

When a person is diagnosed with a chronic illness it can have a profound affect on their self-concept and what's important in life. It is an emotional experience and a period of grieving is commonly needed. People with lupus often go through periods of denial, anger, fear, depression, bargaining and finally, acceptance as they come to terms with their lupus. Coming to terms with the diagnosis and perhaps reshaping your life takes time. Allow yourself to grieve for the loss of your life before lupus, so you can accept and redefine your life with lupus.

This process of re-defining your purpose in life and who you are is seldom easy. Often it is made more difficult by a lack of information about lupus. Understanding what lupus is and what to expect can diminish the fear of the unknown. Developing a wellness-oriented spirit is a process that evolves over time. Just like developing a wellness body, planning is key to developing a wellness spirit. The plan includes:

- adopting a positive attitude
- developing a passion for something outside of yourself; something around which you can focus your life.
- striving to be happy.

In the words of Abraham Lincoln, "Most folks are about as happy as they make up their minds to be."

A richer way of life can be achieved by exploring who you are, why you are here and what you can do. Discovering who you are is a wonderful thing. As a sense of purpose in your life develops and takes form, the mind, the body and your general well-being will benefit.

Summary

Wellness is a philosophy in which one takes responsibility for the positive development of the mind, the body and the spirit. It is your conscious choice to pursue behaviors that enhance and enrich life.

Wellness requires that you develop and use a plan based on your realistic potential. A plan for wellness includes striving to improve each area: the mind—through emphasis on developing positive attitudes; the body—through attention to fitness, nutrition and stress management; and the spirit—through reflection on life.

How can you recognize people who are living well with their lupus? They are individuals who focus on their current talents and abilities. You will rarely hear them dwell on what they used to be able to do. Their life with lupus has new meaning. Making the best of the present and planning for the future is what is important to them. People who are living well with their lupus understand that options and alternatives are available.

They control their life instead of letting lupus control their life. They have successfully navigated through the grieving process, and will tell you it was not an easy trip. Through acceptance, they have reached an understanding that lupus is not their whole life, only a part of it. They take responsibility for their health and wellness and are able to reach outside of themselves to help others.

Adopting a wellness lifestyle can make the difference between enjoying life versus simply surviving life with lupus. The choice is yours.

Chapter 23

Vasculitis

What Is Vasculitis?

Vasculitis is an inflammation of the blood vessels. Inflammation is a condition in which tissue is damaged by blood cells entering the tissues. These are mostly white blood cells which circulate and serve as our major defense against infection. Ordinarily, white blood cells destroy bacteria and viruses. However, they can also damage normal tissue if they invade it. Vasculitis can affect very small blood vessels (capillaries), medium-size blood vessels (arterioles or venules), or large blood vessels (arteries or veins).

Several things can happen to an inflamed blood vessel. If it is a small vessel, it may break and produce tiny areas of bleeding in the tissue. These areas will appear as small red or purple dots on the skin. If a larger vessel is inflamed, it may swell and produce a nodule which may be felt if the blood vessel is close to the skin surface. The inside of the vessel tube may become narrowed so that blood flow is reduced, or the inside may become totally closed (usually by a blood clot which forms at the site of inflammation). If blood flow is reduced or stopped, the tissues which receive blood from that vessel begin to die. For example, a person with vasculitis of a medium-sized artery in the hand may develop a cold finger which hurts whenever it is used; occasionally this can progress to gangrene.

What Causes Vasculitis?

Vasculitis can be caused by:

1. infection of the blood vessel walls, or

2. an immune or "allergic" reaction in the vessel walls.

The first cause is rare. When it occurs, bacteria, viruses or fungi infect the blood vessel. White blood cells move in to destroy the infectious agents and damage the blood vessel in the process. This is a serious condition and requires prompt antibiotic treatment.

The second cause of vasculitis, an immune reaction, is more common. Substances which cause allergic reactions are called "antigens." They cause the body to make proteins called "antibodies" which bind to the antigen for the purpose of getting rid of it. Antigen and antibody bound together are called "immune complexes." Two primary ways in which immune complexes destroy antigens are:

1. by attracting white blood cells to digest the antigen, and

2. by activating other body substances to help destroy the antigens.

Unfortunately, some immune complexes do not serve their purpose of destroying antigens. Instead, they remain too long in the body and circulate in the blood and deposit in tissues. They commonly accumulate in blood vessel walls, where they cause inflammation.

It is likely that some white blood cells which kill infectious agents ("cytotoxic" cells) can also accidentally damage blood vessels and cause vasculitis.

In the vasculitis caused by lupus, the antigens causing the immune complexes are often not known. In some cases, the complexes contain DNA and anti-DNA antigens, or Ro (also called SS-A) and anti-Ro antigens. A recently discovered antibody, ANCA (anti-neutrophil cytoplasm antibody), can cause vasculitis in some individuals.

Diseases Associated with Vasculitis

Vasculitis can occur in many different illnesses. Some of the illnesses that can cause vasculitis are:

Infections
Autoimmune Diseases
- Lupus
- Rheumatoid Arthritis
- Polymyalgia Rheumatica
- Scleroderma
- Wegener's Granulomatosis
- Temporal Arteritis
- Cryoglobulinemia
Erythema Nodosum
Tumors
- Leukemia
- Lymphoma
- Others

Vasculitis can also occur by itself without any obvious associated infection or other illness.

Symptoms of Vasculitis

Vasculitis can cause many different symptoms, depending upon what tissues are involved and the severity of the tissue damage. Some patients are not ill and notice occasional spots on their skin. Others are very ill with systemic symptoms and major organ damage. A list of symptoms based on the tissues in which vasculitis occurs include:

- **Systemic symptoms:** Fever, generally feeling bad ("malaise"), muscle and joint pain, poor appetite, weight loss, and fatigue. This set of complaints can occur in many illnesses and is not specific to vasculitis.

- **Skin:** Red or purple dots ("petechiae"), usually most numerous on the legs. When the spots are larger, about the size of the end of a finger, they are called "purpura." Some look like large bruises. These are the most common vasculitis skin lesions, but hives, itchy lumpy rash, and painful or tender lumps can occur. Areas of dead skin can appear as ulcers (especially around the ankles), small black spots at the ends of the fingers or around the fingernails and toes ("nail fold infarcts"), or gangrene of fingers or toes.

- **Joints:** Aching in joints and a frank arthritis with pain swelling and heat in joints. Deformities resulting from this arthritis are rare.

- **Brain:** Vasculitis in the brain can cause many problems, from mild to severe. They include headaches, behavioral disturbances, confusion, seizures, and strokes.

- **Peripheral Nerves:** Peripheral nerve symptoms may include numbness and tingling (usually in an arm or a leg, or in areas which would be covered by gloves or socks), loss of sensation, or loss of strength (especially in the feet or hands).

- **Intestines:** Inadequate blood flow in the intestines can cause crampy abdominal pain and bloating. If areas in the wall of the intestine develop gangrene, blood will appear in the stool. If the intestinal wall develops a hole (called a "perforation"), surgery may be required.

- **Heart:** Vasculitis in the coronary arteries is unusual in lupus. If it occurs, it can cause a feeling of heaviness in the chest during exertion ("angina"), which is relieved by rest. Heart attacks rarely occur as a result of vasculitis.

- **Lungs:** Vasculitis in this tissue can cause pneumonia-like attacks with chest x-ray changes that look like pneumonia and symptoms of fever and cough. Occasionally, inflammation can lead to scarring of lung tissue with chronic shortness of breath.

- **Kidneys:** Vasculitis is not common in kidneys of people with lupus, even those who have lupus nephritis. It may not cause any symptoms, although most patients with renal vasculitis have high blood pressure.

- **Eyes:** Vasculitis involving the small blood vessels of the retina can occur in lupus. The retina is a tissue at the back of the eye which contains cells that have to be activated to form a visual image. Sometimes, vasculitis of the eyes causes no symptoms. Usually, however, there is visual blurring which comes on suddenly and stays, or a person may even lose a portion of their vision. In other non-lupus types of vasculitis, such as temporal arteritis, there is sudden loss of part or all of the vision in one eye, usually accompanied by severe headache.

Consulting Your Physician

If you suspect that you or a friend or relative has vasculitis you should consult a physician as soon as possible. Remember, vasculitis can be very mild and of little importance, or very severe and life-threatening—or any degree in between. Therefore, an expert should help you decide:

- if you have vasculitis,
- how serious it is, and
- if and how it should be treated.

Doctors trained in several different specialties are taught to recognize and treat vasculitis. These include rheumatologists, general internists, dermatologists, hematologists, nephrologists, gastroenterologists, infectious disease experts, pulmonologists, cardiologists, geriatricians, neurologists, and ophthalmologists.

Diagnosing Vasculitis

The diagnosis of vasculitis is based on a person's medical history, current symptoms, a complete physical examination, and the results of specialized laboratory tests.

Blood abnormalities which often occur when vasculitis is present include an elevated sedimentation rate, anemia, a high white blood count and a high platelet count. Blood tests can also be used to identify immune complexes or antibodies that cause vasculitis in the circulation and measure whether complement levels are abnormal. These tests take several days to complete. The physician may also order a urine analysis.

If there are any symptoms that suggest heart involvement, tests that may be ordered include: EKG, ECHO cardiogram and heart scans. For lung symptoms, the physician may order a chest x-ray, obtain blood from an artery to measure the oxygen content, and schedule a pulmonary function test. A pulmonary function test uses a specialized machine to measure how well the lungs handle air and oxygen as you breathe into it. If there are abdominal symptoms, the physician may order ultrasound or CAT scans of the organs in the abdomen, or other special x-rays to see the intestines. For brain symptoms, CAT scans and magnetic resonance images are frequently useful.

Sometimes, inflammation in medium and large-size arteries or veins can be seen by injecting dye into them and viewing the outlines of the blood vessels on x-ray. This procedure is called an "angiography." It can be done in any area of the body.

The diagnosis is most firmly made by seeing vasculitis in involved tissue. This is done by taking a biopsy of the involved tissue and examining that tissue under a microscope. Your physician may suggest this procedure.

Finally, it may be important for your physician to consult with other medical specialists about your case. For example, if your physician is a rheumatologist and you have visual complaints which could be indicative of vasculitis, you may be referred to an ophthalmologist. It is very important that one physician be in charge of your case, coordinating your cure and helping you with decisions.

Treating Vasculitis

The choice of treatment for vasculitis depends on the severity of the vasculitis, your general health, and your past reactions (positive and negative) to medications.

Many cases of vasculitis do not require treatment. For example, a few spots on the skin now and then (if not combined with other symptoms) may not require any medications.

Most physicians recommend cortisone-type medications, such as Prednisone, Prednisolone, or methylprednisolone (Medrol) as the initial treatment for vasculitis.

Some people with severe vasculitis or vasculitis that does not respond well to cortisone-type drugs will need to be treated with cytotoxic drugs. These medications kill the cells that cause Inflammation in the blood vessels. The two most frequently used are azathioprine (Imuran) and cyclophosphamide (Cytoxan). They are usually used in combination with Prednisone and are often effective in treating vasculitis.

Experimental procedures that have been helpful in treating some cases of vasculitis include: plasmaphereses, intravenous gammaglobulin, and cyclosporin, a medication used to prevent organ rejection in transplant patients. Experimental therapies change frequently. Your physician can provide you with current information.

Outcome

There are various outcomes for people suffering from vasculitis. For many patients, vasculitis, especially if confined to the skin, may be annoying but never life-threatening. For those individuals, life can be normal—or close to it.

On the other hand, a small number of people have severe vasculitis involving major organ systems. In these cases, damage can occur so rapidly that treatment does not have time to work or the condition may be resistant to treatment. An attack of vasculitis can be fatal or permanently disabling for individuals so affected.

For the vast majority of people with vasculitis, treatment is very effective. The vasculitis may disappear only to reoccur later and require treatment again; or it may be suppressed but never really go away, so that some ongoing treatment is always required.

Chapter 24

What Black Women Should Know about Lupus

Do You or Someone You Know Have Signs of Lupus?

Lupus is a serious health problem that affects mainly young women. The disease often starts between the ages of 15 and 44.

People of all races may get lupus. However, lupus is three times more common in black women than in white women.

As many as one in 250 black women will get the disease.

What is Lupus?

Lupus is a disease that can affect many parts of the body. It can affect the joints, the skin, the kidneys, the lungs, the heart, or the brain. Only a few of these parts of the body are affected in most people.

Something goes wrong with the body's immune system in lupus. We can think of the immune system as an army within the body with hundreds of defenders (known as antibodies). They defend the body from attack by germs and viruses. In lupus, however, the immune system becomes overactive and goes out of control. The antibodies attack healthy tissues in the body. This attack induces inflammation, causing redness, pain, and swelling in the affected parts of the body. This tendency for the immune system to become overactive may run in families.

NIH Pub No. 93-3219.

What Does a Person with Lupus Look Like?

Many people with lupus look healthy.

What Are the Signs of Lupus?

The signs of lupus differ from one person to another. Some people have just a few signs of the disease; others have more. Lupus may be hard to diagnose. It is often mistaken for other diseases. For this reason, lupus has often been called the "great imitator."

Common signs of lupus are:

- Red rash or color change on the face, often in the shape of a butterfly across the bridge of the nose and the cheeks.
- Painful or swollen joints.
- Unexplained fever.
- Chest pain with breathing.
- Unusual loss of hair.
- Pale or purple fingers or toes from cold or stress.
- Sensitivity to the sun.
- Low blood count.

These signs are more important when they occur together.

Other signs of lupus can include mouth sores, unexplained "fits" or convulsions, hallucinations or depression, repeated miscarriages, and unexplained kidney problems.

What Causes Lupus?

We don't know what causes the immune system to become overactive. In some people, lupus becomes active after exposure to sunlight, infections, or certain medications.

Can You Catch Lupus From Someone Else?

No, lupus is not catching. You can't give it to someone else. Also, it is not a form of cancer. It is not AIDS.

Does Lupus Run in Families?

Most relatives of lupus patients do not develop the disease, but in some families more than one member gets lupus. If a relative of a lupus patient develops signs of lupus, she or he should see a doctor.

How Serious Is Lupus?

Signs of lupus tend to come and go. There are times when the disease quiets down, or goes into remission. At other times, lupus flares up, or becomes active. Years ago, many people with lupus died. Now, with good medical care, most people with the disease can lead active, productive, and fulfilling lives.

Are There Different Kinds of Lupus?

There are three major types of lupus:

1. lupus that affects certain parts of the body (systemic lupus erythematosus),

2. lupus mainly of the skin (discoid or cutaneous lupus), and

3. lupus caused by medicine (drug-induced lupus).

Systemic lupus erythematosus, sometimes called SLE, is the most serious form of the disease. This type of lupus is the focus of this chapter. Systemic means that it may affect many parts of the body, such as the joints, skin, kidneys, lungs, heart, or the brain. This type of lupus can be mild or serious. If it is not treated, systemic lupus can cause damage to the organs inside your body.

Discoid and cutaneous lupus mainly affect the skin. The person may have a red rash or a color change of the skin on the face, scalp, or other parts of the body.

Drug-induced lupus is caused by a small number of prescription medications. The person with drug-induced lupus may have the same symptoms as the person with systemic lupus, but it is usually less serious. Usually when the medicine is stopped, the disease goes away. The most common drugs that can cause lupus are:

- procainamide used for heart problems,
- hydralazine used for high blood pressure, and
- dilantin used for seizures.

Drug-induced lupus is usually found in older men and women of all races.

Does Sunlight Cause Lupus?

In some people, no matter what shade of skin, an attack of lupus may be brought on by being in the sun, even for a short period of time.

Do Men Get Lupus?

Yes, men get all forms of lupus. However, nine out of ten people who have lupus are women.

Why is Lupus More Common in Black Women Than White Women?

We do not know why the disease is more common in black women. However, research doctors supported by the National Institutes of Health are studying this problem. Researchers are studying why minorities are more inclined to get lupus, what causes it to start, and why is it mild in some and severe in others. Other researchers are studying why the signs of lupus differ between black women and white women.

What Should You Do if You Think You Have Lupus?

You should see a doctor or a nurse and be examined and tested for lupus. They will talk to you and take a history of your health problems. Many people have lupus for a long time before it is detected. It is important that you tell the doctor or nurse about your symptoms. (Photocopy the list of "Signs of Lupus" above and use it as a checklist which you can take to your doctor.)

How is Lupus Treated?

The doctor may treat each lupus patient in a different way because the signs of lupus often differ from one person to another. The doctor may give aspirin or similar medicine to treat the painful, swollen joints and the fever. Creams may be prescribed for the rash, and stronger medicines prescribed for more serious problems.

Is There a Cure for Lupus?

At this point, lupus cannot be cured. However, in many cases, signs of the disease can be relieved. The good news is that with the correct medicine and by taking care of themselves, most lupus patients can hold a job, have children, and lead a full life.

Outlook

The outlook for lupus patients has greatly improved. Research doctors supported by the National Institutes of Health are studying many aspects of lupus, such as what goes wrong with the immune system, why the disease runs in families, how lupus causes damage in the body, and why it can lead to repeated miscarriages. Others are researching why lupus is so much more common in women, especially black women. Researchers have learned a great deal about lupus and are studying new ways to treat and, hopefully, prevent the disease. The future holds great promise for improving the health of all Americans who have lupus.

Awareness

Please share this information with your family and friends. Someone you know or care about may have lupus.

Other Resources

For further information on lupus, see your doctor or health clinic and contact your local chapter of the following organizations:

Lupus Foundation of America, Inc.
4 Research Place
Suite 800
Rockville, Maryland 20850-3226
(301) 670-9292
(800) 558-0121

The American Lupus Society
3914 Del Amo Blvd.
Suite 922
Torrance, California 90503
(310) 542-8891
(800) 331-1802

Both of these groups can provide more detailed information on lupus through free pamphlets and newsletters. They also have pamphlets in Spanish. The two groups also can refer people to doctors and clinics who see a lot of lupus patients.

Additional copies of this chapter are available free of charge as the booklet What Black Women Should Know About Lupus. The National Institute of Health encourages readers to duplicate and distribute this material as needed or to obtain as many booklets as needed from NIAMS Task Force on Lupus in High Risk Populations, National Institute of Arthritis and Muskoskeletal and Skin Diseases, Box AMS, 9000 Rockville Pike, Bethesda, Maryland 20892.

Chapter 25

Multiple Sclerosis

Multiple sclerosis is a disease caused by inflammation and scarring of tissue in the brain and spinal cord. More specifically, the inflammation breaks down myelin, the white, fatty material that provides a thick sheath or covering for nerve fibers in the central nervous system. A healthy myelin sheath enables a nerve cell to send electrical impulses along its fiber at high velocity, a function critical for accomplishing such basic activities as walking, eating, or breathing.

As multiple sclerosis causes more and more of the sheath to be stripped away, a process called demyelination, electrical impulses proceed more and more slowly down the fiber. Depending on which nerves are affected, severe or mild disabilities can occur. If myelin in sensory nerves is lost, for example, a person may have an impaired sense of touch.

Multiple sclerosis gets its name because the demyelination is often followed by sclerosis, or hardening of nervous system tissue, usually at multiple sites. The sclerosis is the result of scar tissue forming in the central nervous system (a process called gliosis). In part because we can not determine in advance which nerve fibers will be affected in a particular patient—the disease can impair any part of the central nervous system—the severity of multiple sclerosis is often unpredictable. Some people may have mild problems, with no significant permanent disability. For others, multiple sclerosis means severe paralysis and confinement to a wheelchair. We do know that the disease often strikes people in the prime of life, most commonly between

NIH Pub No. 90-3015.

the ages of 20 and 40, although some people do not develop multiple sclerosis until their forties or fifties. The disease strikes about twice as many women as men.

Symptoms

Although severe forms of multiple sclerosis can be devastating, the illness shortens a person's average life expectancy by only about five years. Common symptoms of the disease include fatigue and loss of strength. Patients often have increased muscle stiffness due to a condition known as spasticity, or muscle stiffness. There may be loss of sensation in the arms and legs, or an ever-present tingling sensation, like feeling pins and needles. People also may have facial pain. If multiple sclerosis has affected the cerebellum, a portion of the nervous system near the back of the brain, the patient may have poor coordination, loss of balance, or tremors.

If the optic nerve is involved, the patient may have blurred or reduced vision. Patients with demyelination of the brain stem, a region that controls eye movement, commonly have double vision, since each eye may no longer focus on the same object. If the illness has impaired the spinal cord, in addition to losing leg strength, the patient may lose bladder control, become constipated, or become impotent.

One common feature of multiple sclerosis is that many symptoms worsen when patients are exposed to heat. This is because elevated temperatures—whether from a hot bath, exercise, or exposure to the sun—further slow the conduction of electrical impulses in nerve fibers. Conversely, a cold bath can sometimes temporarily relieve symptoms or reduce some of the fatigue multiple sclerosis patients often feel.

Neurologists divide multiple sclerosis into two types. The first, known as *exacerbating-remitting disease*, is characterized by fluctuations in nerve function. Periods of deteriorating ability are followed by periods of recovery, although, as time passes, recovery often becomes less and less complete. The second form of the illness, *chronic progressive disease*, has more of a steady downhill course, typically without periods of temporary recovery. Frequently, people who initially have the fluctuating form of multiple sclerosis go on to develop the chronic form.

The Search for Causes

We do not yet know the cause of multiple sclerosis. Although there is considerable evidence that a virus may trigger the disease, researchers are still uncertain. Genetic factors and an imbalance in the immune system also may help predispose an individual to the illness.

Evidence for a Viral Link

The evidence for a viral or other environmental agent comes from many sources. First, multiple sclerosis is far more common in colder or temperate climates than in warmer climates. Within North America and Europe, there is a higher prevalence of the disease in the north than in the south. Studies of large immigrant populations suggest that people with multiple sclerosis were exposed to some environmental agent at a young age, possibly before age 15. The immigrant studies show that people who emigrated before age 15 had a prevalence of multiple sclerosis similar to that found in the region to which they moved. People who emigrated after age 15 had the same disease prevalence as found in the area from which they came.

Evidence for a virus as the environmental agent comes from studies of two epidemics of the disease in Iceland and the Faroe Islands, the latter an area between Iceland and Scandinavia. Each year for about 20 years immediately following World War II, the incidence of the disease in these regions increased. Both regions were occupied by British troops during the war, and some investigators believe the troops may have inadvertently brought with them a still unknown virus or other disease-causing agent.

Viruses that may be linked to multiple sclerosis include the measles; mumps; rubella, the agent that causes German measles; and the monkey virus known as simian virus 5, or SV-5. Most recently, one of a trio of retroviruses collectively known as Human Immunodeficiency Lymphotrophic Viruses (HTLVs) has been studied for possible association with the disease. Although the virus under investigation, HTLV-I, belongs to the same family of infectious agents as the AIDS virus (HTLV-III), there is no evidence that links AIDS with multiple sclerosis. HTLV-I, however, causes an inflammatory disease of the spinal cord that has many features, including demyelination, in common with multiple sclerosis. The spinal cord disease, found predominantly in the tropics and Japan, is called tropical spastic paraparesis. Thus, although the cause of multiple sclerosis remains unknown, we have discovered that a retrovirus causes a very similar illness. Such knowledge helps pave the way for better understanding and more effective treatment of multiple sclerosis.

Genetic Factors

People generally do not think of multiple sclerosis as an inherited disease, but its prevalence in families of patients with the disease runs somewhat higher than in the general population. For example, the prevalence of multiple sclerosis in the general population is about 5 to 10 cases per 10,000 people (.05 to .1 percent). But in a family with one member who has the illness, the chance of a brother or sister developing multiple sclerosis is about 20 times higher (1 to 2 percent). One could argue that the increased incidence could be due to either genetic factors or an environmental agent since family members share the same environment. But evidence from studies of twins suggests a strong genetic influence. Fraternal (nonidentical) twins had the same higher prevalence for multiple sclerosis as brothers and sisters who were not twins. But if one of a pair of identical twins had the illness, researchers found that the other twin had a far higher likelihood, about a 25 to 50 percent chance, of also developing multiple sclerosis. Because identical twins have the same genes, one or more genetic factors appear important for developing the illness.

Indeed, researchers have found genetic markers associated with the disease—proteins more commonly found in immune system and other cells of people with multiple sclerosis than in the general population. Work has focused on certain classes of proteins found on the surface of white blood cells called leukocytes. Scientists have detected one particular human leukocyte-associated protein, known as HLA-DQN1, in about 90 percent of people with multiple sclerosis. (In contrast, about 70 percent of people in the general population have this protein.) Another protein, HLA-DR2, has been identified in about 60 percent of people with multiple sclerosis, but only in about 18 to 20 percent of the general population. In addition, some forms of another leukocyte protein, known as the T-cell receptor molecule, also appear more prevalent among multiple sclerosis patients than in the general population. Finding more than one genetic marker indicates that more than one gene may be needed to trigger onset of the illness.

The Autoimmune Connection

We also have evidence that a defect in the immune system may predispose an individual to multiple sclerosis. Normally, the immune system fights off infections from foreign invaders such as bacteria or viruses. But in some diseases, for reasons that remain unknown, the immune system attacks the body's own tissues, a reaction known as an autoimmune response. Some studies suggest an autoimmune reaction might cause multiple sclerosis. This research focuses on an animal disease, known as experimental allergic encephalomyelitis, or EAE, that causes demyelination and inflammation similar to that seen in multiple sclerosis. Scientists have induced EAE in animals by making them allergic to a myelin protein called myelin basic protein. The allergy causes the animals' immune systems to attack the nervous system and induce a disease highly similar to multiple sclerosis, without injecting a virus or other infectious agent.

Other studies indicate an imbalance between certain cells in the immune system may set the stage for an autoimmune response that could result in multiple sclerosis. To understand the imbalance requires a bit of explanation about some of the key players in the immune system. Certain white blood cells, called B-cells because they originate in the bone marrow, can transform into plasma cells, which then make antibodies. But the B-cells usually need help from other immune system cells, called helper T-cells, in order to efficiently make the antibodies.

The collaboration between B-cells and helper T-cells is regulated by several factors, including suppressor T-cells. Such regulation is critical because otherwise the collaboration between B-cells and helper T-cells would continue even when antibodies are no longer needed. Without the suppressor T-cells to stop them, the helper T-cells and B-cells could make antibodies against a person's own body tissues. Moreover, studies indicate that multiple sclerosis patients may have impaired function of suppressor T-cells, possibly triggering an immune system attack against body tissue the system normally protects: central nervous system myelin.

Drug studies provide further evidence for an autoimmune role in causing multiple sclerosis. In clinical trials, several drugs that suppress the immune system have been more effective in treating the disease than drugs that boost immune function.

In actuality, a combination of all three effects described above—infection by a virus, genetic factors, and an autoimmune reaction—may explain the occurrence of multiple sclerosis. Some researchers believe that if a viral infection in a genetically susceptible person occurs at a particularly vulnerable time in the development of the immune system, probably in the early teenage years, it could trigger an autoimmune response. This may happen, for example, if proteins on a virus resemble those proteins belonging to body tissue. If the body's immune system has trouble distinguishing between the viral proteins and its own, it may attack both. Scientists speculate that years later such an autoimmune reaction might develop into multiple sclerosis.

Treatment

There are two basic strategies for treating multiple sclerosis. One regimen attempts to reduce the underlying inflammation and the presumed impaired immune attack against the nervous system. The other strategy emphasizes relief of symptoms.

Treating the Causes of Inflammation and Immune System Dysfunction

The choice of drugs to reduce inflammation depends on the type of multiple sclerosis. For people with exacerbating-remitting multiple sclerosis, the more mild form of the illness, physicians often prescribe a pituitary hormone known as adrenocorticotrophic hormone, or ACTH. This hormone stimulates the adrenal glands to produce cortisol and certain other steroids that reduce inflammation. Alternatively, synthetic steroids, such as prednisone or methylprednisolone, may be given to lower inflammation in the nervous system.

Other agents that might more effectively reduce inflammation are under study. Preliminary research indicates that alpha and beta interferon may be of benefit, and ongoing studies seek to determine the optimum dose of these naturally occurring substances. Another promising drug for people with relatively mild multiple sclerosis is copolymer-I. A small study suggests that the drug can help people who take it for an extended period. Unlike many other drugs used to treat multiple sclerosis, copolymer-I appears to have few side effects. A larger, multicenter, controlled study of the drug is underway.

People who have chronic progressive multiple sclerosis, the more severe form of the illness, are much more difficult to treat. Drugs for this illness tend to be stronger immunosuppressive agents and carry more serious side effects. Neurologists debate whether these drugs should be used at all. Some believe that the risks of using these drugs far outweigh their benefits. Others believe that they should treat multiple sclerosis aggressively, even if it means using a drug that can only temporarily stop the disease from getting worse until a better, safer treatment comes along. One of the better known drugs that falls into this category is cyclophosphamide, or Cytoxan. Data indicate that only about a third of people who receive the drug show improvement; another one-third remain stable, neither improving or deteriorating; and one-third deteriorate at about the same rate that would be expected if they did not take the drug.

Another experimental treatment for severe and milder forms of multiple sclerosis is plasma exchange, or plasmapheresis. In this procedure, blood is removed from the body and the plasma portion is discarded before the red and white blood cells are returned. The strategy behind this treatment is that plasmapheresis may remove harmful antibodies or other harmful substances circulating in the blood that may damage the nervous system. A large, multicenter study underway in Canada may determine the effectiveness of the treatment.

Another procedure recently tested in multiple sclerosis patients is total lymphoid radiation. This treatment, which involves radiation of the immune system, has been used successfully for 20 years in treating early stages of a cancer called Hodgkin disease. Preliminary studies at the Medical College of New Jersey suggest that the treatment may help stabilize people with chronic progressive multiple sclerosis for as long as three to four years. A larger clinical trial is planned.

Monoclonal antibodies are one of the more promising experimental therapies for multiple sclerosis, and one which you will be hearing more about in the next few years. Monoclonal antibodies are pure antibodies that can be generated in huge quantities in animals, usually mice. And unlike drugs that suppress the entire immune system, causing unwanted side effects, these antibodies can be directed against specific cells believed to damage the nervous system in multiple sclerosis patients. Various clinical trials are underway or being planned to evaluate monoclonal antibodies directed against all T-cells, against helper T-cells, or against the subset of activated T-cells. Activated T-cells, as opposed to resting cells, are believed to mediate damage to the nervous system in people with multiple sclerosis. Researchers at Stanford University plan to test monoclonal antibodies against HLA-DR2, the genetic marker discussed above. Future studies also are likely to examine the ability to block certain T-cell receptor molecules that may be common in tissue damaged by multiple sclerosis.

Treating Symptoms

We are generally more successful at treating symptoms than the root causes of multiple sclerosis. The drug baclofen (Lioresal) treats such symptoms as painful spasms and stiffness. Another anti-spastic drug, dantrolen (Dantrium), is effective but can cause serious liver damage. Two drugs can reduce fatigue in multiple sclerosis patients: amantadine (Symmetrel) and semoline (Cylert).

The inability to control bladder function is a distressing problem that leaves many people with multiple sclerosis ashamed to leave home. The drug Ditropan helps control bladder function. Constipation, another symptom frequently seen in patients, can be treated with several compounds. A first treatment might be Metamucil alone or in combination with a stool softener such as Colace or Surfak. If these do not work, Milk of Magnesia, Dulcolax or several other agents may be prescribed. An enema may be needed to keep the constipation from causing serious damage.

Facial pain and other painful syndromes can be treated with anticonvulsive medications such as carbamazepine (Tegretol), phenytoin sodium (Dilantin) or Valproic Acid (Depakote). Elavil, originally manufactured as an antidepressant, also helps treat pain originating in the nervous system, as in multiple sclerosis. As a last resort, if severe pain persists and interferes with such basic functions as speaking or chewing, some people may have a section of the nerve surgically removed or blocked. People who undergo this procedure will have numbness over part or much of the face. A surgeon can first reversibly block the nerve to give the patient an idea of the numbness that will be produced. For some, the loss of feeling may be as disturbing as the pain they had before surgery.

Exercise can cause problems for people with multiple sclerosis because the resulting overheating can make neurological symptoms worse. But because cold temperatures increase the velocity of electrical impulses in nerves, which are slowed in multiple sclerosis, exercising in cold water may temporarily help relieve symptoms of multiple sclerosis. The ability to dissipate heat in cold water, combined with the buoyancy that people have in water, allows patients to maintain fitness without suffering the side effects of overheating they would experience if they exercised in more conventional ways. In addition, an experimental drug, 4-aminopyridine, appears to increase the velocity of impulses in demyelinated nerves. This and/or related drugs are expected to become generally available to treat multiple sclerosis during the next few years.

Physical medicine and rehabilitation are important complements to drug therapy for multiple sclerosis. Physical therapists work with the patient on developing strength, coordination, balance, and stamina to perform activities without tiring. Occupational therapists concentrate more on coping with daily living and have introduced several devices that help people function more easily, for example, with dressing and eating. One of the most useful innovations is the motor scooter, a vehicle that has allowed people to maintain their jobs long after they would have had to retire on disability. The device is useful not only for people who can no longer walk, but also for ambulatory people who tire easily due to the disease.

In addition, vocational rehabilitation has taken on greater emphasis. People who can no longer physically perform their jobs can learn new skills in an increasing number of vocational programs, including many sponsored by local chapters of the Multiple Sclerosis Society.

Conclusion

All of these various forms of therapy—established and experimental drug treatments, physical therapy, occupational therapy, and new mechanical devices—have helped to promote a much greater degree of independence among people with multiple sclerosis. Increasingly, people with this disease are leading happier, fuller, and more productive lives. The large number of clinical trials and research studies underway promises to offer even more effective treatments for multiple sclerosis in the future.

Questions and Answers

Do nutritional factors play a role in the disease? Can improved nutrition arrest or reverse multiple sclerosis?

We have no evidence that nutritional deficiencies have anything to do with causing the disease. There is little evidence to suggest that a particular diet or a nutritional supplement can help treat multiple sclerosis. However, relatively few scientific studies have been conducted on nutrition and multiple sclerosis. Most of the recommendations various people make regarding nutritional therapy are based on unproven theories. Almost none of the dietary therapies have been evaluated in standard, double-blind, controlled studies.

Is there any correlation between memory disturbances in Alzheimer disease and multiple sclerosis?

We are becoming more aware these days that people with multiple sclerosis may have some impaired cognitive function, including some memory disturbance. For most people with the illness, it is not a severe problem. Memory impairment is a relatively new area of investigation in multiple sclerosis, and the Multiple Sclerosis Society recently has begun funding this research.

Is multiple sclerosis contagious? Can I catch the disease from working near or living with someone who has it?

Although a virus may be associated with multiple sclerosis, there is no evidence that people with the disease can transmit the illness to healthy individuals. Sexual or other intimate contact with a person that has multiple sclerosis does not appear to increase one's chances of getting the disease. For instance, spouses of patients with multiple sclerosis do not have an increased incidence of the illness.

What effect does pregnancy have on someone with multiple sclerosis?

On average, women with multiple sclerosis tend to have fewer symptoms of the disease during pregnancy. But in the year following pregnancy, symptoms often worsen. Symptoms usually return to pre-pregnancy levels during the second year after pregnancy, but some women who have very severe disease during that first year will not recover fully. They may develop severe, permanent impairment after pregnancy, although often the persistent symptoms may not be as bad as those experienced during the first year after pregnancy.

—by Dr. John Richert, M.D.,
Associate Professor of Neurology,
Georgetown University Medical School.

Dr. John Richert received his medical degree at the University of Rochester School of Medicine in New York. He spent his internship and residency in internal medicine at Strong Memorial Hospital in Rochester. After serving in the Air Force, Richert spent three years as a resident in neurology at the Mayo Clinic. He joined the Laboratory of Cerebral Metabolism at the National Institute of Mental Health in 1977. In 1980, he joined the Neuroimmunology Branch of the National Institute of Neurological and Communicative Disorders and Stroke (now the National Institute of Neurological Disorders and Stroke), where his research focused on immune function in multiple sclerosis. Since 1982, Dr. Richert has been on the faculty of Georgetown University Medical School, where he now serves as an associate professor of neurology.

Chapter 26

A Practical Guide to Myasthenia Gravis

The following summary has been prepared to provide information written in lay language about myasthenia gravis (MG). This is not "the official version," but just a personal view of a complicated and sometimes controversial subject. Each person's experience with it is in some way unique, and this guide can approach the topic only in a general way.

What Is Myasthenia Gravis (MG)?

The distinctive feature of MG is fluctuating weakness of muscles, made worse by use of those muscles and improved at least partially by rest of the same muscles. The muscles affected are called voluntary or striated muscles. Involuntary heart muscle and smooth muscles of the gut, blood vessels, and uterus are not involved in MG.

Muscles which we use all the time, such as the six muscles which move each eyeball and those which hold the eyelids open, are often but not always involved. The muscles of facial expression, smiling, chewing, talking, or swallowing can be selectively affected in some people with MG. We take these muscles for granted until they don't work.

Other muscles which may be affected include those of the neck and limbs. Although MG is said to be painless, pain in the back of the neck and head may be present if neck muscles which hold up the head are weak and in spasm. Symmetrical limb weakness occurs in many other nerve and muscle diseases, but in MG, limb weakness is often not symmetrical, one side being weaker than the other. Shoulder weakness is demonstrated by trouble holding up an arm to comb or shampoo one's hair, or to shave or put on makeup. The grip may become weak opening jars (and child-proof medicine bottles), hips may be weak getting out of deep chairs or the bathtub, and legs may tire climbing stairs or when walking distances.

The "gravis" or seriousness of myasthenia is particularly noticeable when muscles we use in breathing are affected. If breathing or coughing becomes insufficient, the patient is said to be in "crisis," and mechanical breathing assistance in a hospital may be necessary. It is seldom useful to try to determine whether the respiratory insufficiency is a "myasthenic crisis" (weakness from MG exacerbation) or a "cholinergic crisis" (weakness from too much anticholinesterase medication), because most crises have multiple causes and the treatment for any crisis is respiratory assistance. Patients with trouble swallowing and talking are the ones most likely to have trouble breathing also, and usually before a crisis happens there are progressive warning signs that swallowing, talking, and breathing are becoming compromised.

Different muscle groups are affected in different patients with MG. Some have only ocular myasthenia involving the eye muscles and eyelids, others have mainly swallowing difficulties or slurred speech; others have generalized MG affecting many muscle groups. Even though specific muscle fatigue is the hallmark of MG, patients with MG do not often complain of non-specific or general fatigue. Skin sensation is normal.

MG remains confined to the eye muscles in about 15 percent of patients who initially present with only ocular myasthenia. Within the first year after onset about half of the ocular MG patients will go on to experience involvement of other muscles, and another 30 percent do so during the next two years.

The maximum extent of involvement in an individual patient usually manifests itself within the first five to seven years, and thereafter it tends not to be progressive, even though muscle involvement and severity of weakness may still fluctuate from hour-to-hour and day-to-day. The typical untreated patient may feel strong on awakening from a night's rest or a nap, but experiences increasing muscle fatigue as the day progresses. Although MG can be fatal if a respiratory crisis is not immediately treated, normal life expectancy is the rule with proper treatment.

MG occurs throughout the world and in all ethnic groups. Its onset can occur at any age from birth to the ninth decade, although women usually notice it first in the child-bearing ages and men in middle-age. Rarely, infants born to non-myasthenic mothers have myasthenic symptoms on the basis of a genetic defect in neuromuscular transmission. These infants are said to have congenital myasthenia.

However, the vast majority of MG cases are autoimmune, in which the body's immune system mistakenly attacks and destroys special proteins located on the muscle surface where the nerve attaches to the muscle. These proteins respond to the chemical acetylcholine which is released by the stimulated nerve, and this response starts the process which causes the muscle to contract. These special proteins are called acetylcholine receptors.

No one knows what sets off the autoimmune reaction, but if some acetylcholine receptors are missing because of it, the response of the muscle to nerve impulses is poor and weakness may occur.

Twelve percent of babies born to mothers with autoimmune MG develop a feeble cry, poor sucking, respiratory distress and "floppiness" which can be reversed by anticholinesterase medication or blood exchange. These signs of neonatal myasthenia spontaneously disappear over the first few months of life, and no well-documented case exists of autoimmune MG occurring in a child of a mother with autoimmune MG.

Autoimmune diseases such as MG, thyroid disease, lupus, rheumatoid arthritis and juvenile diabetes seem to run in families, and these families statistically (but not invariably) share certain tissue markers. New and promising experimental treatments for autoimmune diseases are based upon the presence of such markers.

How Is the Diagnosis of MG Confirmed?

Weakness and fatigue are such common complaints from a variety of causes that it is not surprising that the diagnosis of myasthenia gravis is often missed in people in whom the weakness is mild or restricted to only a few muscles. Once the possibility occurs to a doctor, however, there are several approaches to confirming the diagnosis.

One way is to test for specific muscle fatigue by repetitive movements of the eyes, arms or legs. This can be done without equipment, or it can be done electrically by recording a weakening muscle response when a nerve to that muscle is electrically stimulated repetitively. Not every person with the disease will show a characteristic response to this repetitive nerve stimulation. A much more sensitive electrical test called single fiber electromyography is more likely to show evidence of neuromuscular malfunction (not specific for MG), but it requires special equipment and skills which are not widely available.

A very specific test for MG is a blood test to look for serum antibodies to acetylcholine receptor. Eighty percent of all patients with MG have abnormally elevated serum levels of these antibodies, but positive test results are less likely in patients with mild or purely ocular forms. The chance of receiving a falsely positive test result from a reputable laboratory is small, although borderline tests should be repeated.

A third approach to MG diagnosis is pharmacological, using drugs which may worsen or improve the weakness. At one time the native South American poison curare was used in very small doses to test for worsening of MG, but this can be dangerous and has fallen out of fashion. Nowadays the short-acting drug edrophonium chloride (brand-name "Tensilon") is used intravenously to try to make the diagnosis of MG by reversing some obvious and measurable weakness, such as a drooping eyelid or a low breathing capacity.

Sometimes all these tests are negative or equivocal in someone whose story and examination still seem to point to a diagnosis of myasthenia gravis. The positive clinical findings should probably take precedence over negative confirmatory tests, each of which has its weaknesses. Some people, therefore, have to be followed by their doctors with a diagnosis of "possible MG" or "probable MG" until the situation clarifies itself. Under such circumstances both the patient and the doctor have to keep an open mind.

How Is MG Treated?

A lot of common-sense things can be very effective in coping with MG. Plenty of rest and a well-balanced diet actually help reverse the weakness. Preference should be given to foods high in potassium, such as oranges, tomatoes, apricots and their juices, bananas, broccoli and white meat of fowl. If possible, one should try to avoid exposure to infections and all forms of stress, but of course that's easier said than done.

It is very important that patients try to pace their activities so that they don't fatigue themselves unnecessarily. This may mean resting the eyes by closing them for a few minutes each hour or lying down briefly several times during the day. Each patient is different and by experience can adopt a daily schedule which optimizes the good times and minimizes the weak times. Support groups of MG patients offer many practical ideas for coping with this condition.

Avoid Exacerbations

Many things can exacerbate myasthenic weakness temporarily, including infections (such as a cold, pneumonia, or even a tooth abscess), fever, excessive heat or cold, over-exertion, and emotional stress. Some women notice increasing severity of their MG during a particular time of the menstrual cycle, during pregnancy, or after delivery. Either too little or too much thyroid activity can worsen MG, as can too little potassium in the body, such as is brought on by diuretics or frequent vomiting. The stress of surgery or radiation therapy can make MG temporarily worse.

The effect of pregnancy on MG follows the "one-third rule": One-third of pregnant myasthenics get better and one-third get worse at some time during their pregnancy, while one-third do not change. The course of MG during previous pregnancies does not predict the course of subsequent pregnancies. MG frequently manifests itself for the first time during a pregnancy. Standard drugs used to treat MG such as anticholinesterase medications or prednisone (see below) are not associated with significant risk for congenital defects, and plasmapheresis (see below) has been carried out safely during pregnancy. Obstetrical problems with myasthenics are uncommon because the uterus, a smooth muscle, is unaffected in myasthenia. Only during the second stage of labor when voluntary "striated" abdominal muscles are used does myasthenic weakness become noticeable. Even many non-myasthenic woman notice increased weakness after delivery, and this may be exaggerated in MG.

People with MG should make sure that their doctors and dentist are aware that many drugs can adversely affect some people with MG. The most common offenders are the very medications used to treat MG (too much anticholinesterase, steroids, or thyroid medication; see below), but anesthetic agents, muscle relaxants, magnesium salts, anticonvulsants and other membrane stabilizers for irregular heart rate, as well as amino glycoside antibiotics, are other drugs generally accepted to unmask or exacerbate MG. Table 26.1 includes drugs which have been reported in medical journals to cause weakness in humans.

Common sense dictates that sometimes an irregular heart beat, for instance, or a severe infection sensitive only to one of the antibiotics on the list will take precedence over the MG, and one of these drugs will have to be used, cautiously. A medical alert bracelet can alert medical personnel to use drug precautions in case of an accident or crisis.

Short-term Treatments

In addition to the above common-sense approaches towards improving health and avoiding trouble, there are some well-known medications and newer treatments which can be tried to counteract the bothersome symptoms of MG.

Anticholinesterases. Anticholinesterases, which boost the body's neuromuscular transmitter acetylcholine by blocking the enzyme which usually breaks it down, include neostigmine (brand-name "Prostigmin") and pyridostigmine (brand-name "Mestinon"). Another drug in this category, ambenonium chloride (brand-name "Mytelase"), is used much less frequently. These medicines don't do anything to cure MG, but they can provide a temporary crutch to help patients function better. Some muscles may improve for a few hours while others may be unresponsive or even get weaker on these medications.

Because muscle involvement and severity vary so much among patients with MG, there is no fixed dose or time schedule for anticholinesterases. For infants and children the dose is based on body weight, starting at one milligram per kilogram for "Mestinon" and 0.3 milligrams per kilogram for "Prostigmin." Generally it is a good idea to try to keep the adult dose somewhere between 1/2 and 2 of the 60 milligram tablets of "Mestinon" or a similar amount of the 15 milligram tablets of "Prostigmin," and to take the medication no closer than every three hours, always keeping on the low side to avoid tolerance (the drug may become less effective with time) or overdosing. These medications produce their maximal effects (good and bad) about one to two hours after ingestion, and these effects wear off after about three hours or sometimes longer. Therefore, patients who have trouble chewing or swallowing are advised to take their medication at a time which will produce optimal strength during meals.

These medicines can cause stomach cramps and gut hyperactivity, so they should be taken with bland food such as crackers or milk to minimize these problems. Increased perspiration, salivation, muscle twitching and muscle cramps are other unpleasant side effects some-times experienced with this type of medication. The presence of these symptoms may be an indication of taking too much medication, in which case Mestinon should be taken at longer intervals or in lesser amounts. "Mestinon" also comes as an 180 milligram "Mestinon Timespan" in which 60 milligrams is released immediately and the remaining 120 milligrams are released over several hours. Timespan is used for patients who require medication throughout the night, but the uneven release by Mestinon Timespan provides less predictable results than with ordinary Mestinon. There is also a liquid " Mestinon" syrup for children and adults who have trouble swallowing pills.

Ephedrine Sulfate. Historically, the drug ephedrine sulfate was discovered to improve myasthenic weakness a decade before the use of anticholinesterases, and it may still come in handy as an auxiliary medication, added to anticholinesterases, for those MG patients who need a little extra strength and are not bothered by its possible side effects of nervousness, palpitations or insomnia. It is taken as 25 milligram capsules two or three times a day.

Plasmapheresis (the drawing off of plasma) is an expensive short-term treatment in which several liters of blood are removed from the patient's vein, spun in a centrifuge, and the red blood cells are re-turned intravenously in artificial plasma (albumin and saline solu-tion). Plasmapheresis is used repetitively (every other day) for two weeks when short-term benefit is critical to the patient, such as in impending respiratory crisis or prior to surgery or irradiation. Some patients get stronger several days following this procedure, but the benefit lasts only weeks.

Intravenous Human Immune Globulin (IVIG). Another expen-sive short-term treatment, intravenous human immune globulin or IVIG, may be thought of as the opposite of plasmapheresis. Instead of drawing off the offending antibodies, IVIG swamps the body with pooled gamma globulin antibodies from many donors. HIV and hepa-titis viruses are removed completely during the preparation of MG. IVIG is thought to have a nonspecific suppressive effect upon the immune system. Like plasmapheresis, the beneficial effects if they occur last only weeks in MG patients. Therefore, its appropriate use at the present time is to avoid or curtail a stay in the even more ex-pensive intensive care unit of a hospital. Allergic reactions sometimes occur, so the first treatment should be given in a hospital or doctor's office. Plenty of fluids should accompany the treatments to minimize the severe headache which can occur.

Long-term Treatments

Usually the short-term treatments above do not completely relieve the symptoms of MG even temporarily, and eventually the patient with more than just mild disease must discuss with her/his doctor the controversial aspects of what to do next to attempt to obtain a long-term remission. This is especially true for patients with serious trouble swallowing or breathing, for whom long-term treatments may protect against rapid deterioration of these functions.

One approach is to do nothing more, and hope to be one of up to 20 percent of MG patients who go into a natural, spontaneous remission which lasts longer than one year. No one knows why MG fluctuates or why natural remissions occur.

Without spontaneous remission, the patient seeking more lasting improvement of generalized MG is faced with two choices:

- Major thoracic surgery (thymectomy), or
- Potentially dangerous drugs.

Each approach has advantages and disadvantages.

Thymectomy

About 15 percent of patients with MG are found by chest x-ray, computed tomography (CT), or magnetic resonance imaging (MRI) of the chest to have a tumor of the thymus gland called a thymoma. Although most thymomas are benign, they are usually removed surgically because of a perceived potential for malignancy. This has led to thymectomy as well for MG patients without thymoma. If most of the thymus gland is removed at surgery, myasthenic symptoms usually lessen and in some individuals go away completely.

The thymus gland is an organ involved in the development of the immune system. It migrates from the neck into the chest during formation of the fetus, and in adults it lies beneath the breastbone (sternum). Like tonsils and adenoids, the thymus is large in infants and gets smaller, to be replaced by fat, as we get older. The thymus gland is not enlarged in patients with myasthenia, but often under the microscope it contains more cells than normal (the pathology term is "hyperplasia"), especially if myasthenia has been present several years.

Some neurologists do not think thymectomy adds to other treatments for MG, but most neurologists recommend it for some patients. In the past, thymectomy was not performed on patients who were over 25 years old (or, more recently, over 45 years old), nor was it offered to MG patients who have had their disease for more than five years. Yet some older patients and some long-standing MG patients have benefited from thymectomy, so now the recommendation for this procedure has to be considered on an individual basis.

Another question regarding thymectomy is, "Which surgical technique is best"? Most surgeons split the breastbone in a transsternal thymectomy, but a few surgical groups have championed a less traumatic approach through the neck, called a transcervical thymectomy. A patient who wants to shop around the country can find practically any surgical gradation between these two techniques, or even (at Columbia University in New York City) both a transsternal and a transcervical thymectomy on the same MG patient.

The results of this double approach are good, but so far not really better than a careful removal of all discernible thymic tissue through a transsternal approach. About 30 percent of MG patients without a thymoma who undergo thymectomy eventually go into complete drug-free remission and another 50 percent experience marked improvement. This improvement usually does not occur immediately after surgery, but may take up to several months or years to reach its peak effect. We are unable to predict beforehand who will benefit from thymectomy, and even after benefit occurs there is still a small possibility of subsequent relapse. However, thymectomy itself rarely worsens the long-term course of MG.

Even invasive thymomas are not always detected with imaging tests and have been discovered serendipitously during thymectomy surgery. Such experiences would argue in favor of eventual thymectomy over immunosuppressive drug therapy in otherwise healthy young or middle-aged MG patients, once the patient is up to the surgery. The possibility of an eventually complete symptom-free remission after thymectomy without the need to take any drugs, compared to a remission dependent upon the continued treatment with immunosuppressive drugs, is another significant advantage of thymectomy.

Immunosuppressive Drug Therapy

These drug alternatives consist of a group of general suppressants of the body's immune system, although no one really knows how they work in MG. In decreasing order of their frequency of use in MG, they are prednisone, azathioprine ("Imuran"), cyclophosphamide ("Cytoxan") and cyclosporine ("Sandimmune"). Except for prednisone, none of these drugs is endorsed by its manufacturer specifically for treatment of MG.

Prednisone. Prednisone is a synthetic drug taken by mouth which resembles natural hormones produced by the cortex of human adrenal glands. The body depends upon these hormones, called corticosteroids or "steroids," during stress. When prednisone is taken in doses higher that 20 milligrams daily for longer than a week, the body's natural production of adrenal hormones begins to decrease. This is called "adrenal suppression," and is an undesirable but inevitable effect of taking high doses of a synthetic steroid. Once this occurs, prednisone cannot be stopped all at once but must be slowly tapered down over several months to give the adrenal glands a chance to "wake up" and begin producing natural adrenal hormones again.

Prednisone has a great many potential undesirable effects, usually related to dose and duration of drug use. It can cause mood changes, weight gain, decreased resistance to infection, increased susceptibility to diabetes, high blood pressure, osteoporosis, glaucoma, lens cataracts and stomach ulcers, as well as a host of uncommon "side" effects. Unique to MG is the possibility of increasing weakness during the first two weeks of prednisone therapy. This necessitates close medical supervision of MG patients when prednisone is instituted, either on an out-patient or in-hospital basis.

Some physicians try to avoid this initial weakening by starting with a low dose of prednisone and gradually working up to a recommended amount of 50 to 60 milligrams every day for several months. Onset of improvement in muscle strength usually occurs within 2 weeks but may take as long as 2 months. In order to lessen the chance of undesirable effects, a gradual transition to alternate-day therapy is made after about two months of daily therapy, so that eventually twice the usual dose is given every other day for several more months. As soon as is feasible (3 to 12 months), the drug is very slowly tapered over many months to a long-term maintenance dosage (ideally, 5 to 10 milligrams every other day) sufficient enough to keep myasthenic symptoms in abeyance. The choice of prednisone therapy is thus a long-term commitment lasting several years.

Thirty percent of MG patients on high-dose prednisone therapy experience a drug-dependent symptom-free remission, and another 50 percent obtain marked improvement on prednisone. One out of four MG patients also experiences serious complications from this drug. Patients on prednisone should watch their weight, keep as active as possible, eat a balanced diet (high in protein, calcium and potassium but low in salt, free sugar and fat), stay out of crowds in enclosed areas in order to avoid people with infections, and see their physicians regularly.

Azathioprine. Azathioprine (brand-name Imuran) was used to treat MG in Europe for years, but U S. experience is relatively recent, since it was introduced as an accompaniment to plasmapheresis. It is being used mainly for patients who cannot tolerate or do not respond to prednisone, or as an aid to decreasing the dosage of prednisone which a patient requires. The undesirable effects of azathioprine are less varied than those of prednisone but they can be very serious. Young women who may want to have children should avoid this drug, because it has a known potential for producing fetal deformities. Complete blood counts must be obtained periodically at the beginning of azathioprine therapy to detect rapid drops in the number of white and red cells in the blood, and periodic liver function tests must also be obtained to detect potential toxicity to the liver. Sometimes a systemic reaction occurs in the first few weeks of azathioprine therapy, consisting of fever, nausea, vomiting, loss of appetite, and abdominal pain. The drug must then be discontinued.

While most of the undesirable effects of azathioprine make themselves known early on, the beneficial effects seem to take months to occur and often emerge so slowly and subtly that they are apparent only in retrospect. Remissions which occur on azathioprine, like prednisone, are drug-dependent, and symptoms of MG recur when the drug is discontinued. There is still much to learn about azathioprine, including answers to such worrisome questions as whether it may increase the risk for cancer many years later.

Cyclophosphamide. Cyclophosphamide (brand-name Cytoxan) is considered only for the most severe cases of MG when other therapies have failed. Hair loss is an almost universal occurrence on the drug, and the risk of bladder hemorrhage and bladder cancer are of great concern. However, experience from the Philippines reported complete drug-free remission for a year and a half in three out of four MG patients who were treated with cyclophosphamide. Experimental regimens in which cyclophosphamide is given intravenously or orally once a week—instead of daily—may reduce the occurrence of adverse effects. This drug usually requires the assistance of a rheumatologist or oncologist who is more familiar with it than are most neurologists.

Cyclosporine. Cyclosporine (brand-name Sandimmune) has recently been tested in clinical trials at one-third the dose which is used for immunosuppression during organ transplantation. It was tested for its potential ability to allow MG patients on prednisone to take less prednisone (a "steroid-sparing" effect). The results of this study are not yet available, although a preliminary study without prednisone suggested that such a dose of cyclosporine could produce significant improvement in some MG patients if they could tolerate the side effects of this medication, the most prominent of which are elevated blood pressure, headaches, and increased body hair.

Although cyclosporine is currently the gold standard for evaluating several new immunosuppressive agents, current pharmacologic approaches to nonspecific immune suppression of MG leave much to be desired. It is hoped that future treatment strategies will employ more specific regulation of immunity focused on selected molecules or cells, approaches which are at present experimental.

There is still much to learn about myasthenia gravis, its diagnosis and its treatment. There is no one recipe for all situations, so the choice of treatment for an individual patient requires judgment and experience. Patients and their doctors are often required to make decisions even when the evidence is inconclusive. Patients need all the support which doctors, family and friends can offer.

Acknowledgments: Special thanks are due to the Director of Pharmacy, Horace B. Williams, Jr., Ph.D., and the Assistant Director of Pharmacy, Donald J. DeFazio, Pharm.D., at Methodist Hospital of Southern California, Arcadia, California, for their assistance with the Table of Drugs Which Affect Myasthenia.

—by John C. Keesey, M.D. and Rena Sonshine.

A. Drugs generally accepted to unmask or exacerbate MG:

Excessive anticholinesterases	Neuromuscular blocking agents (including botox)
Adrenocorticosteroids &ACTH	Anesthetic agents (including alcohol)
Thyroid preparations	Magnesium salts, Epsom salts

Antiarrhythmics:
- lidocaine (Xylocaine) intravenously but not locally
- quinidine (Quinaglute, Quinidex, Quinora, Cardioquin)
- procainamide (Procamide, Procan SR, Pronestyl)
- phenytoin (Dilantin)

Antibiotics

Aminoglycosides
- gentamicin (Garamycin)
- tobramycin (Nebcin)
- amikacin (Amikin)
- kanamycin (Kantrex)
- neomycin (Mycifradin, Neobiotic)
- streptomycin
- paromomycin (Humatin)

Polypeptides
- polymyxin B (Aerosporin)
- colistin (Coly-Mycin, Mycin)
- colistimethate (parenteral Coly-Mycin)

Tetracyclines
- chlortetracycline (Aureomycin)
- oxytetracycline(Terramycin)
- tetracycline (Achromycin, Tetracyn)
- demeclocycline (Declomycin)
- methacycline (Rondomycin)
- doxycycline (Vibramycin, Doryx)
- minocycline (Minocin, Vectrin)

Miscellaneous
- clindamycin (Cleocin)
- ciprofloxacin (Cipro)
- ampicillin—very high doses
- intravenous erythromycin (E-Mycin, Erythrocin)

B. Drugs or toxins which can induce MG by precipitating an autoimmune reaction:
- D-penicillamine (Cuprimine)
- trimethadione (Tridione)
- wasp stings
- coral snake bite

C. Other drugs implicated in isolated instances of MG exacerbations (Not every patient with MG is expected to react adversely to these medications):

cimetidine (Tagamet)	meglumide diatrizoate (Reno-M-dip)
citrate	propanolol (Inderal)
chloroquine (Aralen, Avloclor, Rosochin)	quinine
cocaine	timolol maleate drops (Timoptic)
diazepam (Valium)	trihexyphenidyl (Artane)
lithium (Lithotabs, Eskalith, Lithane)	

Table 26.1.

Chapter 27

Get Hooked on Seafood Safety: Important Health Information for People with Immune Disorders

Protect Yourself: Only Eat Fish That's Been Thoroughly Cooked

This chapter is to inform people with immune disorders of the hazards they face if they eat raw molluscan shellfish like oysters, mussels, clams, and whole scallops. It also contains useful information about safe handling and consumption of seafood in general.

Fish—fin fish and shellfish—have many of the qualities that health-conscious food shoppers look for. They are generally low in saturated fat and are excellent sources of protein, vitamins, and minerals, although nutrition values differ depending on the type. Properly handled and thoroughly cooked, fish is tender, easy to digest, and safe to eat.

But sometimes shellfish, especially mollusks—oysters, clams, mussels, and whole scallops—area eaten raw, as in oysters-on-the-halfshelf. Eating raw or undercooked shellfish can be a serious problem for persons with:

- liver disease, including cirrhosis, hemochromatosis, and chronic alcohol use
- diabetes mellitus
- immune disorder, including AIDS, cancer, and reduced immunity due to steroid or immunosuppressant therapy

DHHS Pub No. (FDA) 92-2261.

- gastrointestinal disorders, including previous gastric surgery, and low gastric acid (for example, from antacid use or achlorhydria).

The problem occurs because raw mollusks sometimes carry bacteria called *Vibrio vulnificus* that may multiply after the shellfish are caught, even with refrigeration. **These bacteria are completely killed when the shellfish are thoroughly cooked, removing all danger of bacteria causing food poisoning.**

But if mollusks are eaten raw or partially cooked, the bacteria remain alive and may make you very sick. Symptoms include sudden chills, fever, nausea, vomiting, and stomach pain. ***Vibrio vulnificus*** **can cause blood poisoning, a condition that could be fatal in up to half the people who get it.** Death usually occurs within two days.

Certain viruses known as Norwalk viruses also could contaminate oysters, clams, and mussels and cause severe diarrhea in those who eat them. Here again, thorough cooking kills the virus.

How Do Mollusks Get Contaminated?

Mollusks usually live where rivers and seas meet. Because many cities are located near those places, the waters are more likely to be polluted than offshore waters. For this reason, shellfish harvesting is prohibited in areas contaminated by sewage. To enforce this, these areas are patrolled by state health and fishery agencies.

Mollusks feed by filtering water through their systems, so they are more likely to pick up and store bacteria or viruses from the water, including those that can cause illness in humans. If you eat mollusks raw, you eat the live viruses and bacteria too.

Another source of contamination of shellfish can come from naturally occurring algae blooms called "Red Tides." Waters are closely monitored for these blooms to prevent shellfish poisoning in humans. The Food and Drug Administration and the coastal states all test for these blooms, and when they appear, the waters are closed to all fishing.

Is Raw Fin Fish Safe to Eat?

Raw fish dishes, such as sushi and sashimi, can be safe for most people to eat if they are made with very fresh fish, commercially frozen (at temperatures lower than in home freezers), and then thawed before they're eaten. This kills any parasites that may be present.

Parasites are also killed by thorough cooking, and, once killed, they are no longer a danger to you. But people with immune disorders should not eat raw fin fish because freezing does not kill bacteria. **Persons with immune disorders need to take extra precautions to thoroughly cook all fish.**

Seafood Safety Tips

Shopping

* Fresh seafood should not smell unpleasantly "fishy." It should smell like a "fresh ocean breeze."

* Fresh fish steaks and fillets should be moist, with no drying or browning around the edges. The eyes of the fresh whole fish should be bright and clear, not cloudy or sunken. Scales should not be "slimy" and should cling tightly to the skin. Gills should be bright pink or red. Frozen fish should not be freezer burned or have damaged packaging.

* **Mollusks in the shell should always be alive when you buy them.** When a clam, oyster, mussel, or scallop is alive, the shells will be tightly closed or will close when tapped lightly or iced. A test for freshness is to hold the shell between your thumb and forefinger and press as though sliding the two parts of the shell across one another. If the shells move, the shellfish is not fresh. Throw away any that do not close tightly.

* **Buy seafood only from reputable dealers.** You can't know what you're buying from the back of a pickup truck. It could have been caught by someone not subject to FDA or state inspection.

* Ask to see the shipper's tag for molluscan shellfish which will show the harvest date and location and certificate number.

* Cook fish no later than two days after purchase.

Storing

- Keep fresh fish cold—in the coldest part of your refrigerator, usually under the freezer or in the meat drawer, until it's ready to cook and serve.

- Store fresh fish in your refrigerator in the same wrapper it had in the store.

- Store live mollusks in your refrigerator in containers covered loosely with a clean, damp cloth. Do not store live shellfish in airtight containers or in water.

- Canned fish should be refrigerated after opening.

- Smoked fish, pickled fish, vacuum-packed fish, and modified-at-mosphere-packed fish products should always be refrigerated.

- **Keep cooked and raw seafood separate.** It's not safe to put cooked seafood back in the original container used for raw seafood, or to store raw and cooked seafood together.

Cooking

- The safest way to thaw frozen seafood is in the refrigerator in its own container. Allow about one day for defrosting.

- For fin fish (baked, broiled, poached, fried, or stewed): allow 10 minutes cooking time for each inch of thickness. Turn fish over halfway through the cooking time unless it is less than a half-inch thick. Add 5 minutes to the total cooking time if the fish is wrapped in foil or cooked in a sauce. **Properly cooked fish will flake easily with a fork and should be opaque and firm. It should not be translucent.**

For molluscan shellfish:

- **Boiled**—shells will open during boiling. After shells open, boiling should continue for 3 to 5 more minutes.

- **Steamed**—cook 4 to 9 minutes from the start of steaming. Use small pots to boil or steam shellfish. If too many shells are cooking in the same pot, it's possible that the ones in the middle won't get thoroughly cooked. **Discard any clams, mussels, or oysters that do not open during the cooking.** Closed shells may mean they have not received adequate heat.

- **Shucked oysters**—Boil or simmer for at least 3 minutes. Fry in oil for at least 10 minutes at 375 degrees Fahrenheit. Bake for at least 10 minutes at 450 degrees Fahrenheit.

Following these steps for buying, storing, and cooking will protect you and still allow you to enjoy seafood.

Danger Zone

Keep cold seafood cold: 40 degrees F. and below.

Keep hot seafood hot: 140 degrees F. or above.

Avoid the Danger Zone.

Part Four

Neuroimmunology: Immunity and the Nervous System

Chapter 28

The Brain and Immunity

"We're going to see a lot of commonalities between these two systems." —Michael B. Prystowsky.

The notion that the mind can affect overall health is not new. Ancient Eastern writings, particularly from India, espouse a healthy mind to keep the body robust. Nearly two millennia ago, Galen, a Greek physician, wrote that melancholy women are more susceptible to breast cancer than are cheerful women. A number of modern investigators have reported that positive mental attitude improves survival rates in cancer patients.

The scientific literature is filled with both anecdotal and concrete evidence that the mind has a powerful influence on the body. Stresses of all kinds—mental and physical—can reduce the body's ability to fight disease, yet a positive outlook can help patients battle even the most serious illnesses, including acquired immune deficiency syndrome (AIDS) and cancer.

This connection between the mental and the physical works both ways. Infection in the body has well-known effects on behavior and mental state. Everyone is familiar with the lethargy, gloom, and irritability that accompany a cold or flu. Patients infected with the human immunodeficiency virus (HIV) often show subtle behavioral changes before any other symptoms appear. As they develop full-blown AIDS, subtle behavioral problems often turn into debilitating dementia.

NIH Pub No. 94-3774.

Today, spurred on in part by the tragedy of AIDS and also by the progress made on a number of scientific fronts, researchers from a wide variety of disciplines are giving new meaning to the old adage, "Laughter is the best medicine."

A Multidisciplinary Field of Study

Neuroscientists and immunologists, along with molecular biologists, virologists, epidemiologists, developmental biologists, and others, are uncovering the myriad connections between our mental and physical states. Armed with a host of new biochemical, genetic, immunological, and imaging tools developed over the last two decades, these researchers are pushing the boundaries of psychoneuroimmunology—the study of the interrelationships among behavior, the nervous system, and the immune system.

Heretofore, researchers have focused on individual systems in the body, seeing them as distinct, self-contained, and self-regulated entities. Now, they are finding that the nervous and immune systems have much more in common than previously thought, work together efficiently, and are in constant communication with each other (See figure 28.1). Psychoneuroimmunology focuses on this integrated, interacting whole.

Investigators in this relatively new field are struggling with the ever-present problem of having to conduct most of their experiments on bits and pieces—cells and molecules—or on specially bred animals. *In vitro* studies involve isolating a type of cell, gene, molecule, or other entity, placing it in an artificial environment, and watching how it reacts under a variety of exposures and conditions. These findings then have to be related to the much more complex human body. For example, new chemical mediators are being discovered in the laboratory that appear to play important roles in activating both the immune system and the nervous system. Now investigators must determine if these substance perform the same way *in vivo*—in the body—where they may be parts of several complicated systems and interact with numerous other chemicals. Psychoneuroimmunologists happily embrace such challenges, for this type of intellectual obstacle drives science forward.

Three Interacting Components

To appreciate the interrelationships among behavior, the nervous system, and the immune system requires some understanding of each entity alone. Their differences in structure and apparent function make it easy to see why they were studied independently for so long.

Behavior

Thought and behavior still mystify us. The connection between intelligence, emotion, and the body is so elusive that separate concepts are used—an ephemeral thing called the mind and a concrete, physical thing called the brain. Whether the mind controls the brain or vice versa is beyond the scope of this report.

Behavior arises from both internal and external cues. For example, individuals may be so engrossed in thinking about something that nothing disturbs their train of thought, or so distracted by whatever is going on around them that they cannot think clearly. Emotions may be so strong as to seem out of control.

Extreme disorders in thought and mood are labeled mental illness, and some success in treating them has been attained through the body by giving the patient various chemical substances. Some depressions have been controlled by light therapy.

Some mental and emotional distress is alleviated by the presence of caring people. Loving caregivers and support groups made up of people sharing the same problem have brought noticeable improvement in many mental and physical conditions. Sometimes, simply the presence or absence of family or friends is the determining factor.

Things that impinge upon a person's present mental or emotional state are lumped together under the generic term "stress." These can be positive or negative events and can arise from within the person or come from the environment. The effects of stress depend on the nature of the stress and its duration. Being startled by something that turns out to be non-threatening will have little or no impact, while facing an ongoing, serious threat for an appreciable time can be quite deleterious.

On the other hand, positive stress, such as preparing for a happy event like a wedding, can have positive effects on mental and emotional well-being. Athletes under the stress of competing in an important, major event can become so incredibly focused that play seems automatic, and they perform better and more effectively than ever before (or since) in their lives.

Several approaches have been used to alleviate the effects of longstanding negative stress. These include prescribing drugs such as tranquilizers, teaching relaxation techniques, and providing group psychotherapy.

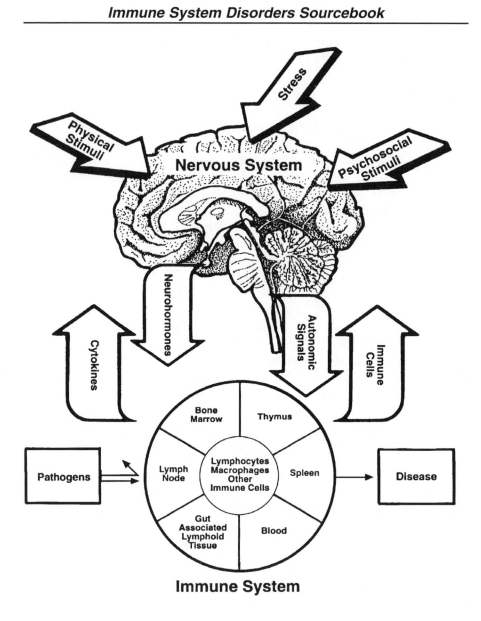

Figure 28.1. *Bidirectional communication between the nervous and immune systems. Some organs comprising the two systems interact to ward off pathogens and prevent disease while the organism is responding to external stimuli. The unimaginable complexity of the interactions is being slowly but surely unravelled at the cellular and molecular levels. [After D. Felten.]*

The Nervous System

The brain, spinal cord, and peripheral nerves—those branching out from the spinal cord to various tissues and organs—are the chief components of the nervous system. Part of the peripheral nervous system, called the autonomic system, controls the internal organs. The peripheral system relays commands from the central nervous system—the brain and spinal cord—to the rest of the body and conveys information about the body and the external world to the brain. While cells in the central nervous system also perform such communications functions, they have integrative and analytic abilities that cells in the peripheral nervous system lack.

The two main classes of cells in the nervous system are neurons and glia. Neurons send and process information in the form of electrical and chemical signals. Glia have a host of support functions. During development, far more neurons are produced than are needed in the mature brain, and about 40 percent of them die. Many theories have been put forth for this normal neuronal death, but neuroscientists still do not fully understand the reasons behind this overproduction.

Neurons

A neuron consists of a cell body, containing the nucleus and metabolic apparatus, and long extensions, much like the branches of a tree, called dendrites. Also projecting out of the cell body is a single fiber called an axon, which can be three or more feet long in humans and has many terminals branching from its end. Information, in the form of an electrical pulse, comes into the nerve cell via the dendrites and goes out from the cell through the axon, which passes that signal to the dendrites of neighboring neurons. Large axons are surrounded by a fatty sheath of myelin, which acts as an insulator.

Neighboring neurons do not actually touch but are separated by a thin gap known as the synaptic cleft. Electrical signals cannot cross this gap, so the neuron releases a chemical, called a neurotransmitter, from a terminal at the end of the axon. Neurotransmitters diffuse across the synapse and attach themselves, or bind, to sites (receptors) on the neighboring dendrites that will accept only that specific type of chemical. This binding triggers a chain reaction within the dendrite that produces an electrical signal that moves up the dendrite to the body of the neuron.

Other compounds, known as neuropeptides and neuromodulators, are also released from terminals of the axon. These substances modulate or attenuate the effects of the primary neurotransmitter active at a particular synapse. Once the signal has been passed, the neurotransmitter is taken up by the dendritic nerve terminal, while neuropeptides and neuromodulators are cleared from the synaptic cleft by neighboring glia.

Glia

The central nervous system has between 10 and 50 times more glial cells than neurons. Glia are smaller than neurons and do not generate electrical signals. Like neurons, however, they secrete a host of chemicals that trigger actions by other cells. Some of these chemicals may prove to be critical links between neurons and the immune system. Most glia provide structural support for neurons, a scaffolding upon which neurons grow and make connections with one another.

Glial cells come in several forms, and the functions of many of them are yet to be discovered. Astrocytes, oligodendrocytes, and ependymal cells are large cells known collectively as macroglia. One known function of oligodendrocytes is to form the myelin sheath insulating axons. Astrocytes absorb toxic substances in the fluid surrounding neurons and produce biochemicals, such as neurotransmitters, that enable the neuron to function (See Figure 28.2). They are the most important regulators of homeostasis in the brain. Astrocytes are capable of displaying various phenotypes when examined in isolation, but their precise phenotypes in the living body are unknown.

Microglia include a variety of cells capable of engulfing and digesting cellular debris after injury, infection, or disease. These cells are also capable of moving through the brain under certain circumstances.

The Immune System

The immune system is made up of cells and molecules whose main function is to distinguish the body (self) from foreign matter (non-self) and to defend against foreign organisms or substances. The lymphoid system, including the spleen, thymus, and bone marrow, plays an important role in the development of immune system cells (lymphocytes), and these cells produce many of the molecules that detect and respond to invaders. Lymphocytes may further develop into helper cells, suppressor cells, or killer cells.

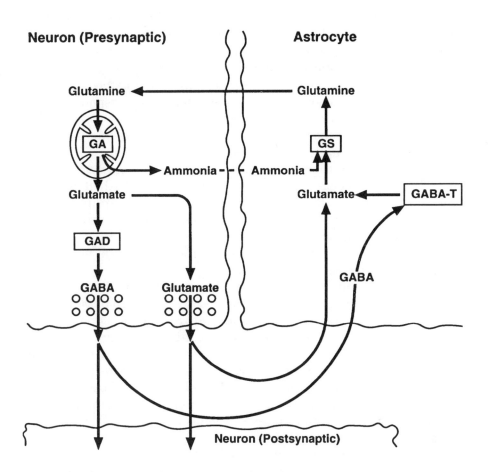

Figure 28.2. How astrocytes facilitate neuronal functioning. Astrocytes synthesize glutamine using ammonia, a toxic substance, in the brain. Ammonia is removed from the body by biochemical reactions called the urea cycle, which does not operate in brain. Glutamine is taken up by neurons and converted into glutamate, a major excitatory neurotransmitter. Glutamate is then used either for neurotransmission or converted into gamma-aminobutyric acid (GABA), an inhibitory neurotransmitter. Excess neurotransmitter molecules, if present in the synaptic cleft, are "mopped up" by astrocytes. Enzymes catalyzing these reactions are compartmentalized between astrocytes and neurons. They are glutamine synthetase (GS), glutaminase (GA), glutamate decarboxylase (GAD), and GABA transaminase (GABA-T).

On occasion, the mechanisms that control the ability to discriminate between self and non-self fail; immune tolerance (nonreaction) is lost, and the immune system attacks the body's own tissues. This failure is known as autoimmune disease. In addition, damage to healthy tissue can occur in the normal process of eliminating pathogens.

When the immune system detects non-self, it can respond in a variety of ways. The complement reaction, for example, consists of a complex series of biochemical steps (a cascade) involving a number of molecules circulating in the blood and recently detected in brain tissue that among other things poke holes in an offending cell and kill it. Large phagocytes (cells that engulf and digest) called macrophages migrate to the site of an infection or injury and capture the material that requires elimination. Complement proteins and macrophages, along with other cells called neutrophils and monocytes (the precursors of macrophages), are components of the nonspecific immune response (see figure 28.3).

The humoral immune response is characterized by the production of molecules called antibodies. Antibodies are produced by cells called B-lymphocytes that are formed and matured in the bone marrow. These cells usually react when they encounter particular molecules, called antigens, on the surface of invading bacteria and viruses. Each B-lymphocyte and its offspring recognizes and responds to one type of antigen by producing antibodies that bind to, or neutralize, that antigen. The antigen-antibody reaction triggers other immune system cell activity that culminates in the destruction of the cell or organism containing the antigen.

Cell-mediated immunity is carried out by immune cells called T-lymphocytes that start out as progenitor cells in the bone marrow and mature in the thymus. T-lymphocytes act against viral and fungal infections, reject grafts of foreign tissue, and fight malignancies. T-lymphocytes themselves, along with all the other cells of the immune system, produce a variety of biologically active substances known as cytokines, which include interferons and interleukins.

Key players in both humoral and cell-mediated immunity are the members of the major histocompatibility complex (MHC) of gene products. These large molecules—proteins with attached sugars—are found on the surfaces of many types of cells and play a role in signaling B-lymphocytes and T-lymphocytes. There are two classes of MHC molecules. MHC Class I molecules are found on virtually all cells in the body, though there is still some question as to how widespread they are in the central nervous system. These molecules help T-lymphocytes recognize cells infected by a virus. MHC class-II molecules are confined largely to immune system cells and play a critical role in the recognition of foreign antigens by both B-lymphocytes and T-lymphocytes.

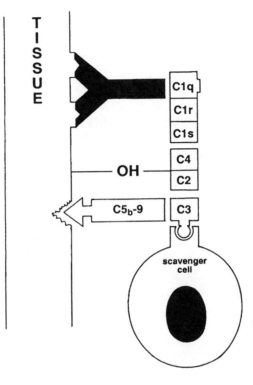

Figure 28.3. Schematic diagram of various interactions between diseased tissue components and complement proteins. The first interaction is mediated by an antibody molecule (in black) binding to an antigen in the tissue, and complement proteins C1q, C1r, and C1s (top). The second interaction is between -OH groups on proteins in the tissue and the complement proteins C2 and C4 (middle). The third interaction is between the membrane of a cell comprising the tissue and complement proteins $C5_b$-9, called "membrane attack complex" (bottom). Activation fragments of C3 serve as chemotactic signals for a scavenger cell, such as a macrophage, microglial cell, or possibly an astrocyte, to approach diseased tissue and remove the damaged parts. Complement proteins may mistakenly facilitate healthy brain tissue destruction (arrow). [Courtesy J. Rogers.]

Two Systems With Many Similarities

It is a common observation that nature is redundant: what works in one situation, whether it be a behavior or a chemical reaction, is often used with only slight modification in another situation. Nowhere is this more true than in the nervous and the immune systems. Certainly, the brain is unlike the thymus or bone marrow, and neurons and glia differ in many significant ways from lymphocytes and macrophages. Nevertheless, both systems engage in a constant survey of the local environment—internal and external—and both analyze and respond to constantly changing conditions.

Moreover, research is continually turning up ways in which these two systems are more similar than different, at both the cellular and molecular levels. For example, these are the only two systems endowed with the ability to "remember" and "learn" from their experience and then modify their "behavior" based on past exposure.

Cells With Similar Functions

In the nervous system, neurons may be the main actors, but they do very little without the support of glia. Similarly, T- and B-lymphocytes are in many respects the cornerstone cells in the immune system, yet they could not function without the support of macrophages.

The similarities go beyond this simple analogy. Until recently, microglia were largely a mystery, but now there is increasing evidence that these normally quiescent cells likely play the same role in the brain that macrophages play outside the central nervous system: scavenging cellular debris. When neurons are damaged, during infection or following physical trauma such as stroke, microglia appear to interpose themselves between synaptic processes and the neuron cell body. There, they clear the site of cellular fragments by the same process that macrophages use, while also releasing cytokines such as interleukin-1, which may stimulate a variety of actions within both the brain and the immune system.

Shared Molecules

Interleukin-1 is just one example of a molecule used by both the nervous system and the immune system. In fact, many scientists now argue that neurotransmitters, the molecules used by nerve cells to communicate with one another, and cytokines, the molecules used by immune cells to communicate with one another, are all part of a complex, but unified, system of chemical communication.

Cytokines and neuropeptides, for example, both bind to specific receptors thought to be on only one kind of cellular surface. But research has also found neuropeptide receptors on the surfaces of lymphocytes and other immune cells, while neurons and glia have cytokine receptors.

This is not to say that these molecules and receptors have identical functions, but it does suggest that they may share common chemical pathways, extending perhaps to the level of gene expression, that ultimately produce a tissue- or cell-specific response appropriate for a particular environment. Examining these possibilities could lead to a unified theory of biological signaling, which could have profound implications for treating infection, inflammation, tumor development, mental illness, and other immunological and neurobehavioral problems.

MHC molecules, key players in the immune system, are found in the nervous system on microglial and perivascular cells. In some areas of fully developed pathology, a few astrocytes may express MHC molecules. Only recently, researchers have discovered one of the latest in a group of genes that are activated in both T-lymphocytes and neurons exposed to cytokines. This gene, named F5, responds to interleukin-2 stimulation by producing a protein of still unknown function in growing, or proliferating, T-lymphocytes as well as in all areas of the brain, particularly where neurons have long axons and many connections, such as the hippocampus, motor cortex, and cerebellum. Furthermore, F5 is active only in neurons, not glia, and its expression is greatest when neurons are forming synapses with other neurons rather than when the neurons are replicating.

Plasticity

One of the hallmarks of the immune system is its ability to adapt to constantly changing conditions and to remember how it responds to each of those conditions. Much of this memory is expressed in the way the immune system responds to antigens that it has seen before.

Conversely, the nervous system was long thought to be static, with little ability to change once its billions of neurons were in place. One of the more important discoveries in neuroscience was that the brain, too, is constantly changing and adapting in response to changing conditions. For example, it is now clear that behavioral modification during learning results from functional changes in the connections between nerve cells and in the way they respond to neurotransmitters.

Behavior and Immunity

The connections between behavior and the immune system are perhaps best established in the body's response to stress. Research has clearly shown that psychological stress can lead to increased susceptibility to disease by suppressing the immune response. Yet, studies in both humans and laboratory animals show that mild stress actually increases the activity of various immune cells. In one set of experiments, researchers subjected animals to a mild stress and found that natural killer cell activity, interleukin-2 production, and other measures of immune system activity increased over the next hour.

Even when the stress is moderate to severe, changes in immune cell function do not always translate into increased susceptibility to illness. However, researchers studying the effect of chronic stress, such as long-term caring for a relative with Alzheimer's disease, found decreased immune cell function and increased incidence of illness in the caregivers; when the stress was removed, immune system function did not always return to normal. Clearly, much more research is needed to explain this range of responses.

Stress and Susceptibility to Disease

Considerable evidence from studies of humans shows that naturally occurring stressful events and negative moods such as anxiety and depression are associated with changes in immune function. Whether these changes have implications for susceptibility to infection and other immune-mediated diseases is less clear.

A recent study examined whether persons experiencing stress were at greater risk for developing a common cold. Volunteers were exposed to nasal drops containing one of five viruses known to cause a cold. Before exposure, the subjects filled out three questionnaires designed to assess their current level of stress. A life-events scale measured the occurrence of stressful events—divorce, death of a relative, problems at work or school, and the like. Another scale gauged perceived stress-feeling that the demands of life exceed one's ability to cope. A third measure assessed negative moods, including depression, anxiety, and anger.

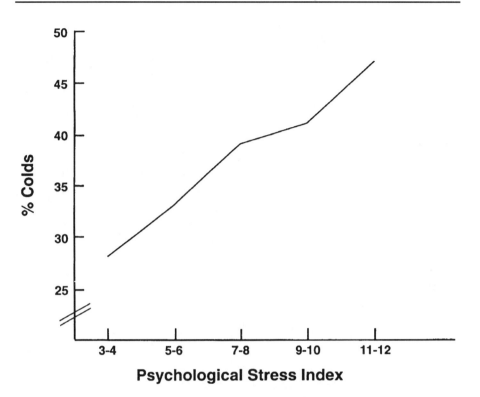

Figure 28.4. *Susceptibility to a cold is directly proportional to the intensity of psychological stress. Healthy volunteers were exposed to one of five viruses known to cause colds. The probability of getting sick increased with the severity of psychological stress the person reported experiencing. [Courtesy S. Cohen.]*

The researchers found that the higher the level of reported stress, the greater the probability of developing a cold. This association held whether the three stress measures were considered alone or together and across all five viruses tested (See figure 28.4). Although functional measures of immunity were not assessed in this study, researchers are currently examining the possible role of immune factors in linking stress to infectious susceptibility.

Medical students were studied to compare immune system function during intermittent periods of stress (comprehensive examinations) and no stress. These studies gathered data on both psychological factors and immune measures, and the results show clearly that these students, though they are expert test-takers, have significant downregulation (slowing) of the cellular immune response at examination time and recover immune function after exams are completed. The one caveat of these studies is that all indicators of immune function were measured *in vitro*, which may not correlate with the actual overall health of an individual. However, a correlation was found between the time of examination, negative changes in the immune parameters, and upper respiratory tract infections.

Since some people handle stress better than others, investigators refined their analysis and looked at how different levels of anxiety, one measure of the psychological response to stress, correlated with immune system response to a specific challenge, such as exposure to hepatitis B vaccine. In this case, the more anxious medical students had a smaller immune response to vaccination than did students who were less anxious.

This finding suggests that vaccinations may be less effective if administered when a person is feeling the effects of stress. For example, soldiers about to go oversees—a potentially stressful situation—are often vaccinated, but they may not build up full immunity as rapidly as under more relaxed circumstances.

The Protective Effects of Social Support

One clinically relevant finding of the medical student vaccination study was that the low anxiety group, who had the strongest immune response to vaccination, also had the highest level of social support from their peers. This suggests that providing social support to those vulnerable to stress may be an effective means of improving overall health.

More direct evidence for the beneficial role of social support comes from a study of the effects of social environment on the cellular immune response of monkeys. After two years, animals whose social groups were continuously disrupted by the researchers had poorer T-cell response to experimental stimulants than animals whose social environments were stable over the course of the study. However, when the investigators distinguished between individual animals who were affiliated with other animals and their more isolated counterparts, the picture changed. The immune suppression found among the socially disrupted group occurred only among the more isolated animals. Affiliative animals showed no immunosuppressive effects of the unstable social environment.

Unanswered Questions

Researchers are now trying to determine an appropriate model for judging the effect of stress—or any environmental change—on the variety of immune responses. Some theoretical structure is needed to make sense of the wealth of data now being generated in the Nation's laboratories. These findings raise important methodological and clinical questions: What is an appropriate model for judging the effect of environment and stress on a variety of immune responses? Is mild, intermittent stress more relevant than chronic, severe stress? Is *in vitro* immune cell function a relevant measure of the immune system's ability to fight disease? Does the immune system function best under some optimal level of stress?

We have no clear answers to these questions, but investigators are beginning to come to grips with these issues, and their awareness will certainly lead to future advances in this important area of research. They may have to develop a new model for environmental pressure on an organism that will be more useful scientifically than the nebulous concept of stress.

Maintaining Homeostasis

The many ways the nervous and immune systems communicate with one another give the body its remarkable ability to maintain itself in equilibrium while existing in an ever-changing environment. This robust homeostasis may actually define life, as every minute of every day the human body attempts to maintain this precarious state despite the ever-present burden of inherited and acquired biochemical defects, including those induced by infectious organisms Thus, a major goal of psychoneuroimmunology is to understand the psychobiology of defense and repair. Learning how the mind, via the nervous system, affects all of the systems that defend or repair the body—and is in turn affected by them—may provide significant breakthroughs in treating psychiatric, neurological, and immune disorders.

Recommendations for the Future

- Establish whether behavioral, cognitive, and emotional states affect immune system function by conducting careful, quantitative studies with sufficiently large numbers of subjects to yield clear-cut results.

- Identify behavioral, neuroendocrine, and immune pathways that link psychosocial factors to the onset and pathogenesis of infectious disease in humans.

- Explore behavioral conditioning and/or vaccinations as therapeutic modalities for treatment of behavioral dysfunctions.

- Discover novel mediators of mechanisms of neuro-endocrine-immune-behavior interactions.

- Identify the changes in the immune system occurring outside the central nervous system that impact on or affect behavioral states, and determine cellular and molecular mechanisms underlying these effects.

- Elucidate how immune tolerance is established and maintained in the brain as compared to other nonlymphoid tissues.

- Determine physiological, pathophysiological, environmental, and sensory factors that stimulate elaboration and release of molecules common to the central nervous and immune systems (e.g., cytokines) within the brain.

- Analyze common aspects of the nervous and immune systems' structure and function in general, and identify and functionally characterize common or related receptors and these receptors' antagonists, in particular.

Further Reading

Paul, W.I. *Fundamental Immunology*. 3rd ed. New York: Raven Press, 1993.

Ader, R., Felten, D.L., and Cohen, N., eds. *Psychoneuro-immunology*. 2nd ed. San Diego: Academic Press, 1991.

Cohen, S., et al. Psychological stress and susceptibility to the common cold. *New England Journal of Medicine* 325:606-612, 1991.

Kandel, E.R., Schwartz, J.H., and Jessell, T.M. *Principles of Neuroscience*. 3rd ed. New York: Elsevier, 1991.

Chapter 29

Nervous System Interactions in the Immune System

"If you look at the totality of the way the system works, you have a constant conversation going on at every level within the body, and this conversation really forces you to think in a more integrated sense." —Seymour Levine

The immune system, like the nervous system, was once thought to be a self-contained and self-regulated entity. As the evidence mounted that mood and stress can affect the ability of the immune system to ward off disease, researchers began looking for the pathways by which the central nervous system could influence the immune system. In searching for these links, investigators hope to find out how stress, depression, behavioral conditioning, and other psychological factors may be related to susceptibility or resistance to infectious and autoimmune diseases and how behavioral or neuropharmacological interventions might be used to either boost or attenuate the immune response.

Multiple Pathways From Brain to Immune System

So far, research has shown that the immune system reacts to powerful hormones released by the brain in response to stress. It is widely accepted that the hypothalamus releases the hormone called corticotropin-releasing factor, which travels to the anterior portion of

NIH Pub No. 94-3774.

the pituitary gland and causes it to secrete two other hormones, adrenocorticotropin (ACTH) and p-endorphin. ACTH acts on the adrenal gland to release hormones known as glucocorticoids.

Low levels of glucocorticoids are necessary for normal immune system function, and high levels have the opposite effect. Some of this may have to do with complex feedback loops. Cytokines, including various interleukins and tumor necrosis factors, and prostaglandins are part of the feedback loop stimulating corticotropin-releasing factor release by the hypothalamus. Each point in this loop—there are dozens, with more being discovered—may be vulnerable to disruption by infectious agents or other insults.

This is certainly one of the major routes by which the brain coordinates immune function. It is well established, for example, that removing the adrenal gland markedly reduces the effect of stress on certain parts of the immune system, providing strong support for the idea that steroid hormones made by the adrenal gland play a critical role in the connection between the nervous and immune systems.

However, other pathways also play a role in fine-tuning the immune system's reaction to various challenges. Some of these pathways may involve direct connections between nerves and the organs associated with the immune system, or even the immune cells themselves.

Multiple pathways may seem to be a waste of resources, but with the critical role that the nervous and immune systems play in maintaining homeostasis, such redundancy may be important for keeping both systems operating at optimal levels under a variety of ever-changing conditions. Working out these pathways is a critical challenge in the field of psychoneuroimmunology, one that investigators are now pursuing with all the tools at their command.

Direct Neural Connections in Lymphoid Organs

Investigators are now mapping neural circuits in the lymphoid organs. These studies are necessary to understand the link between behavior and immunity. Already, mapping efforts have found that neurons often follow pathways set down by blood vessels. Several such neural circuits, each using a different neurotransmitter, have been tracked into the spleen. Neural circuits in bone marrow may help immune cells make their way to various target organs, a phenomenon known as homing.

Administering a compound that blocks the sympathetic nervous system's ability to stimulate the spleen eliminates the detrimental effects of stress on lymphocytes in the spleen. The lymphocytes do not show suppressed activity under stress, presumably because the nervous system can no longer send some important suppressive signal to the spleen.

Neurons may directly stimulate developing lymphocytes in lymph nodes as well as in the spleen and thymus. Nerve terminals are found just a few millionths of an inch from both T-lymphocytes and macrophages, the smallest gap yet found between a nerve ending and its target cell. During development of the spleen, nerve terminals appear first in the regions where lymphocytes mature. Only later do they grow into the spleen's parenchyma. In fact, such innervation may play a role in the proper development of the spleen as a lymphoid organ.

Assuming that these nerves are targeting lymphocytes, researchers are now studying the effects on nerve endings of removing these cells as well as the effect on lymphocyte development of destroying the nerve terminals. Following treatment with a drug that eliminates lymphocytes from the spleen, the nerves seem to retract within the spleen, though they remain capable of transmitting nerve signals. However, using various antigens to challenge an animal with a depopulated spleen causes the nerves to degenerate. Further study has shown that this is probably a result of interleukin-1 somehow interacting with the nervous system.

This remarkably stable system, therefore, turns out to be stable in the face of loss of target cells but not so stable during an immune response, an effect that may be driven by cytokines. This seems to imply that the immune system might lose some of its ability to react to antigen challenge after repeatedly responding to such challenges. In fact, an experiment with animals supports this idea. One group of animals was constantly challenged with various antigens, while the other lived in a pristine environment. After 26 months, there were 50-percent fewer nerve endings in the spleen and thymus of the challenged animals than in the protected animals.

Investigators have also examined this effect in a strain of mouse that is born without T-lymphocytes and B-lymphocytes, though it has natural killer cells and macrophages. Surprisingly, the density of nerve endings in the spleen and thymus of these animals is normal. The reason may be that the macrophages are responsible for maintaining innervation in these lymphoid organs.

These findings may help researchers solve some critical questions concerning autoimmune diseases, such as arthritis. For example, animals with drug-induced arthritis and with the nerve terminals in their lymph nodes destroyed have far greater swelling and faster tissue degeneration than those animals with normal innervation of the lymph nodes. However, if only certain nerve terminals are destroyed—those that use the neuropeptide known as substance P—the animals fail to develop autoimmune arthritis. This suggests that susceptibility to autoimmune disease is not only an immune phenomenon, but is at least in part a neural one.

Neurally Derived Substances Affect Immune Cells

If the immune system is regulated by substances released from the nervous system—neurotransmitters or neurohormones—then there must be receptors for those neurally derived substances either on the surface or inside of immune cells. These receptors may be present at all times or they may appear only when the immune cells are activated by exposure to antigen, cytokine, or both. In all likelihood, the biochemical events triggered when a neurally derived substance binds to its receptor will not themselves activate an immune cell but will instead play a modulatory role in the development of a mature immune cell.

The hormones prolactin and growth hormone, for example, bind to receptors that belong to the same family as those to which many cytokines bind. In addition, the folding of growth hormone is similar to that of interleukin-2, even though the two molecules have different amino acid sequences (See figure 29.1). Both molecules have a bundle of four helices as a major structural motive. These similarities have prompted investigators to look at the possibility that two seemingly dissimilar molecules produced by different systems may be interacting with the same cell-surface receptors.

Such molecular cross-talk could lead to chaos in the immune system as a lymphocyte or macrophage struggles to decipher the wave of incoming chemical signals. But immune cells appear to have a sophisticated mechanism for using this information in directing their development. This mechanism, used throughout the nervous system, is called the second messenger system. When an extracellular molecular signal, be it a cytokine, neurotransmitter, neuropeptide, or hormone, binds to its receptor embedded within the cell wall, a cascade of molecular events begins that produces another molecule within the cell—the second messenger. This, in turn, triggers further events, such as a change in gene expression, enzyme activity, or ionic balance. Each receptor on a given cell type, though it binds a unique substance, is

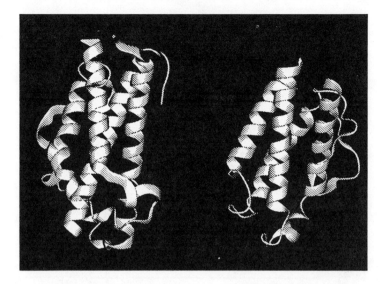

Figure 29.1. *The three-dimensional similarity between growth hormone (left) and cytokine interleukin-2 (right) is revealed by "ribbon diagrams" of these distinct molecules. These computer-generated images were created using Protein Data Base files (denoted 1HUV and 31NK) of the Brookhaven National Laboratory. [Courtesy V. Novokhatny.]*

tied into a number of messenger systems, providing a means of integrating multiple incoming signals through the transduction mechanism of the receptor.

The molecule cyclic-AMP (cAMP) is a common second messenger, and investigators have found that the timing of cAMP production within a lymphocyte is critical for activating that cell. The accumulation of cAMP in lymphocytes can occur through the activation of receptors on these cells by certain naturally occurring substances such as neurotransmitters called catecholamines. If cAMP production is increased in lymphocytes in the absence of immune signals, it is unlikely to have a profound or long-lasting effect. However, when cAMP production is increased at or about the same time as the lymphocyte receives an immune signal, lymphocyte function is greatly altered. Because it is difficult to predict when or where these two signals will reach the lymphocyte, spatial and temporal concerns become important. In the living body, lymphocytes may receive signals from two or more neurally derived substances as well as the immune signal, adding further complexity to how lymphocyte function is altered (See figure 29.2).

297

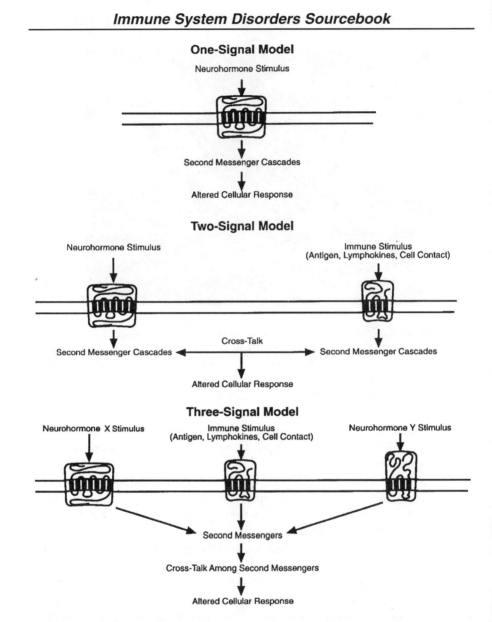

One-Signal Model

Neurohormone Stimulus

Second Messenger Cascades

Altered Cellular Response

Two-Signal Model

Neurohormone Stimulus

Immune Stimulus
(Antigen, Lymphokines, Cell Contact)

Second Messenger Cascades ◄── Cross-Talk ──► Second Messenger Cascades

Altered Cellular Response

Three-Signal Model

Neurohormone X Stimulus

Immune Stimulus
(Antigen, Lymphokines, Cell Contact)

Neurohormone Y Stimulus

Second Messengers

Cross-Talk Among Second Messengers

Altered Cellular Response

Figure 29.2. Models of one-, two-, and three-signal transduction mechanisms in lymphocytes. Note the increase in complexity with the increasing number of signals simultaneously affecting a single cell. The cell depicted here is a lymphocyte, but it could be any other type. Most cells, but particularly those in the brain, simultaneously respond to an unknown but certainly large number of signals. Signal receptors are predominantly proteins positioned in the cellular membrane, depicted here by a fence-like structure. [Courtesy T. Roszman.]

A New Mediator?

Recent experiments suggest that factors other than neurotransmitters and steroid hormones may be able to suppress immune system activity. One such candidate, still unidentified, is a large molecule present in the blood of stressed animals that can suppress the activity of lymphocytes removed from animals that had not been stressed. This suppressive factor also downregulated cytokine production by lymphocytes as well as *in vitro* activity of natural killer cells and was able to keep immune cell function suppressed even 24 hours after exposure. Thus, this soluble factor may play a role in forming what could be considered a molecular memory of stressful events, perhaps by blocking expression of interleukin receptors on the surface of lymphocytes.

What is certain is that there are multiple pathways by which the brain can signal—and affect—the immune response. Uncovering these pathways and determining their relevance to specific behavioral and immunological conditions is a daunting challenge. Surely, such redundancy has important biological consequences, and it will take a concerted effort by researchers in many fields to make sense of this complex communication system.

Recommendations for the Future

- Determine how neuroimmune interactions may be skewed in different individuals depending on their previous behavioral and immune experience.

- Identify synaptic interactions by which cortical limbic signals alter autonomic, endocrine, and behavioral responses that affect the immune system.

- Characterize functional changes occurring *in vivo* in immunocytes elicited by hormones and neurotransmitters.

- Elucidate how hormones, neurotransmitters, and neuropeptides affect immunocytes' functions at the molecular and cellular levels.

- Elucidate local effects on immune activity reflecting neurotransmitter usage in a particular location outside the central nervous system.

- Determine whether locally elaborated immune modulators affect the peripheral and central nervous system, producing a global feedback response.

Further Reading

Pribyl, T.M., et al. The human myelin basic protein gene is included within a 179-kilobase transcription unit: Expression in the immune and central nervous systems. *Proceedings of the National Academy of Sciences USA* 90:10695-10699, 1993.

Blalock, J.E., ed. *Neuroimmunoendocrinology, Chemical Immunology*. Vol. 52, 2nd ed. Basel: S. Karger, 1992.

Ader, R., Felten, D.L., and Cohen, N., eds. *Psychoneuroimmunology*. 2nd ed. San Diego: Academic Press, 1991.

Chapter 30

Immune Interactions in the Nervous System

"Four or five years ago, it was apparent that this system was complex. All I can say is, it's become infinitely more complex since then." —Samuel M. McCann

The brain is the most privileged organ in the body. It takes precedence over other organs for nutrients and oxygen and is highly selective in what it allows to enter. Even substances circulating in the blood are prevented from reaching the brain by the blood-brain barrier, which permits only specific cells and molecules to cross over.

Until recently, investigators thought that immune cells did not enter the brain. A healthy human brain has few signs of antibodies, lymphocytes, or any other immune system components. However, research has now shown that the immune system can mount a significant response to infection or damage in the brain. In addition, some substances released by the immune system to fight infection elsewhere in the body are known to enter the brain and may play one or more roles in the mood changes and other behavioral symptoms that commonly accompany illness.

It is also clear that the immune system can malfunction in the brain, just as it can in the rest of the body. The immune response can be inadequate, allowing invading organisms to damage brain cells or even use them as a reservoir for later release and infection. The immune system may also mistakenly attack healthy brain tissue.

NIH Pub No. 94-3774.

Communication between the immune system and the brain is crucial for regulating the immune response throughout the body. Investigators have found that cytokines can stimulate the stress-response system in the brain and, conversely, that the hormones released in reaction to stress can suppress the immune system under some circumstances. Apparently, this interaction with the brain helps keep the immune system in check.

A Normal Immune Response

Activation of the immune system produces a host of physiological and psychological changes, including altered blood flow and hormone levels, a rise in body temperature, loss of appetite, and lethargy. One such change, fever, appears to result when neurons in the hypothalamus, the part of the brain that regulates body temperature, are activated by cytokines such as interleukin-1, interleukin-6, and tumor necrosis factor-α and probably other molecules still to be discovered.

Experiments have shown that extremely low levels of both interleukin-1 and interleukin-6 can activate the fever response. Injecting an exceedingly tiny amount (0.6 picomoles) of interleukin-1 directly into the brain triggers a fever; few if any other neuroactive substances are this potent. The same effect is seen when a fever-inducing component of bacterial cell walls, known to stimulate interleukin-1 release, is injected into brain.

The levels of stress-response hormones also increase in the bloodstream following administration of a small quantity of either interleukin-1 or the bacterial cell wall component. The amount of corticotropin-releasing factor, which triggers the body's response to stress, traveling from the hypothalamus to the pituitary rises significantly. This leads to an increase in the release of other stress-response hormones such as cortisol and ACTH.

Interestingly, elevated levels of corticotropin-releasing factor are found in the extracellular fluid of the brain in depressed individuals. When rats are subjected to stress, this hormone is concentrated particularly in the region of the brain called the locus ceruleus, where changes in neuronal activity are associated with depression. These observations suggest that corticotropin-releasing factor plays a role in depression precipitated by stressful conditions. The precise regions of the brain where corticotropin-releasing factor exerts its effect in depression are presently under investigation.

Cytokines in the Brain

Investigators now believe that cytokines from outside the brain act on the brain at certain "windows," places where these molecules have access to the central nervous system. These windows are thought to be at sites along the edges of the ventricular system that lack a blood-brain barrier and where neurons have the opportunity to respond to cytokines circulating in the bloodstream. One such window lies next to the hypothalamus, though it is far from certain that this site plays any role in the ability of cytokines, particularly interleukin-1, to produce fever. However, the discovery of compounds that can block interleukin-1 by binding to its receptor should make it possible to test this hypothesis.

Cytokines may act directly on neurons, much as if these substances were neuropeptides. In fact, antibodies specific for interleukin-1 bind to neurons in the hypothalamus and brain stem, indicating that this cytokine is present in those neurons. At least some of these neurons project to hypothalamic cells that produce corticotropin-releasing factor. Studies in mice have found another cytokine, tumor necrosis factor-α, in many of the same neurons, particularly those in the hypothalamus.

In all likelihood, researchers will find that interleukin-1 is produced in many regions of the brain and acts by mechanisms specific to each region. In the hypothalamus, for example, interleukin-1 appears to act on neurons that release corticotropin-releasing factor. Studies have shown that interleukin-1 turns on the genes that code for corticotropin-releasing factor. This effect is eliminated if corticotropin-releasing factor antiserum—antibodies that bind to the hormone—is administered prior to interleukin-1. Presumably, interleukin-1 still induces the hypothalamus to produce and release corticotropin-releasing factor, but the antibodies bind to and neutralize this hormone as soon as it is released into the blood stream.

This antiserum also blocks the effects of the cytokines interleukin-6 and tumor necrosis factor-α, suggesting that interleukin-1 activation of corticotropin-releasing factor release is a necessary first step in any cytokine-induced activation of the stress-response system. The effect of this activation, if strong enough, may be to downregulate an ongoing immune response. Within 15 minutes after interleukin-1 is administered in the brain, a number of immune system cells outside of the brain show marked decreases in activity.

This downregulation may play a role in the immune suppression characteristic of AIDS. Studies have shown that infusing the protein gp120, found on the surface of HIV, into the brain stimulates interleukin-1 release in brain tissues. It also provokes a rise in plasma steroids—part of the stress-response system—and a decrease in natural killer cell activity. Injecting compounds known to interfere with interleukin-1 activity blocks these effects.

One of the most potent inhibitors of interleukin-1 is actually produced in the brain—a peptide called melanocyte-stimulating hormone. On a molecule-by-molecule basis, melanocyte-stimulating hormone is 25,000 times more potent for reducing fever than aspirin, a well-known fever reducer, presumably by blocking the effects of interleukin-1 in the hypothalamus. In fact, a number of studies have now shown that administering this hormone blocks the release of corticotropin-releasing factor from the hypothalamus. At least some investigators now believe melanocyte-stimulating hormone could prove therapeutically valuable in eliminating the effects of excessive production of interleukin-1 and cytokines with similar action, such as interleukin-6 and tumor necrosis factor-α.

Alternative Pathways

Though it is still unclear how the interleukins interact with neurons in the hypothalamus, neuroscientists have found that prostaglandins play a key role in the process. Prostaglandins are involved in many important biochemical processes, at least some of which are inhibited by aspirin. Prostaglandins are made from the lipid arachidonic acid via a long series of chemical reactions. Blocking a key enzyme in this series of reactions blocks the release of corticotropin-releasing factor.

A search for prostaglandins and this key enzyme in brain tissue revealed some surprises. One was that only neurons, and apparently not glia, produce prostaglandins. Another interesting finding was that the enzyme was more prevalent in areas of the brain associated with higher cognitive functions, including the hippocampus and limbic system (which plays a role in controlling mood and affect), than in lower brain centers.

Interleukin-1 may also work by stimulating the release of the hormone vasopressin. This idea is supported by experiments showing an increase in the expression of vasopressin messenger ribonucleic acid (mRNA) levels—a measure of gene activation—following interleukin-1 administration into the brain. In addition, injecting either antibodies against vasopressin or vasopressin antagonists prior to interleukin-1 blunts the stimulatory effect that interleukin-1 (injected into brain ventricles) has on the pituitary gland's secretion of the stress hormone ACTH. Thus, it appears that vasopressin may represent a second pathway by which interleukin-1 activates the release of ACTH.

A new element in this picture is nitric oxide, which only recently was found to be an important modulator of many biochemical processes, including gene expression in neurons. (Nitric oxide is different from nitrous oxide, the chemical commonly used as an anesthetic.) A number of studies have shown that interleukin-1 stimulates the release of nitric oxide by turning on production of an inducible form of the enzyme that synthesizes nitric oxide, so-called inducible nitric oxide synthase (iNOS). A more recent experiment found, though, that blocking nitric oxide release boosted the ability of blood-borne interleukin-1 to increase ACTH secretion. This augmenting effect, interestingly enough, is seen with one other stimulus: cocaine. The implications of these results are presently unclear, but they are providing researchers with another lead for studying the link between the immune system and the brain.

Immunoprotection in the Brain

Much is still unknown about what happens when the central nervous system itself is infected or damaged. Instead of thinking of the brain as immunologically privileged, researchers today find it more useful to consider the brain as being immunologically quiescent, or downregulated, under normal circumstances and immunologically active, or upregulated, in disease states. This is not unique to the brain, for the same holds true for most other organs in the body. Healthy muscle, for example, is not infused with lymphocytes either.

Under normal conditions, lymphocytes and other immune system cells circulate (traffic) through the brain and spinal fluid and back out to the periphery, that is, outside the central nervous system, seeking any foreign antigens or signals indicating significant cellular abnormalities. When necessary, immunocyte trafficking increases in frequency. There is evidence that stimulated lymphocytes secrete enzymes that enable them to cross the blood-brain barrier, just as they can cross through other tissues elsewhere in the body.

It also appears that chemical attraction signals, released from still-unknown sources, somehow direct lymphocyte movement into, within, and out of the brain. Some of these signals may involve cytokines. Other molecules, such as integrins and other cell-adhesion molecules, that are expressed on the surfaces of cells may also play a role in bringing lymphocytes into the brain. Understanding this interface between the brain and the immune system represents a major research challenge and is an important priority among neuroscientists and immunologists.

Another unknown is the role that binding proteins play in helping cytokines enter the brain and reach their targets. These cytokine-binding proteins normally render cytokines inactive, but when released from these carriers—the triggers are unknown—the cytokines can activate a host of biological actions.

In recent years, investigators have learned that microglia and astrocytes can release cytokines to stimulate an immune response. These cells may also display on their surfaces the same antigen-presenting MHC molecules that immune system cells express to signal the presence of an invader.

Interest in the contribution of astrocytes to immunological abnormalities in the central nervous system came about from studies of multiple sclerosis, which is a central nervous system disease of unknown etiology, though it certainly has an immunological component. In multiple sclerosis, the number of T-lymphocytes and the amount of various cytokines in the central nervous system show a noticeable increase. The number of cells expressing major MHC class-II molecules, which target cells for attack by T-lymphocytes, also increases. Researchers studying multiple sclerosis thus focused on astrocytes surrounding brain lesions in the patients. These astrocytes, when stimulated, express MHC class-II antigens and produce a wide array of cytokines, including interleukin-1, tumor necrosis factor-α, and interleukin-6.

While cells in the central nervous system do not normally express MHC class-II antigens, experiments in animals have shown that the cytokine γ-interferon will stimulate such expression. Certain viruses induce the same result. This expression is enhanced, but not turned on, by tumor necrosis factor-α. How this happens is still unclear, though it may be that tumor necrosis factor promotes more efficient expression of the MHC class-II antigen genes turned on by γ-interferon.

Using cultured astrocytes, investigators have learned that MHC class-II expression is induced by γ-interferon and certain viruses. Tumor necrosis factor-α has no effect on MHC class-II expression but can synergize with either γ-interferon or virus for enhanced MHC class-II expression. The researchers have also found that MHC class-II expression is more easily downregulated on astrocytes than on microglia, implying that different modes of regulation occur in these two cell types.

Three regulatory elements (boxes), W, X, and Y, in MHC class-II genes have been studied. These elements are important for constitutive expression (i.e., always expressed) of the gene in some cells, such as B-cells and macrophages, and inducible expression (i.e., only expressed when stimulated by some factor) in other cell types. To further probe this system, investigators took the portion of the MHC class-II gene containing the W, X, and Y boxes, linked it to a reporter gene, and inserted it into rat astrocytes. If the boxes were functional, the reporter gene product would be made and would be identifiable after treating the astrocytes with γ-interferon.

To probe the regulatory elements, the investigators mutated specific conserved regions (i.e., sequences in the gene that are the same across species) in the W, X, and Y boxes. Key mutations in any of these three regions knock out inducibility by γ-interferon. The investigators then looked for the protein in the cell nucleus that might be binding to these regions and mediating the induction; they found a protein that bound specifically to the X box. Mutations in the X box prevented the protein binding. Mutations in the W and Y box did not prevent this protein from binding to the X box, but blocked the ability of tumor necrosis factor-α to enhance γ-interferon-mediated induction of MHC class II.

Based on these studies, the researchers proposed that γ-interferon alters the binding ability of X-binding protein, perhaps by triggering enzymatic phosphorylation of the protein. Modifying the protein somehow turns on the MHC class-II gene. Tumor necrosis factor-α may augment whatever changes in the X-binding protein are triggered by γ-interferon.

Interestingly, similar experiments conducted in rat microglial cells reveal the presence of γ-interferon-induced X-binding protein; however, tumor necrosis factor-α does not amplify expression in these cells. These results emphasize that expression of MHC class-II genes is differentially regulated in astrocytes and microglia.

Investigators are keenly interested in finding the biological stimuli that induce MHC class-II genes in the nervous system, because glial cells expressing these genes may play a critical role in triggering an immune response within the central nervous system. The X-binding protein may represent a new class of transcription factor, which may give investigators an insight into the earliest steps of immune responses by glial cells.

Host of Possibilities

Clearly, researchers are just beginning to touch on some of the important questions about the actions of the immune system in the brain. The exquisite potency of interleukin-1 in the brain, for instance, suggests that this cytokine may, in fact, be a neuromodulator, a compound that attenuates a nerve's response to a neurotransmitter. Indeed, it brings into question whether cytokines and neuromodulators are really one and the same—compounds whose functions are determined by the environment in which they are released. Current research also raises the issue of redundancy, that is, whether multiple systems might be controlling the same end effect. This idea is supported by the finding that interleukin-1 seems to act in the brain through at least two intracellular mediators. On one level, interleukin-1 can induce a cytokine cascade in glial cells. At another level, interleukin-1 triggers production of signaling molecules and intracellular mediators. Further work is needed to tease out the nature of this redundancy and to understand how different systems, if they do exist, might work together to regulate both immune responses and behavior.

Recommendations for the Future

- Elucidate mechanisms of immunocyte trafficking through the central nervous system and develop ways to alter this trafficking.

- Determine whether immune cells function in qualitatively different ways in the brain than in other non-lymphoid organs.

- Determine exogenous cellular (e.g., pathogens, tumors) and molecular (e.g., psychoactive drugs) factors that enhance/inhibit passage of immunocytes into the central nervous system.

- Elucidate immune reactions in the brain directed at answering the following questions:

1. How do immune effector cells and molecules gain access to their neuronal target antigens?

2. Which subcellular compartments in a neuron are accessed by an antibody, and what are the effects of the antibody's entry into these compartments on neuronal function?

3. What effector mechanisms can protect neurons from viral infection?

*   Analyze the antigen-presenting potential of endogenous brain cells other than neurons, how antigen presentation is regulated in the brain, and how antigen-presenting cells in the brain compare with those of other tissues.

*   Determine mechanisms by which immune stimuli (e.g., cytokines) act on the brain to cause changes in behavior and in autonomic and endocrine responses.

*   Analyze the effects of microglial and macroglial secretory factors known to be capable of affecting both immunocytes and neurons.

Further Reading

McCann, S.M., et al. Induction by cytokines of the pattern of pituitary hormone secretion in infection. *Neuroimmunomodulation* 1:2-13, 1994.

Ehrhard, P.B., et al. Expression of nerve growth factor and nerve growth factor receptor tyrosine kinase trk in activated CD4-positive T-cell clones. *Proceedings of the National Academy of Sciences USA* 90:10984-10988, 1993.

Life, death and the immune system. *Scientific American* Special Issue 269:52-144, September 1993.

Steinman, L. Connections between the immune and the nervous system. *Proceedings of the National Academy of Science USA* 90:79127914. 1993.

Kent, S., et al. Sickness behavior as a new target for drug development. *Trends in Pharmacological Sciences* 13:24-28. 1992.

Ader, R.; Felten, D.L.; and Cohen, N., eds. *Psychoneuroimmunology.* 2nd ed. San Diego: Academic Press, 1991.

Chapter 31

Autoimmunity and Neuroimmunological Diseases

"Autoreactivity does not always mean pathology." —Keith A. Krolick

Recent research has raised the possibility that some autoimmune diseases may be as much a neural as an immune problem, opening new avenues of inquiry that may lead to novel therapeutic approaches to these devastating diseases. In similar fashion, investigators are learning more about the immunological mechanisms that are involved in various central nervous system diseases, such as multiple sclerosis and Alzheimer's disease, again raising the possibility of clinical breakthroughs in the not too distant future.

Normally, the immune system is programmed not to recognize self molecules that are present in or circulate through the thymus. Any self-responsive T or B cells that come into contact with their specific target antigens are programmed to die. However, some autoreactive immune cells are not exposed to their specific self molecules during development, especially to organ-specific antigens such as those found in the central nervous system, peripheral nervous system, connective tissue, and pancreas. These autoreactive cells are not removed from circulation and are present at low levels even in normal healthy individuals.

Under abnormal conditions, for example, when viral infections induce inflammation and damage the organ, the number of autoreactive cells may be selectively expanded. When these cells reach a critical

NIH Pub No. 94-3774.

311

threshold level, they may attack the self antigen in the tissue, leading to autoimmune diseases such as multiple sclerosis, Guillan-Barré syndrome, rheumatoid arthritis, and diabetes.

Alternatively, an invading foreign antigen may possess a particular molecular moiety that "looks like" part of a self protein to the immune system. This is the concept of "molecular mimicry." Thus, in attacking the invader, the immune system may mistake self for nonself.

Multiple Sclerosis

One of the first brain diseases thought to be caused by an autoimmune response, multiple sclerosis (MS), manifests itself as impaired sensory or motor performance; this latter defect occurs infrequently. MS is thought to result from altered neurotransmission caused by T-lymphocytes specific for myelin antigens. Thus, T cells specific for basic protein (BP) or proteolipid protein (PLP) may cross the blood-brain barrier to produce central nervous system inflammation and destruction of the myelin sheath that wraps axons. Oligodendrocytes, which lay down the myelin sheath, are initially spared but may eventually be destroyed, thus limiting myelin regeneration. In most patients, MS is progressive, although it is common for symptoms to improve spontaneously and then later reappear and worsen.

An Animal Model

An autoimmune disease similar to MS, called experimental autoimmune encephalomyelitis (EAE), can be induced in laboratory animals by injecting BP or PLP with adjuvants that enhance immunization and increase the number of myelin-specific T cells. Within two weeks, the animals develop progressive paralysis and some demyelination. The extent of demyelination varies with the species of animal and occurs predominantly in the central nervous system. Thus, EAE has become an important animal model for multiple sclerosis.

T cells that cause EAE tend to use receptors very similar to those involved in MS. By immunizing animals with a peptide representing a conserved region of the pathogenic T-cell receptor (TCR), it has been possible to induce TCR-specific T cells and antibodies that can neutralize the harmful T cells and prevent later induction of EAE. Perhaps more importantly, as least concerning possible clinical applications, immunizing animals that already have EAE with this

TCR fragment stops the disease process. This therapeutic effect is rapid and dramatic, causing a decreased number of T-lymphocytes that can recognize basic protein. More work is needed to clarify the role of TCR in EAE. This work is progressing along well-defined lines, as outlined in Table 31.1.

Another approach to prevention and treatment of EAE involves oral administration of the basic protein. Investigators have shown that orally administering BP to rats or mice before or at the first sign of clinical disease suppresses clinical symptoms. The mechanism underlying oral tolerance has been shown to be clonal anergy of BP-specific T cells or suppression of specific T cells through elaboration of suppressive cytokines.

EAE can also be suppressed in rats and mice when animals are exposed to restraint stress. Such stress, which produces elevated levels of adrenal glucocortocoids and catecholamines, results in decreased clinical signs and depressed systemic immune responses to neuroantigens.

TABLE 31.1
Role of T cell and its receptor in experimental autoimmune encephalomyelitis, an animal model of multiple sclerosis.

What We Know

1. T cell-receptor (TCR) peptides prevent and alleviate experimental autoimmune encephalomyelitis.

2. Effects are mediated by anti-TCR peptide-specific T cells and antibodies.

3. Effective TCR protein sequences represent natural idiotopes.

4. Treatment with TCR peptides decreases functional response to the basic protein but does not delete a subset of T cells, called Vγ8.2+ T cells, from the outside or within the central nervous system, suggesting anergy (diminished reactivity to specific antigens).

5. The TCR/anti-TCR regulatory network is independent from and can be superimposed upon natural recovery mechanism(s).

What We Do Not Know

1. Why is neonatal tolerance to TCR idiotopes not induced *in vivo*?

2. How does natural immunization to TCR sequences take place *in vivo*?

3. Is cell-cell contact required for regulation to occur, or can soluble cytokines mediate the effects?

4. Are other cell types (e.g., CD8+ T cells) involved in regulation?

5. How and where does regulation occur, and what is the fate of the regulated T cells?

Future Directions

1. Identify functional defects in anergized T cells.

2. Generalize and optimize anergy induction in specific T-cell subsets.

3. Develop approaches for depletion of autoreactive T cells.

4. Develop strategies for identifying autoreactive pathogenic T-cell specificities.

[After H. Offner]

T-Lymphocyte Response in Humans

While TCR peptide therapy in animals offers hope for clinical advances, two important questions must be addressed in order to apply this strategy to MS: Is there evidence for T-lymphocyte response to myelin antigens in multiple sclerosis patients? If so, will immunization with the receptor fragments boost the immune system's ability to prevent T-lymphocytes from attacking myelin?

Longitudinal analyses revealed that MS patients had an elevated frequency of T cells specific for BP, both in the blood and the cerebrospinal fluid. Like MS itself, the T-cell response was episodic and reached levels similar to those found in animals with EAE. Moreover, as in EAE, the T cells tended to utilize common TCR molecules. A conserved region was identified from two such TCR sequences, and corresponding peptides were synthesized for use in a clinical trial.

As in EAE, injection of the peptides successfully boosted TCR-specific T cells in a majority of the progressive MS patients tested, and in some patients, the response to BP was reduced. The effect was selective, in that responses to other microbial antigens were not affected, and no toxicity could be detected from the treatment. These encouraging results have prompted further studies in a larger group of MS patients to assess clinical efficacy.

A small clinical trial was also conducted testing the efficacy of administering myelin orally to patients with relapsing-remitting multiple sclerosis. Those individuals receiving oral myelin showed fewer declines in performance than those receiving placebo (an inactive pill made to look like an experimental drug). Interestingly, male patients showed greater clinical improvement than female patients. A larger trial is planned.

At the same time, researchers are still looking for the molecular trigger that induces such myelin-reactive T-lymphocytes. Unlike the situation in EAE, where encephalitogenic lymphocytes form in response to immunization with BP, some other event, for example, an infectious organism, must trigger the disease process in MS patients. Once a causative agent can be identified, it will be possible to target the organism and prevent MS. Meanwhile, the TCR peptide strategy, as well as other antigen-specific tolerance protocols, may provide selective regulation of autoreactive T cells to inhibit the MS disease progression.

Alzheimer's Disease: An Overaggressive Immune Response?

Alzheimer's disease is an age-related, progressive neurodegenerative disorder that has become increasingly identified with inflammatory mechanisms. Although there is no clinical test for Alzheimer's brain, samples collected at autopsy reveal several hallmarks of pathology that provide a definitive diagnosis. These include profuse fibrillar deposits of a molecule called amyloid ß peptide and widespread formation of abnormal filaments (neurofibrillary tangles) in neurons. There is also substantial loss of neurons and their connections. These phenomena particularly occur in brain areas thought to subserve higher cognitive functions such as memory.

Evidence has accumulated over the last decade that inflammatory mechanisms may play a significant role in the brain damage characteristic of Alzheimer's disease. Initially, research on inflammation and Alzheimer's disease concentrated mainly on cataloging inflammatory markers and cells present in brain samples of affected patients. Among the most important of these were cytokines, such as interleukin-1, and complement proteins, a group of some 20 or more proteins that interact in a cascade to damage or destroy cells. The complement proteins were readily detectable in Alzheimer's brain samples and absent or greatly reduced in brain tissues from normal elderly people. They also appeared to be most prominent in those regions of Alzheimer's brain where damage to nerve cells occurs—the higher cognitive centers.

Subsequent studies have begun to elucidate mechanisms by which these processes might arise. In some respects, there are clear parallels to immunologic activity in other parts of the body and other human disorders. For example, virtually all the complement proteins have been found in Alzheimer's brain tissue, as have complement regulatory proteins, such as membrane inhibitor of reactive lysis and sulfated glycoprotein 2. The latter are upregulated outside the central nervous system as a means of controlling ongoing inflammatory attacks. Their presence in the Alzheimer's brain, and not in samples from normal elderly controls, strongly suggests that a functionally relevant inflammatory attack is ongoing in Alzheimer's disease.

In other respects, the immune activity in Alzheimer's disease may differ significantly from that in other organs and other disease states. Edema and neutrophil invasion, which are hallmarks of inflammation outside the brain, are not present in Alzheimer's. The activation of complement also appears to have an unusual source. Classically, complement reactions are initiated by antibodies. In Alzheimer's brain, amyloid ß peptide appears to activate complement, as has been shown *in vitro* and confirmed in several independent laboratories. This, plus the continuing difficulty in unequivocally demonstrating brain-reactive antibodies in Alzheimer's patients, suggests that Alzheimer's may be an inflammatory disorder but not an autoimmune disorder.

Inflammation is an inherently destructive process. This would be particularly true in the brain, an organ that is heavily invested in neurons, a cell type that cannot be replaced, as many cells in other organ systems can. Inflammation may arise in the Alzheimer's brain as a response to previous damage. Once initiated, however, there is a high potential for a vicious cycle in which inflammation breeds more damage which breeds more inflammation. Whether as a primary event or not, the great weight of accumulated evidence strongly suggests that inflammation becomes a cause of damage in Alzheimer's disease.

If nothing else, it should be clear from Alzheimer's research that a better understanding of immunologic mechanisms in human neural diseases may be expected to bear fruit. If inflammation can arise in Alzheimer's, then it is likely that it can arise under other conditions. Microglial activation, for example, is rampant in Alzheimer's disease, a phenomenon that may prove relevant to AIDS dementia.

Clinically, several retrospective studies have suggested an inverse relationship between Alzheimer's disease and a prior history of anti-inflammatory drug use. Perhaps the most compelling of these reports is a Duke University study of identical twins, one of whom had Alzheimer's and the other either did not or developed it significantly later. The twins were found to be significantly different on prior use of anti-inflammatory drugs.

Finally, a recent clinical trial was performed on Alzheimer's patients with encouraging results. Although very small, the study found that, on average, patients taking a placebo declined almost 10 percent on memory tests during the trial period. By contrast, patients taking an anti-inflammatory drug, indomethacin, that crosses the blood-brain barrier did not deteriorate and, in fact, showed nearly 2-percent improvement.

Perhaps because of the outworn dogma of the immunologically privileged brain, neuroimmunology may have become best known for showing how the nervous system affects the immune system. Like almost all relationships in the body, however, brain/immune interactions are probably a two-way street. Alzheimer's disease and multiple sclerosis make this abundantly clear.

Stiff-Man Syndrome

Stiff-man syndrome (SMS) is a rare disease of the nervous system characterized by progressive muscular rigidity and painful spasms. The symptoms result from the simultaneous activation of agonist and antagonist muscles, which, in turn, is the consequence of the continuous firing of α-motor neurons. Symptoms are partially improved by drugs that potentiate the action of the inhibitory neurotransmitter gamma-aminobutyric acid (GABA), such as benzodiazepines and baclofen. For this reason, it is believed that GABA-ergic neurons that are involved in the control of α-motor neuron activity are somehow affected in this syndrome.

Investigators studying a patient who had both SMS and insulin-dependent diabetes mellitus found that this patient's cerebrospinal fluid and serum contained autoantibodies directed against the GABA-synthesizing enzyme glutamic acid decarboxylase (GAD). This enzyme is localized in neurons around the tiny sacs called synaptic vesicles that store GABA for release when needed.

Further studies of more than 100 patients with SMS established that more than 50 percent of them had anti-GAD autoantibodies. In addition, many of these SMS patients had insulin-dependent diabetes mellitus, a well-established autoimmune disease. Interestingly, both GAD and GABA are present in pancreatic cells that secrete insulin and are destroyed in the autoimmune attack leading to diabetes.

These findings raised the possibility that autoimmunity directed against GAD may have some role in insulin-dependent diabetes mellitus. Subsequent studies of insulin-dependent diabetes mellitus patients without SMS demonstrated that the large majority of these patients had autoantibodies directed against GAD and that GAD is identical to the so-called 64 kD autoantigen of insulin-dependent diabetes mellitus, a previously identified dominant antigen of diabetes.

Although the autoantibodies found in SMS and insulin-dependent diabetes mellitus are similar, differences show up in certain analytical tests. Furthermore, the titre of anti-GAD autoantibodies in SMS patients is much higher than in insulin-dependent diabetes mellitus patients, suggesting that different types of autoimmune response to GAD may correlate with different clinical conditions. To date, investigators do not know the role of these autoantibodies in producing the neurological symptoms of SMS.

Not all who have SMS develop this specific antibody, and researchers have been examining this smaller group of patients as well. A few of these patients, all women, had autoantibodies against another neuronal protein called amphiphysin. This protein, like GAD, is localized in proximity to neuronal synaptic vesicles as well as other areas. Strikingly, all these SMS patients also suffered from breast cancer. In two cases, the search for (and detection of) an occult breast cancer was triggered by the previous identification of the anti-amphiphysin autoantibodies. Removal of the tumors was always followed by an improvement in the neurological symptoms.

Again, it is not clear how anti-amphiphysin autoantibodies are involved in producing muscle rigidity, and researchers are intrigued by the fact that the same neurological condition is related to two distinct sets of autoantibodies. Yet the two autoantigens share the property of being associated with synaptic vesicles. One possibility is that autoimmunity to both GAD and amphiphysin may somehow impair the efficiency of neurotransmitter release from synaptic vesicles.

"Autoreactivity Does Not Always Mean Pathology"

Autoreactivity may appear to be a universally pathogenic event, and immunologists once held that idea as fact. But in recent years, it has become clear that autoreactive antibodies are present in nearly everyone, and these antibodies do not cause any apparent harm.

This idea led researchers studying the neuromuscular disorder myasthenia gravis to look more closely at the autoantibodies against the acetylcholine receptor that characterize this disease. In myasthenia gravis, antibodies against this receptor interfere with the ability of acetylcholine to act as a neurotransmitter at the junction between motor neurons and muscle cells. These antibodies can, in some instances, also trigger the complement reaction, which attracts macrophages and other immune cells to the neuromuscular junction, exacerbating damage. One observation that baffled clinicians is that the measurable levels of acetylcholine receptor antibodies do not correlate with disease severity in myasthenia gravis patients. In other words, some myasthenia gravis patients with high antibody levels have exceedingly mild symptoms, while some patients who have died from the disease have marginally detectable antibody levels. This has led investigators to propose that not all anti-receptor antibodies are equally capable of interfering with acetylcholine receptor-dependent neuromuscular function.

A corollary to this hypothesis is that antibody levels and disease severity will only correlate when the disease-causing antibody subsets approach 100 percent of the total anti-receptor antibody level. A second corollary is that disease severity will not be determined by total anti-receptor antibody levels, but rather by the level of a specific subset of autoantibodies that are able to interfere with neuromuscular function. Furthermore, it should be possible to identify those autoantibodies that are pathogenic using an *in vitro* assay of motor neuron function; only those autoantibodies that are pathogenic will block nerve signal transmission between neuron and muscle cell.

Immunizing an animal with acetylcholine receptor fragments causes B-lymphocytes to generate autoantibodies against the receptor and symptoms of myasthenia gravis to develop. Investigators are now using this model to identify the pathogenic antibodies and determine how they interact with the receptor. It appears that between 10 and 20 different antibodies react with the receptor, only some of which, as expected, are capable of producing disease symptoms when injected into healthy animals. All antibodies that are pathogenic could bind to the receptor in intact cells.

Now that they have identified the pathogenic autoantibodies, investigators are trying to determine what molecular event triggers their formation. Others, meanwhile, are looking at antibody heterogeneity in a variety of autoimmune diseases, trying to determine the role that both pathogenic and nonpathogenic autoantibodies play in the immune system's ability to function properly.

Studying Neuronal Death

Little is known at present about the mechanisms that trigger the nerve degeneration seen in disorders such as Parkinson's disease and amyotrophic lateral sclerosis. What is characteristic of all of these illnesses is that neurons in specific anatomical and functional groups die off with no evidence of prior pathology, and the disease appears secondary to the loss of these neurons. One way to study neuronal death is to use neurotoxic drugs. One such drug, guanethidine, induces the destruction of sympathetic neurons in the superior cervical ganglion (SCG) that innervate organs physically above the diaphragm, including the thymus. One interesting property of guanethidine-induced cell death is that it happens quickly, within five days. Moreover, it is associated with chronic inflammatory response in the SCG. This is too fast for the typical T-lymphocyte-driven process that characterizes most chronic inflammatory processes.

This observation led researchers to look for a different mechanism, one involving some other immune component. The search was fruitful, leading to the discovery that natural killer cells were responsible for guanethidine-induced neuronal death (See figure 31.1). Never before had researchers found an instance in which natural killer cells functioned as the primary effector cell in a neurodegenerative condition. Eliminating natural killer cells with an antibody that specifically binds these cells totally prevents guanethidine-induced neuronal death.

Having shown that natural killer cells can kill neurons directly in laboratory animals, investigators wondered if the same thing might

Normal Neuron – no interaction with NK cells

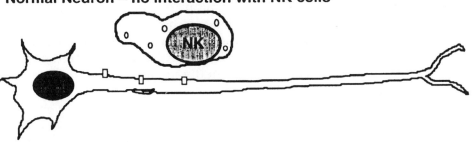

Guanethidine Exposed Neuron – novel or altered expression of cellular moiety attacked by NK cells

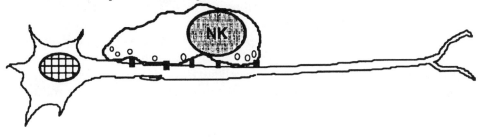

Figure 31.1. Neuronal degeneration mediated by natural killer (NK) cells.

hold true in some neurodegenerative diseases. Guanethidine and its close chemical relative guanacline were once used as drugs for treating hypertension, so investigators poured through the medical literature to see if there were any reports of neuronal death in patients receiving these drugs. Sure enough, there were scattered cases of unremitting orthostatic hypotension in a small group of patients who had received therapeutic doses of guanacline. It may be that neuronal death was responsible for this irreversible side effect.

This has led investigators to propose a new mechanism by which neurodegenerative disorders might occur. Under normal conditions, natural killer cells and neurons coexist peacefully. At some point, though, a group of neurons is exposed to a toxin, be it a particular drug or some substance in the natural environment. This substance in and of itself is not toxic, and it would not affect most of the people who encounter it. But in a subset of individuals this toxin finds its way into neurons and in some fashion alters the molecular composition of the neuronal membrane, making it "visible" to natural killer cells and triggering an attack that leads to neuronal death.

An interesting sidelight to this research is that researchers do not know what natural killer cells actually recognize or fail to recognize. This research may open the door to finally identifying the targets of these key immunocytes.

Cytotoxic T-Lymphocytes

One subset of T-lymphocytes, called cytotoxic T-lymphocytes, is capable of suppressing viral replication by killing the cells that play host to the virus. Recently, investigators have found that this usually protective mechanism can have a pathological side to it. For example, disease symptoms might develop if the cytotoxic T-lymphocytes, in killing infected cells, also damaged healthy cells that happen to share some recognition molecule on their cell surfaces with the infected cells. Cytokines released by the cytotoxic T-lymphocytes might also produce pathological consequences.

Tropical spastic paraparesis is a neurodegenerative disease that occurs in less than 1 percent of all people infected with the human T-lymphocyte leukemia virus-1 (HTLV-1). Most of them never develop any illness caused by this virus. Researchers have been interested in determining why such a small proportion of people infected with HTLV-1 ever become sick, while everyone infected with HIV, a related virus, eventually develops AIDS and dies. One of the hallmarks of HIV infection is that the levels of cytotoxic T-lymphocytes in the blood stream are extremely high. It appears that a similar situation may hold true in those HTLV-1-infected people who develop tropical spastic paraparesis. These cytotoxic T-lymphocytes are equally distributed in both blood and cerebrospinal fluid.

To date, little is known about the role that cytotoxic lymphocytes play in producing, as opposed to curing, disease. In one clinical trial, however, treatment with high doses of the steroid prednisone, which suppresses the production of cytotoxic lymphocytes, produced some improvement in patients with tropical spastic paraparesis. Accompanying the improvement was a drop in the number of cytotoxic lymphocytes specific for the HTLV-1 virus. Lymphocyte counts did not fall in patients who showed no clinical improvement.

Recommendations for the Future

- Develop better ways of identifying potential autoimmune components of psychiatric disorders than the usual screening for "markers."

- Determine whether recognition of neural antigens influences brain development and function.

- Study how T-cell-mediated inflammation may lead to autoimmunity in the nervous system.

- Identify and characterize novel or rare nervous system disorders associated with the immune or autoimmune response as revealed by family studies and/or unusual clinical presentations.

- Stress the importance of probing molecular mechanisms of an entire process, recognizing that multiple points could provide opportunities for therapeutic intervention.

- Develop better ways of distinguishing primary immune etiology from secondary or from exacerbating effects of the immune/inflammatory cascade.

- Create an animal model of autoimmune disease directed against a neuronal antigen, such as is found in human paraneoplastic syndromes.

Further Reading

Life, death and the immune system. *Scientific American* Special Issue 269:52-144, Sept. 1993.

Rose, N.R., and Mackay, I.R. *The Autoimmune Diseases*. San Diego: Academic Press, 1992.

Chapter 32

Neurovirology and Mental Disorders

"The impact of viral infections is determined by behavior."
—Linda S. Crnic

Viruses have long been suspected of causing behavioral problems, including severe mental illness. This idea has gained new force with the advent of AIDS and AIDS-related dementia. Further evidence comes from the repeated finding that many viruses (neurotropic viruses) infect neurons and can remain dormant in them for years. In addition, the symptoms of neurotropic viral infection share many similarities with both behavioral and neurological disorders. Manic depression and multiple sclerosis, for example, are both relapsing disorders, and the association between these two diseases is tenfold higher than chance.

Moreover, at least some neurotropic viruses display a pattern of latency and reactivation similar to the cyclic pattern of these two disorders. Still, it has proven difficult to confirm the connection between viral infection and behavioral disorders, in large part because such disorders may occur years or decades after exposure to the virus.

Investigators have pondered the many ways in which viruses can cause behavioral disorders. One hypothesis is that a common virus, one that infects a large proportion of the population, could injure the nervous system in some extraordinary way in only a few susceptible individuals. Animal studies have shown, for example, that viruses can

NIH Pub No. 94-3774.

325

produce a range of effects, from none to severe, in different inbred strains of laboratory rodents. Other studies have found that the age of an animal or its gender can determine the severity of damage produced by viral infection.

Another possibility is that the host's immune response, and not the virus per se, damages neurons, which would also make it difficult for researchers to link the initial viral infection to the eventual behavioral change. For example, there is sound epidemiological evidence that some viruses trigger the immunological changes that produce multiple sclerosis. Yet many good investigators have spent significant parts of their careers searching unsuccessfully for the offending virus. Researchers must also deal with the fact that while the eventual effects of a viral infection on behavior might be severe, the underlying damage to the central nervous system could be subtle. Viral infection may produce changes in neuronal organization, for example, or slight up- or down-regulation of certain host genes. Viruses might also stimulate autoimmune reactivity if viral proteins share antigenic features with important host molecules (molecular mimicry).

Viruses Produce Cognitive Defects

Behavioral changes are often the first sign of viral infection. Though most adults try to deny this, viruses can have major effects on mood, behavior, and mental ability, a fact appreciated by anyone who has cared for a 2-year-old with a cold. In fact, many investigators now believe that pathogens, including viruses and bacteria, must have played a very important role in evolution. While it is more common to think of predators as playing a dominant role in natural selection, more selective pressures were probably exerted by pathogens than predators. Therefore, animals have developed behaviors that lead them to avoid infecting others with pathogens or becoming infected themselves.

When an animal is sick, its temperature rises, it stops eating, curls up to conserve heat, and lowers its activity level to conserve energy. These responses reduce its interactions with other animals, limiting the spread of the pathogen. At least some of these changes are linked to the release of interferon-α that occurs during the immune system's response to viral infection. In primates, interferon-α produces changes in sleep patterns reminiscent of those seen in human depression. To some investigators, this suggests that each person is programmed to experience depression in response to viral infection. If this is indeed the case, then perhaps clinical depression is a normal response inappropriately and excessively activated by some wayward biochemical process. Whether this notion proves true or not, it opens heretofore unconsidered avenues of investigation into the etiology of a major mental illness.

A Model for Hyperactivity

Can the aftermath of a viral infection yield a fairly normal animal with a discrete lesion that generates a specific behavioral disorder? Investigators have used a mutant strain of herpes simplex virus to study this question. Newborn mice were infected with the mutant virus, and those that survived became hyperactive. The principle neural lesion in these mice was an alteration in migration of neurons into the cerebellum, producing abnormal development of this part of the brain.

Though the neurobehavioral effect of infection was significant, the infection itself was mild, and the animals' growth was normal in all other respects. All traces of the virus were gone after 20 days, though the hyperactivity was permanent.

The hyperactive mice exhibited the same daily rhythm of normal and uninhibited behavior seen in hyperactive humans. Even with the threat of touching an electrified grid, the animals could not resist walking around. These animals could, however, master all other learning tasks, indicating that the viral infection had not diminished their intellectual abilities

These findings are important for at least two reasons. First, it was not widely considered before that the cerebellum was involved in controlling activity. Second, cerebellar organization occurs fairly late in human development, extending as long as seven months after birth, and thus could be particularly vulnerable to a variety of insults, such as neurotropic viruses. On the other hand, it is possible that very subtle pathological alterations in other brain regions may be partially or largely responsible for hyperactivity.

Schizophrenia and Influenza: Epidemiological Evidence

Further evidence that viruses can disrupt normal brain development, and thus cause major behavioral difficulties long after infection, comes from epidemiological studies of schizophrenia. This research, conducted largely with the detailed medical records kept by

Scandinavian health departments, strongly suggests that an important part of the predisposition to schizophrenia consists of a disruption in fetal brain development. This probably occurs in the second trimester of gestation; some studies have even more closely pinpointed the sixth month of gestation.

The hypothesized disruption of brain development may involve errors in the migration, positioning, orientation, and connection of young neurons. These errors of development may be triggered by exposure to teratogens, such as maternal viral infection, that occurs during a critical period of gestation. The chief viral culprit identified so far is influenza virus.

The first of numerous studies that support these hypotheses focused on women who had been pregnant during the **Helsinki influenza epidemic** that ran from October 8 to November 14, 1957. This was the first appearance of a new strain of influenza known as A2. For comparison, the researchers also studied women who had been pregnant in the six preceding years.

Using psychiatric records kept by the eight mental hospitals in the vicinity of Helsinki, the researchers found a significant increase in the rate of schizophrenia for those individuals who had been exposed to A2 influenza during their second trimester of fetal development. Those individuals who had been exposed to the epidemic in their first or third trimesters of gestation, and the controls born in the six preceding years, showed no increase in rate of schizophrenia. When the exposed individuals reached 30 years of age, their rate of schizophrenia was more than double the normal lifetime risk for schizophrenia.

A review of the excellent antenatal clinic records in Helsinki revealed that these "second-trimester schizophrenics" were not only exposed to the virus but that obstetrical nurses had noted that the mothers had actually suffered an influenza infection during the second trimester. The antenatal clinic files also made it possible to determine the stage of fetal development based on date of last menstruation. In previous studies, the stage of gestation was estimated from date of birth; this estimate would be thrown off by premature births, which are more numerous among schizophrenics.

These scientists then replicated their findings in a larger investigation involving all births of schizophrenics and all influenza epidemics during a 40-year period (1911-50) in Denmark. Access to data on births of schizophrenics was made possible by Denmark's Institute for Psychiatric Demography, which houses the world's most complete and accurate national psychiatric register. The scope of the study

Author	Nation	Finding
Mednick et al. 1988	Finland	Second trimester
Kendell & Kemp 1989	Scotland	Replication for females
		Replication (6th month effect)
Bowler & Torrey 1990	U.S.A.	Nonreplication
O'Callaghan et al. 1991	U.K.	Replication (6th month effect)
Kunugi et al. 1992	Japan	Replication (6th month effect)
Waddington 1992	Ireland	Replication
Crow & Done 1992	U.K.	Nonreplication
Machon & Mednick 1993	Finland	Replication (6th month effect)
Fahy et al. 1993	U.K.	Replication
Welham et al. 1993	Queensland	Replication
Kendell et al. 1993	U.K., Denmark	Replication
	Scotland	Replication
Beckmann et al. 1993	Germany	Replication

Table 32.1. Replication Tests of the Helsinki "Second Trimester" Effect.

Author	Country	Period covered	Finding
Barr et al. 1990	Denmark	40 years	Replication (6th month effect)
Sham et al. 1992	U.K.	22 years	Replication
Morris et al. 1993	Ireland	50 years	Replication (3rd trimester effect)
Takei et al. 1993	U.K.	27 years	Replication
Welham et al. 1993	Australia	3 large epidemics	Replication

Table 32.2. Replication Studies Covering Several Epidemics.

enabled the researchers to further narrow the time of viral insult to the sixth month of pregnancy. The findings of these two studies have been replicated in different parts of the world by several independent investigators (See Tables 32.1 and 32.2).

Perhaps not coincidentally, the second trimester is a critical time for development of the hippocampus, part of the brain's limbic system. Scientists have long thought that a defect in this area plays a role in schizophrenia. Now, they are using magnetic resonance imaging to see if the brains of Helsinki second-trimester schizophrenic patients show anatomical defects in the hippocampus. They are also examining 6-month-old infants of mothers who have suffered a second-trimester influenza infection to determine whether the infants are defective in neurointegrative functioning.

Chronic Fatigue Syndrome: Repeated Viral Assaults?

Major, persistent, debilitating fatigue is the hallmark symptom of chronic fatigue syndrome, a condition with no known cause or cure. Diagnosis is difficult, based more on the absence of other overlying problems that might cause fatigue, such as HIV infection or Lyme disease, than on a positive laboratory test for some pathogen. Other symptoms include sore throat, headache, chest pain, depression, and dyslogia.

Theories to explain the origins of chronic fatigue syndrome have come and gone, but recent research suggests that the condition begins with an acute viral infection. According to this theory, the initial infection, which may be an influenza-like disease, produces an immune dysfunction. This is not a full-blown immunodeficiency as seen in HIV infection, but rather a small change in the immune system. Subsequent infections—most likely by viruses other than the initial culprit—or other stressors further change the activity of the immune system. The end result is chronic fatigue syndrome.

The evidence that a viral infection has occurred is sketchy, and the literature does not give universal support to any one virus being either the initial or secondary insult. At various times, retroviruses, enteroviruses, and several herpes viruses have been linked to chronic fatigue syndrome.

Apparently strong evidence seemed to favor roles for retroviruses and enteroviruses in chronic fatigue syndrome, but recent studies of specific viruses have shown that probably neither of these virus families is involved. Double-blind experiments with an HTLV-II-like agent and a human spumavirus found that chronic fatigue syndrome patients did not differ from control subjects on the presence of virus or antiviral antibodies. Similarly, the study of appropriate controls in enteroviral assays indicates that the presence of viral RNA in muscle is not a specific property of chronic fatigue syndrome patients. Thus, the most promising viral candidates for association with chronic fatigue syndrome are currently the lymphotropic herpes viruses.

Epstein-Barr virus, a member of the herpes family, was the leading candidate in the mid-1980s considered to cause chronic fatigue syndrome. However, investigators came to the conclusion that if Epstein-Barr virus was involved in the syndrome, its involvement was not invariable. Since then, investigators have found some evidence, also not consistent, of a second herpes virus (HHV-6) in the tissues of chronic fatigue syndrome patients. These viruses share several characteristics that would be consistent with their being involved in this disorder. All, for example, produce primary infections leading to persistent infection, which can reactivate to produce another acute infection after immune system activation.

With the evidence of viral involvement equivocal at best, researchers have been asking if viruses play any role at all in chronic fatigue syndrome. While the answer is unclear, there is certainly no proof linking any one virus to the syndrome. However, the immunological evidence remains that people with chronic fatigue syndrome have more antibodies to viruses as a whole than normal individuals. One patient might have a high titer of antibodies to Epstein-Barr virus, while another may have elevated levels of antibody against HHV-6. The numbers of certain subtypes of antibodies and natural killer cells are frequently lower than normal in chronic fatigue syndrome patients. However, since no single measure of immune system status is consistently changed in all patients, researchers are being forced to look further, at cytokine levels, for example, for the underlying cause of this disorder.

A Compromise Response

When cells in the periphery become infected with a virus, the most common response is for the immune system to attack those cells, kill them, and clear them from the body. This is less of an option in the central nervous system, because killed neurons would not be replaced. Evidence suggests instead that the virus is merely inactivated in infected neurons, but at the cost of always having a virus' genetic material present in those cells.

Studies of the **Sindbis virus** provide support for such a compromise. Sindbis belongs to a family of viruses that are spread by mosquitoes and cause encephalitis. These viruses infect mostly neurons, providing investigators with the opportunity to study the immune response that follows a neural infection within the central nervous system. Upon inoculation into mice, Sindbis virus replicates throughout the brain, and an immune system response occurs. Adult mice recover within a week with little evidence of neuronal damage, while newborn mice suffer major nerve cell destruction and die within three to four days after infection. Because the virus is the same in both cases, the key to this problem must lie in the neurons themselves.

Investigators suspected that a particular gene might be involved in protecting mature neurons. This gene codes for a protein, found in the inner membrane of mitochondria (part of the cell), that by some unknown mechanism inhibits the normal neuronal death that occurs during the later stages of brain development. When inserted into cultured cells that would otherwise die from Sindbis infection, the gene protects the cells from death, though the virus itself is not killed. In fact, the virus continues to replicate in the protected cells, albeit at a low level, and the infection remains persistent for months, during which time the cultured cells continue growing and dividing. Researchers are now looking for evidence of differential gene expression in mouse neurons as well as for the function of this protein.

The other mystery with Sindbis virus is that genetically inbred mice that lack T- and B-lymphocytes do not show any symptoms of Sindbis encephalitis, though they develop a persistent infection in the nervous system. T-lymphocytes infused into these mice do not clear virus from infected neurons. This may happen because neurons do not express antigen-presenting MHC class-I or MHC class-II molecules on their cell surfaces to signal the need for T-lymphocytes.

What does seem to have an effect on the virus is adding antibodies removed from normal mice that have previously recovered from Sindbis infection. These antibodies seem to suppress viral replication in infected cells, though the mechanism involved is unclear. What is known is that the antibodies get inside infected neurons. In addition, viral gene expression continues at low levels in infected neurons, even those treated with antibodies that can prevent active viral production or those removed from normal adult mice that had recovered from the infection. Using a new technique that allows amplification of genes in cells, researchers have recently found single copies of other viral genomes in latently infected neurons.

From these results, investigators have postulated that neurons can protect themselves from death only at the expense of maintaining a store of suppressed viral genetic material. B-lymphocytes, producing antibodies against key viral antigens, keep viral replication suppressed for the life of the animal, which might explain why many antiviral antibodies remain in the central nervous system for life—they may be necessary to prevent latent virus from reactivating. If this eternal vigilance fails, the virus may once again appear, which could be a mechanism by which some conditions, such as **postpolio syndrome**, reappear long after recovery from the original viral infection.

Establishing Infection

The development of viral latency has three stages:

• establishment,
• maintenance, and
• reactivation.

Investigators have found evidence that the first step is a function of the neuron itself. This was shown using a strain of **herpes simplex virus** that lacks a key regulatory gene. This mutation renders the virus harmless; though it infects neurons, killing a few, it does not kill the animal and will not produce new viruses. To the surprise of investigators studying this mutant, it does establish a latent infection within neurons but without expressing any of its own genome. For some reason, certain neurons not all will take in viruses and incorporate their genomes into their own. This mysterious process is now under active study.

Another virus that establishes latent infection in neurons is the **varicella zoster virus**. It causes chicken pox during initial infection and can reactivate to produce **shingles, zoster**, or **postherpetic neuralgia**, a condition of long-term debilitating pain. Unlike herpes simplex virus, which is harbored in sensory neurons, varicella zoster virus hides in the satellite cells that surround sensory neurons. Another difference is that latent herpes simplex virus expresses only one gene when it is incorporated in the host genome, while varicella zoster expresses several genes. Investigators are now studying these genes to determine their role in the latency and reactivation processes.

Some viruses persistently infect neurons and remain active at all times, rather than entering a latent stage. One example is **Theiler's virus**, a common virus in mice. This virus enters brain tissue and remains active there for the lifetime of the host, producing a demyelination syndrome. The virus also infects other organs, but the immune system clears the virus from those locations within a few weeks.

Neural Damage Through the Production of Free Radicals

Many neurotropic viruses indirectly kill neurons by inducing cell-mediated immune responses in the central nervous system. For example, **Borna disease virus (BDV)**, which primarily affects horses and sheep but also might infect humans, stimulates an immune response that inadvertently causes neural damage. At the peak of infection, tremendous tissue damage occurs, which investigators have correlated with levels of expression of proinflammatory cytokines, including interleukin-T, interleukin-6, and tumor necrosis factor-α. The expression of these cytokines coincides with the peak levels of enzymatic activity for inducible nitric oxide synthase (iNOS) in the brain, supporting the notion that certain cytokines may produce central nervous system damage by stimulating macrophages or resident microglia to produce free radicals such as nitric oxide.

During the disease process initiated by BDV, the activity of iNOS dramatically rises in brain regions where viral RNA expression occurs. The correlation of iNOS expression with the development of neurological signs in Borna disease, as well as enhanced expression within brain regions with inflammatory lesions, may indicate that the production of nitric oxide as a toxic substance contributes to virus-induced neural damage.

The action of nitric oxide, however, is paradoxical; it can be neurodestructive as well as neuroprotective. **Nitric oxide-mediated neurotoxicity** is engendered by reaction with the superoxide anion that leads to the formation of peroxynitrite, a highly reactive oxidizing agent capable of causing tissue damage. The recent finding that expression of xanthine oxidase, which provides a source of superoxide anions, is also highly upregulated in the brain during Borna disease, supports the concept that free radicals such as nitric oxide may mediate virus-induced neurodegeneration.

Preliminary studies of compounds that either inhibit nitric oxide synthase or scavenge nitric oxide show that a reduction of nitric oxide concentration decreases the severity of BDV infection as measured by the loss of body weight. If further studies confirm these findings, investigators would have a new lead to therapeutic strategies that might ameliorate the effects of neurotropic viruses.

Lentiviruses: Infectious Chameleons

HIV is a member of the lentivirus family, whose members all cause diseases that involve infection of macrophages and microglial cells within the central nervous system. Lentiviruses are capable of replicating in nondividing, terminally differentiated cells, unlike other RNA viruses that can only grow in dividing cells. This suggests that lentiviruses may have a unique set of the genes required for growth and replication genes normally active in growing cells but quiescent in terminally differentiated cells that would be good targets for intervention. Such intervention could involve blocking the expression of those genes or interfering with the function of the gene products.

Lentiviruses are also species specific, suggesting that they require specific host cell proteins in the early stages of viral replication. In addition, lentiviruses express significant genetic diversity once infection has occurred. However, investigators have found that those viruses that go to the brain may have a much narrower genetic diversity than do those that infect tissues outside the central nervous system.

In addition to regulatory genes, all lentiviruses have auxiliary genes that are not required for growth in tissue culture but are necessary for infection *in vivo* and pathogenesis. Some investigators now believe that these viruses, over the course of their evolution, have acquired genes from their hosts that are critically involved in disease progression. These genes may have little in common structurally, but they are similar functionally across all members of the lentivirus family. As such, understanding their role in the viral life-cycle may prove important in understanding the pathogenicity of these viruses.

Using the simian immunodeficiency virus as a model, investigators have begun probing the role of genetic heterogeneity in an AIDS-like disease. The researchers started with a variant of this virus that only infected T-lymphocytes and did not enter the central nervous system. As this virus progressed from one animal to another, its cell-type specificity broadened, first to include macrophages, then eventually to include brain and lung tissue. Accompanying this evolution were changes in two regions of the viral genome. One of these regions coded for viral envelope proteins, which determine the virus's ability to enter a given cell. The other was a regulatory region that controls viral replication once it has infected a cell. These changes were relatively minor, but they were enough to enable the virus to cross the blood-brain barrier, perhaps via infection of endothelial cells, and enter and replicate in neurons.

Human Immunodeficiency Virus

Two key targets of HIV are the immune system and the brain. Not surprisingly, then, individuals with AIDS often show neurobehavioral symptoms in addition to profound immunological deficiencies. However, HIV's effects on the brain and the immune system are not independent of one another. To begin with, HIV appears to enter the brain in infected monocytes/macrophages. In addition, the brain and immune system are linked by a variety of neural and hormonal signals, some of which may be altered by HIV infection.

Autopsy studies have found that the majority of AIDS patients have HIV infecting the central nervous system. However, only a fraction of AIDS patients develop what is known as AIDS dementia complex, characterized by progressive impairment of motor and cognitive functions. The possibility exists, however, that HIV may exert physiologic effects in the brain, via the many connections between the brain and immune system, that influence the course of the systemic infection without impairing brain function.

During the early stages of HIV infection, few if any symptoms of neurological damage are evident. But even then, neuropsychologists can often measure subtle deterioration in thought processes, including reasoning, memory, and reaction time, and patients themselves report slight problems in performing everyday tasks. In this stage, neuropsychological testing may be more sensitive than neuroimaging (such as magnetic resonance imaging scans) in identifying the early and often mild effects of damage in the central nervous system. Recent studies of HIV infection have found a loss of large neurons in the cortex, the brain region involved in many cognitive functions. Other studies have reported that the density of neuron-to-neuron connections is reduced in HIV-infected brain tissue.

Recently, investigators have found that a portion of the HIV's coat protein is toxic to some animal neurons *in vitro*. This protein, called gp120, appears to affect the flow of calcium ions out of neurons, which can cause cell death. This suggests that drugs that block calcium flow might prevent this toxic effect. Researchers are also finding that other viral proteins can alter immune cell function. One protein, known as gp41, stimulates antibody production by B-lymphocytes. This might explain why many AIDS patients develop **hypergammaglobu-linemia**—a nonspecific activation of B-lymphocytes that then produce large amounts of immunoglobulin with no protective influence. Another viral protein, called gag, inhibits *in vitro* lymphocyte and natural killer cell activity, an effect countered by interleukin-2.

Summary

The past 15 years have seen a renewed focus on the role that viruses can play in producing neurobehavioral disorders, and as a result, it is now clear that viruses infect the central nervous system, damage neurons, and trigger a host of physiological changes in both the nervous system and the periphery. Many of these changes appear to involve the links between the brain and the immune system, and thus viruses are proving to be useful tools in further probing these connections. Learning more about the mechanisms by which viruses interact with the central nervous system will certainly provide new insights into many areas of brain function, including gene expression in neurons, the cross-talk between cytokines and neuropeptides, and development and organization of neural networks within the brain.

Recommendations for the Future

- Determine whether viruses are involved in the etiology of mental disorders and chronic diseases of the nervous system; investigate human populations that have been prenatally exposed to viral infections.

- Elucidate brain-specific mechanisms regulating viral replication: tropism, need for viral diversity for infection, latency, activation, and cellular factors continuing viral infection in the brain.

- Determine whether lack of particular immune reactions in the brain may permit propagation of viruses and other pathogens in this organ.

- Analyze how the interaction of the nervous system and the endocrine axis in the immune system determine susceptibility to particular outcomes of virus infection.

- Study viral pathogenesis in animal models to evaluate the differential effects of viruses on the adult and developing nervous system.

- Develop an understanding of how astrocytosis and microgliosis relate to pathological states caused by viruses in adult and developmental models.

- Study the effects of common, mild viral infection on behavior and behavioral adaptations that help to avoid or fight infections.

Further Reading

Price, R.W., and Perry, S.W., ed. *HIV, AIDS, and the Brain.* New York: Raven Press, 1994.

Life, death and the immune system. *Scientific American* Special Issue 269:52-144, Sept. 1993.

Chapter 33

Technical Opportunities and Problems

"Science plus public-health needs equal opportunities."
—Frederick K. Goodwin

Many consider this period in scientific history to be the Age of Biology, when biological knowledge has reached that critical mass that suddenly propels all fields forward at breakneck speeds. Much of this newfound wisdom and intellectual energy has been made possible by the development of new tools—ranging from the polymerase chain reaction to high-field magnetic resonance imaging—that investigators now have at their disposal. The technical advances embodied in these tools are themselves a product of the Age of Biology, and certainly, further knowledge will only lead to newer, more powerful tools, which will, in turn, propel understanding of biological systems even faster.

Not that these advances will be a panacea. Often, new information, gathered with new tools, raises more questions than it answers. For example, new analytical techniques now enable investigators to detect and measure minute amounts of biologically active substances, such as cytokines or neuropeptides. But finding these substances in increasing numbers of places in the body tells little about what role these substances may be playing, if any, in a particular tissue. Likewise, immunologists have developed ever more sophisticated measures of immune cell activity *in vitro*. However, the relevance of *in vitro* activity to an *in vivo* immune response is not necessarily clear. Thus, investigators not only have to learn what to do with new tools,

NIH Pub No. 94-3774.

but also must determine the proper interpretation of the data they may be able to gather with such technological advances.

In this context, the National Institute of Mental Health's advisory panels on psychoneuroimmunology and neurovirology were asked to identify key technical opportunities, methodological problems, and potential breakthroughs in knowledge that are emerging now and will mature over the next five to ten years.

A Need for Functional Anatomy

A key piece of information needed to better understand the links between the nervous and immune systems is the circuitry that connects them. Amazingly enough, very little is known about these anatomic and biochemical connections. For example, substance P is known largely as a sensory neurotransmitter, that is, it is a neurotransmitter in sensory neurons. However, there are substance P-containing neurons in the autonomic nervous system that innervate the spleen, though not much is known about the function of these neurons.

It is far from easy to trace neural and biochemical circuits through the body. Many biochemicals, for example, are able to diffuse a considerable distance through the intracellular matrix from their point of release. Therefore, localizing a store of neurohormone, for example, does not always pinpoint those neurons or immune system cells where that substance acts. Therefore, mapping studies must include efforts to determine the distribution of both biologically active substances and their receptors.

A Possible Vector Into the Brain

Investigators studying the interaction between neurons and the **herpes simplex virus** have discovered a mutant virus that establishes a latent infection in neurons but does not replicate in or kill these cells. The mutant virus is called the **HSV4-minus virus**. In addition, the virus only infects neurons. Even though this virus is not pathogenic, it does incorporate itself permanently into neuronal DNA. Thus, this variant of herpes simplex is the first nonpathogenic virus known to target nerve cells and could serve as a vector for delivering genes into the nervous system.

One useful trait of this virus is that it can carry relatively large amounts of extra DNA into a cell. It may be possible, then, to incorporate not only structural genes that code for one or more proteins, but also the natural regulatory genes that control the expression of the structural genes. The structural genes that scientists would want to increase the "dosage" of are, for example, those encoding proteins that increase the survival of aging neurons.

Model tests, using a reporter gene coupled to a regulatory segment from another gene, showed that the recombinant virus latently infects spinal neurons. Furthermore, the reporter gene does turn on, and the infected cells do make reporter gene product for extended periods of time. Currently, investigators are working to couple the gene for nerve growth factor with a regulator gene and inserting the combination into HSV4-minus. Augmenting nerve growth factor in neurons could perhaps help protect neurons against the damage associated with Alzheimer's disease and other neurodegenerative disorders.

The stumbling block at present is finding a promoter element that will remain active when the viral infection passes from the acute to the latent stage. Investigators working with these viruses believe that there are no theoretical constraints; they just have not found the correct combination of promoter and placement within the viral genome.

Mouse Model for Studying HIV Gene Expression

As its name implies, the human immunodeficiency virus only grows in humans, presenting a challenge to investigators looking for weaknesses in the virus' defenses against elimination. Using the techniques of genetic engineering, investigators have inserted several of HIV's regulatory genes into mouse nerve cells and are now attempting to determine what molecular events trigger expression of these genes and how these genes' products affect cells that make them.

The investigators were interested in how changes in promoter elements might affect replication of HIV in the central nervous system, so they inserted into the mouse genome a reporter gene coupled to promoters from three different HIV strains—one that only infected T-lymphocytes and two that were isolated from brain and cerebrospinal fluid of a patient who died with AIDS dementia. They can now use these transgenic mice to study the molecular events that lead to HIV activation.

Early experiments showed that the promoter region taken from the HIV strain that only infects lymphocytes did not turn on in brain cells. This suggests that a virus' apparent tissue specificity, or tropism, involves more than its ability or inability to infect a particular type of cell. Indeed, a virus with a narrow tropism may infect many cell types, but its genome may then fail to express itself once the infection process is complete. In this case, some molecular factor in neurons, as opposed to lymphocytes, may be preventing the promoter taken from a lymphocyte-tropic HIV strain from working outside of its normal environment.

In contrast, promoters from the two neurotropic strains did express in brain cells, and were most active in areas rich in neurons, such as the hippocampus and the nuclei of the visual system. Regional patterns of expression between the two neurotropic strains differed.

Investigators pursing these leads are now hoping to identify the factors that influence gene expression in different strains of HIV and to determine which regions in regulatory genes are activated. In this way, they hope to uncover the cellular factors in the central nervous system that are important for activating latent HIV. This information may, in turn, suggest ways of shutting down the transcriptional process, and thus, the virus' pathogenicity.

A New Kind of Genetic Analysis

A standard method of separating proteins from a mixture is to apply a sample to a gel and electrophoretically separate the proteins in two dimensions. Now, the same principle has been applied to nucleic acid fragments. In two-dimensional "electrophoretic genetics," nucleic acid fragments are separated in the first dimension according to fragment size and in the second dimension according to sequence through the use of a chemical denaturing agent. This technique can simultaneously separate thousands of nucleic acid fragments covering millions of base pairs. The difference between fragments can be as small as a single nucleic acid.

As a result, investigators will be able to more easily study genetic polymorphism—the natural variation across individuals of a species or even across cells within the same individual—that occurs in the base-pair sequence of a particular gene. When combined with amplification techniques, such as polymerase chain reaction, two-dimensional electrophoretic genetics will enable investigators to study gene expression in individual cells.

Using this new technique, investigators should be able to map multigene defects that are implicated in many mental diseases. The exquisite single-nucleotide resolution should also make it possible to look for mutations involved in producing changes seen in nerve degeneration and aging. In addition, it should now be much easier to study the genomic rearrangement that occurs as part of the maturation of both B-lymphocytes and T-lymphocytes and may, if recent experiments are confirmed, also occur in the nervous system during neuronal differentiation. This technique may also prove to be a complete way of looking at total cellular gene expression.

The ability to examine genetic expression in single cells should be a boon to investigators, for it should enable them to discover whether viral and cellular genes are being expressed in single cells in a particular disease state. Researchers will also be able to examine individual neurons and glia to look for evidence of viral latency in regions of the brain that are relevant to a particular disease.

In Situ *Polymerase Chain Reaction*

In the 1980s, molecular biologists developed a powerful method for making millions of copies of nucleic acid fragments from as little as one copy, thus providing a way of "amplifying" DNA and RNA. This technique, known as polymerase chain reaction (PCR), enables investigators to study the genetic makeup of single cells and is proving to be a powerful new tool for finding viral DNA incorporated into neurons and immune cells. In fact, researchers have already used PCR to detect HIV *in situ* in individual lymphocytes and macrophages.

In the past, latent viral genomes, such as those of HIV, herpes simplex, and other neurotropic viruses, have been invisible, both to the cell and to biologists searching for evidence of infection. That is no longer true, because PCR enables investigators to make millions of copies of a single cell's genetic material and then probe this relatively vast quantity of material for viral DNA using standard gene probes; these probes are not capable of identifying a single copy of a nucleic acid fragment.

Combining PCR with immunocytochemistry, a technique called *in situ* PCR, will enable investigators to visualize these cells in tissues as opposed to isolating the cells and testing them *in vitro*. This can have several applications. Detecting mRNA produced from viral genes will give investigators insight into the processes of latency and reactivation by allowing them to identify those gene products necessary for the various stages of the viral life-cycle. In addition, *in situ* PCR will identify types of cells that are infected with a virus, providing information about the ways different cell types restrict/permit viral expression. PCR-amplified mRNA, in combination with two-dimensional electrophoretic genetics, can also aid in the phenotypic characterization of individual neurons and immune cells by providing a fingerprint of a cell's genetic expression.

Problems with Reproducibility

Often, when a new technique spreads throughout the scientific community, each investigator personalizes the method to reflect the instruments and reagents at hand. Though these changes may seem minor, they can introduce confounding factors that can make comparisons among laboratories difficult if not meaningless. This seems particularly true with both neurochemical and immunological measures, many of which attempt to quantify small differences in naturally variable systems. To address this problem, a number of scientists have suggested that standards be developed for various neurochemical and immunological assays against which all researchers could compare their results.

Such an effort has been started with cytokines. The National Institutes of Health has had a longstanding program for exchanging reference reagents. A researcher can, for example, obtain a reference standard of interleukin-2 with which activity of laboratory samples can be compared.

Another problem in assessing immunological variables is that differences in the overall state of an animal's health may have a greater effect on immune cell activity, cytokine levels, and other measures than any experimental manipulations. Animal care facilities are well maintained, but it is impossible to have each facility exactly as clean as all others. Such variations could confound some inter-laboratory comparisons, even those done on the same strain of inbred mice with the same reagents.

Recommendations for the Future

- Create animal models that recapitulate some signs and symptoms of psychiatric disorders.

- Define molecules that reflect brain-immune interactions to study the linkages between these systems and behavior.

- Study immunodeficient mutant mice with characterized genetic defects to determine whether common genes control functioning of the central nervous and immune systems or whether defects in the immune system then affect the central nervous system.

- Develop methods for physiologically (as opposed to genetically) knocking out certain specific cell types, hormones, or cytokines.

- Develop stable lines of phenotypically homogeneous, terminally differentiated neurons, suppressor T cells, microglial cells, and astrocytes that approximate the normal cells.

- Establish standard assays *in vivo* and *in vitro* to evaluate mechanisms of neuronal damage and destruction with a goal of identifying specific molecular pathways that mediate neuronal damage and correlating the damage with electrical, physiological, and behavioral dysfunction.

- Develop stable, covalent receptor ligands that would permit not only identification, but perhaps modulation of these receptors.

- Establish banks of rapidly obtained tissues and sera from humans with viral infections (e.g., HIV-1, CMV, HSV, HZV, enteroviruses, measles, shingles) accompanied by medical histories, cognitive evaluations, and routine pathological stains of tissue sections.

- Analyze the presence and functional significance of sexual dimorphism at critical points of neuroendocrinimmune circuits.

Chapter 34

New Perspectives

Over the past decade or so, investigators in a host of disciplines have been generating new, exciting findings about the many links between the nervous system and the immune system. As this knowledge base grows, it becomes increasingly clear that understanding the physical connections between these two systems, as well as the barriers that keep them separate, has tremendous implications for improving human health. Already, the field of psychoneuroimmunology has generated novel therapies, both behavioral and biochemical, that are being tested in humans. One example is the use of social support therapy to help patients combat breast cancer. Another example is a current trial using nonsteroidal anti-inflammatory agents in treating Alzheimer's disease. Many more are in the pipeline for future clinical trials.

Despite the tremendous strides forward, more is unknown than known about the two-way interactions between the body's two great integrative systems, the nervous system and the immune system. At the molecular level, investigators are almost overwhelmed by the dozens of chemicals that pass messages among the different components of these two systems. Researchers speak of a "unified field theory of chemical communication," one that would reveal the common mechanism used by hormones, neurotransmitters, neuropeptides, cytokines, and their receptors. It is hoped that such a unified theory would make sense of the seeming redundancy and overlap among the various chemical messengers and uncover new avenues for therapy.

NIH Pub No. 94-3774.

At the cellular level, scientists are struggling to sort out the roles that the various cell types play in mediating interactions between the two systems. In at least some ways, neural cells resemble immune cells in both function and form, suggesting a common evolutionary beginning. Both classes of cells have the ability to form memories of experiences of the world outside the organism, a property that is seemingly unique among these cells of the body.

At the behavioral level, the meeting ground between the outside and the inside worlds, researchers are more certain than ever that common mechanisms exist to translate experience into action, whether it be the firing of a neuron or the activation of an immune cell. Then again, they are perhaps more uncertain about what those mechanisms may be. What is undeniable, though, is the tremendous variety and richness in the way the body translates stress, be it immunological or psychological, into biochemical actions intended to protect the body from harm. On occasion, these biochemical actions can have the exact opposite effect, causing illness. Again, elucidating these mechanisms, and their weaknesses, offers the promise of great therapeutic advances.

This promise, as well as the formidable intellectual challenge, pushes investigators to answer these and other questions. The challenge is so great because, by themselves, the nervous and immune systems are incredibly complex. Each is a hierarchical system in which the various components are able to receive data from several sources, analyze them in an integrative way, and produce an action that represents more than just the sum of individual molecular and cellular events. Then, these two systems coordinate their actions in yet another integrative interpretation of incoming data, producing a situation that is many orders of magnitude more complex than if one were simply studying the actions of one cell or one neural circuit.

A good example of this complexity is the remarkably redundant network by which stressful events suppress a variety of immune responses. This network has multiple pathways by which the same effects on these immune responses are mediated. The network effectively preserves this suppressive response in the face of a variety of situations that might block one particular pathway or another. Evidently, this response is somehow important to the organism, as indicated by the power and redundancy built into the network. Studying one pathway in this network may provide a coherent picture of the relationship between stress and immune responsiveness, but it would in no way be the complete picture.

Development and Function

Because the nervous and immune systems have so much in common, investigators hope to gain some insights into the mechanisms they share by comparing how these two systems developed throughout evolution. One hypothesis holds that these two systems began with the evolution and diversification of the family of genes that control immunoglobulin, or antibody, formation. There are hundreds of members of this family. Parts of these genes are conserved throughout the family, while other segments are variable, enabling the system to interact quickly with a wide range of foreign proteins and other molecules that are not identified as self. The gene products themselves are unique because they resist the actions of enzymes that degrade most proteins, making them suitable for their role of sitting on the outside of cells and mediating intracellular communication. As evolution proceeded, this family of genes diversified, producing many key molecules, such as receptors, in both the immune and nervous systems.

Another evolutionary avenue may have led to the development of the genes for the major histocompatibility complex and other recognition molecules thought to play key roles in both the immune and nervous system. In the immune system, recognition molecules and cell adhesion molecules are central to the separation of self from non-self and for directing the immune response. In the nervous system, such molecules are thought to control the development of the brain itself by controlling the migration of neurons and glia and the formation of connections between neurons. Understanding the development of such a complex cell-recognition system has great importance in understanding the functions of both the immune and the nervous systems and should provide new insights into shared features and common mechanisms.

Multiple Pathways

Another common feature of the nervous and immune systems is that of multiplicity. At the system level, there are usually multiple pathways by which a given action, be it an immune or behavioral response, can occur. Indeed, many pathways seem to connect these two systems, as shown by how the effects of stress are transmitted from brain to immune system and back. At the molecular level, both neurons and immune cells are able to integrate multiple chemical signals into an eventual action. In fact, it takes many chemical signals to fully activate a lymphocyte, just as it takes many incoming neurotransmitter and neuropeptide signals, some stimulatory and others inhibitory, to fully activate a neuron.

Much is unknown about these different levels of multiplicity. Investigators have found some of the common mechanisms and duplicate systems. However, no one believes that they have found all the mediators—be they cytokines, neurotransmitters and neuropeptides, or hormones—and the receptors for these substances used by the two systems. Nor have they uncovered all the neural and hormonal pathways that connect the brain and immune system. A key effort, then, must be to identify all the actors involved in this complex dance within each system and between the two.

Researchers also face the task of sorting out genesis and function of these molecules and receptors. When immunologists first discovered cytokines, their initial idea was that one cell type would make one class of cytokine-lymphocytes would make lymphokines, monocytes would secrete monokines, and so on—which would then act on another particular cell type, regulating one particular gene. Today, they know that this is wrong and that there is tremendous overlap in the production of cytokines, the targets they activate, and the actions that result from those interactions. Despite this duplication, it appears that common pathways, mediated by so-called second messengers operating inside cells, translate cytokine binding to a target cell to that cell's activation. Therefore, understanding these second-messenger systems could help unscramble some of the confusion resulting from the overwhelming number of molecules and pathways that investigators are now characterizing.

The same can be said of the nervous system. For example, investigators have found that in one small section of the frontal cortex, a subset of astrocytes expresses the gene for interleukin-1, others express transforming growth factor beta one, a third subset expresses both genes, and a fourth type expresses neither one of these cytokines. Such findings raise the questions: What makes this heterogeneity? What controls it? Is this heterogeneity biologically significant, or is it just an artifact of researchers' inability to subtly probe and detect small amounts of cytokines in some cells in the functioning central nervous system?

In Vitro *Versus* In Vivo

As in most areas of biological research, investigators carry out the majority of their experiments by isolating a process under study *in vitro.* Whereas working *in vitro* is certainly necessary, the problem is to interpret these results in relation to other processes occurring simultaneously *in vivo.* In other words, does a change in T-lymphocyte activation detected by a particular *in vitro* assay have anything to do with a change in the body's ability to fight a pathogen that the body was exposed to before the T-lymphocytes were isolated?

The answer to this question is currently unclear, but this concern for biological relevance is constantly nagging those researchers who study complex systems such as the immune and nervous systems. These investigators are well aware that *in vitro* studies are essential for elucidating possible physiological mechanisms, but they also know that it is critical to continually check these results against biologically relevant human health outcomes, such as the ability to ward off an infection. It is now clear, for example, that the immune system is relatively stable; that is, it takes a number of factors to trigger its activity. Thus, the relevance of any one change measured by an *in vitro* assay is unclear, and placing too much importance on one such measure may take research down the wrong path.

In fact, this is a major problem in psychoneuroimmunological research. So many variables are changing at any one time in either the brain or immune system, let alone in both at the same time, that it is extraordinarily difficult to understand how the individual pieces fit together. There is a critical need to find ways of both integrating individual findings and studying multiple physiological events at the same time.

Fortunately, there are ways of approaching these complex problems. Breakthroughs in molecular biology and genetics offer researchers the opportunity to alter entire systems at once with various genetic lesions. For example, a genetically altered strain of mouse that lacks those lymphocytes that respond to antigens provides investigators with the ability to study other parts of the immune system with one fewer confounding factor. Antisense genetic probes, which can bind to and inactivate targeted mRNA, thereby knocking out a specific protein from key biochemical processes, provides investigators with a new probe of that protein's function. Similarly, chemical agents capable of destroying specific peripheral neural circuits allow researchers to probe subtle, but widespread, changes in immune function that may occur as a result of such neuronal cell loss. These studies may also identify redundant systems that were previously unknown.

But such studies must again be brought back to issues concerning biologically meaningful outcomes, for example, those relating to human health. One way of doing that would be to examine patients with

351

rare neurological, immunological, or psychological disorders for some of the same genetic or biochemical defects being studied in animals. These patients may offer researchers unique opportunities to connect animal models to human disease states.

The key to all of these efforts is to remember that no one technique will provide all answers to all questions. Instead, investigators need to take a variety of approaches, getting as much information as they can from intact animals, isolated organs, cultured cell lines, and disassociated receptors. Multidisciplinary research such as this requires a broader knowledge base than many scientists now possess; it is difficult at best to keep up with results and techniques used by one's peers. Thus, it may be necessary to create new modes of training researchers, enabling them to learn about advances made by researchers outside their limited disciplines. At the same time, investigators must remember that what happens *in vitro* or even in the most cleverly designed animal model may not hold true in humans. This is probably most true when it comes to studying behavior, for it is extremely difficult to develop animal analogs that truly represent some human behaviors. To accomplish this, investigators will have to determine what processes need to be modeled and then try to create animals with those traits. Again, those with the broadest knowledge of techniques developed across the biological sciences will have the greatest chance of developing such models.

Extreme Versus Moderate Stimuli

Perhaps the hallmark of the majority of complex biological systems is their ability to respond to subtle changes in their surroundings. This is particularly true of both the immune and the nervous systems. Yet it is beyond the ability of most experiments, particularly those done *in vivo*, to recreate subtle stimuli whose effects can be measured. For example, many important studies involve knocking out the particular genes or even entire neural circuits—the former with antisense probes, the latter with neurohormone toxins—and measuring the effect on an animal's health. Certainly, those studies are important, and they may even provide insights into some human disorders. However, it is likely that most human maladies result from slightly abnormal changes in the normal response, and these "brute force" experiments may not help get at the root cause of these maladies.

Another aspect of this problem is the difficulty researchers have in measuring minute quantities of biochemicals *in vivo*, or administering physiologically important concentrations of such compounds into biologically relevant regions of the brain. This is a particular concern when studying such potent compounds as cytokines and neurotransmitters. In all likelihood, these compounds are produced close to where they act. Therefore, infusing cytokines into the cerebrospinal fluid may produce biological effects that have no bearing on real circumstances simply because the effects of flooding the brain with a cytokine might overwhelm small, but real, biological effects. However, as biological techniques improve, investigators will be able to measure smaller, more localized effects, and most believe that further advances will soon enable investigators to conduct such experiments on a physiologically relevant scale.

Defining Stress

Stress has become chief psychological variable in the field of psychoneuroimmunology, and the effects of stress on immune competence have provided some of the most compelling evidence supporting the link between the brain and immune system. But stress is a broad, inexact concept, with no firm definition. As a result, many investigators in the field are concerned that without a standard definition of stress, it is difficult at best to compare results from different experiments and laboratories.

For example, stress can be chronic or acute. It can be physical or psychological. What is stressful for one animal might not be for another, in the same way that some humans cope better with stress than others. Investigators themselves are now trying to cope with the stress of not having good operational definitions of stress.

Some say that the problem with stress is that the biological response has nothing to do with the stressor itself, but rather with an animal's characteristic way of coping with the stressor. In some situations, the coping response might be activation of the hypothalamic-pituitary-adrenal axis, whereas in a different situation—or even the same situation at a different time in the animal's life—the response might involve suppression of the sympathetic nervous system.

Measuring Appropriate Behaviors

An equally pressing problem involves deciding what behaviors are appropriate to study in the context of psychoneuroimmunology. Behavior can be affected by factors that are only indirectly affected by stress or illness. A sick or stressed animal, for instance, may not eat, and nutritional imbalances may affect behavior. Sophisticated behaviors are often influenced by sensory, motor, or motivational deficits, common sequelae of various infections.

Often, researchers use learning as a behavior that they can alter with some experimental paradigm. But learning may, in fact, be extremely insensitive to manipulation because it is so important to the survival of an animal; one that cannot learn where to find food will soon die. Instead, a more useful measure, though one that will take more resources to acquire, might be to simply observe an animal throughout the day in its acclimated environment and see how various manipulations change those overall behavior patterns.

Gender Differences

Physicians have long noted profound gender differences in the occurrence of many disorders, but particularly autoimmune diseases—an indication that hormonal differences may affect those disease processes. Yet few investigators account for or use sex as an experimental variable, and thus they may be missing an important opportunity, for sex hormones are one of the best understood and most easily manipulated systems in biology. Changing levels of sex hormones early in development, for example, can have profound influences on neuronal organization and thus could serve as an important, well-defined probe for neuroscientists and immunologists.

Some responses are independent of gender, while others are not. Probing these differences may provide important clues to mechanisms involved in communicating within and between the nervous and immune systems. It is also important to relate sexual dimorphism to human illness in order to shed light on how sex hormones may affect response to immunological or neurological stimuli. Ultimately, better understanding in this largely unexplored area may lead to more effective therapeutic approaches to various illnesses.

Therapeutic Possibilities

There is tremendous excitement among those studying the interface between the brain and immune system as they see their research offering new approaches to disease therapy. Recently, for example, investigators found that the hormone prolactin enhances the immune response and have evidence implying that this hormone may aggravate autoimmune diseases. This suggests that a drug blocking prolactin's effects on the immune system may benefit sufferers of multiple sclerosis or rheumatoid arthritis. Similarly, researchers now believe that excess cytokine production may be producing some, if not all, neurobehavioral symptoms associated with AIDS. Since α-melanocyte-stimulating hormone is known to block the effects of cytokines in the central nervous system, it might be possible to use this natural peptide to ameliorate at least one set of symptoms of this devastating disease. With the discovery that the complement system may be involved in producing the cell death associated with Alzheimer's disease, investigators are now searching for drugs that can block this pathogenic mechanism in the central nervous system.

Examples such as these, though just the beginning of the process of moving from discovery to clinical use, have encouraged researchers to begin thinking of likely targets for intervention. High on the list of many investigators are the autoimmune diseases, since many neurochemically and immunologically important mechanisms involved in these diseases have already been identified. Efforts to target key receptors and chemical mediators involved in these illnesses are already underway.

As researchers learn more about the genes and receptors involved in certain disorders, it may be possible to develop ways of controlling the expression of those genes and receptors. Antisense RNAs, which bind to messenger RNA and block the translation of genetic information into protein, may prove to be useful drugs. So, too, might antibodies or other compounds that bind to particular receptors or regulatory proteins.

Behavioral Interventions

Since behavior affects immunity, it is likely that behavioral intervention could provide a relatively simple and inexpensive method of augmenting the immune response when needed. Already, investigators have shown that social support boosts immunity against various viral infections and also prolongs survival in certain cancer patients. The old expression, "Take two aspirin and call me in the morning" might become "Take two aspirin and call your best friend right now."

What is needed to corroborate these results are long-term longitudinal studies that carefully examine the effect of behavioral therapy by itself or in combination with pharmacological interventions. The recent finding that the placebo effect is larger than previously thought highlights the urgency of this matter. Only with further study, which will require significant commitment of time and money, can the likely benefits of behavioral therapies be realized and used with confidence.

An increasing number of Americans are already convinced that the mind can hold significant control over the rest of the body. These everyday citizens, many highly educated, are turning to alternative forms of medicine that promote the use of behavioral adjustments as a means of maintaining health. It behooves the research community to assess these therapies, for if they work, not only will new avenues of research open up for further studying the interactions between the nervous and immune systems, but all people will benefit.

Recommendations for the Future

There is little doubt that uncovering the connections between the brain and immune systems is one of the foremost challenges of the medical sciences, one that will require the best and brightest applying all their combined knowledge. Already, interdisciplinary teams of scientists have made important discoveries of how HIV, for example, attacks cells in the brain, goes dormant, and becomes activated again by cytokines; how the body's stress response system influences and is influenced by he immune system; and how cognitive therapy can induce changes in biochemical functions that then prolong survival of patients with cancer. Investigators have discovered a few of the many forms of cross-talk between the body's two great integrative systems, and they are learning that there may be a unified form of chemical communication that operates throughout the body. Perhaps as importantly, with each of these discoveries, researchers are breaking down the intellectual barriers that once kept apart the many disciplines that today form psychoneuroimmunology.

Yet these are just beginnings that have aroused the curiosity of the biomedical research community. After all, the nervous system and the immune system provide the means by which the body interacts with and reacts to the outside world. Somehow, these two systems enable each organism, itself a complex being, to maintain its robust homeostasis, that stability in the face of an ever-changing world that is a hallmark of life. Probing the links between these two systems enables investigators to more closely examine key questions facing all biologists, such as: How do cells communicate with one another? How do they recognize one another, bind to one another, or avoid one another? How do genes, via mRNA and protein, affect not only what goes on inside a cell but how that cell interacts with all other cells in its universe? How do cells, or collections of cells, integrate information and produce the complex reactions that constitute life? We have yet to see the answers to these questions, but if progress continues at the current pace, those answers may come sooner than we ever thought possible.

For progress to continue, the advisory panels made some recommendations requiring cooperation of several institutes and agencies:

- Determine the behavioral effects of immune modulators on humans enrolled in either ongoing clinical trials or in small trials set up for that purpose.

- Introduce appropriate behavioral testing batteries in phase I clinical trials.

- Verify the biological and functional importance of specific gene products.

- Analyze the genetic polymorphism of laboratory strains of rats and mice so that neurobiology being done in rats and immunology being done in mice can be reconciled.

- Overcome undue restrictions on distribution of and access to mutant animals, reagents, cloned genes, and so forth that have been generated with public funding and thus should be in the public domain.

- Develop an inventory and/or repository of available transgenic and knockout mutant mice and rats so that all investigators would have ready access to them.

- Create and distribute standardized materials and methods for easy use of established animal models in a variety of laboratories for verification and elaboration of findings.

- Train graduate students and postdoctoral fellows to integrate the traditional medical disciplines of virology, pathology, contemporary molecular biology, genetics, and neuroscience.

Part Five

Treatments and Therapies

Chapter 35

Adults and Primary Immunodeficiency Diseases

"Adults with primary immune deficiency live in the real world. They work, play, and many have families like other people. There is no reason why their immune deficiency should alter this."

Although the first primary immunodeficiency diseases were identified in children, there has been a growing awareness that adults, too, may have a number of primary immunodeficiency disorders. Because of the advances in medicine, earlier diagnosis and treatment of the childhood immunodeficiency diseases has allowed many patients who were born with primary immunodeficiencies to grow into adulthood. In other cases, many adults who were born with apparently normal immune systems go on to develop a primary immunodeficiency late in adolescence or even in adulthood. It is important to distinguish between the adult onset primary immunodeficiencies and AIDS. Because some of the primary immunodeficiency disorders have their onset in adulthood they are sometimes called "acquired" immunodeficiencies even though they are not caused by the virus that causes AIDS.

The most common immunodeficiencies to affect adults include: the antibody deficiency diseases (Selective IgA deficiency, Common Variable Immunodeficiency, Immunoglobulin G subclass deficiency, and X-linked Agammaglobulinemia) and less commonly disorders of the phagocytic cells (Chronic Granulomatous Disease) and disorders of the complement system. Details of these specific immunodeficiency disorders are covered in other chapters. There are several features of immune deficiency diseases of which a newly diagnosed adult should be aware. In most cases, the well informed patient, working with attentive medical staff should be able to pursue a career and live a full life.

The following chapter reviews the types of problems that adults with primary immunodeficiencies develop, discusses how you and your doctor can coordinate care, and outlines some of the psycho-social aspects of living as an adult with these disorders.

Common Symptoms

Recurrent infections are the most common problem that patients with immune deficiencies experience. Typically, patients will have recurrent infections in the sinuses (sinusitis) and in the chest (i.e., bronchitis and pneumonia). Early recognition of illness is important to allow rapid treatment before infections become severe. Some early signs may be as obvious as changes in color or consistency of drainage from the nose or changes in sputum coughed up from the chest, or as subtle as easier fatigability or a shortened temper.

It is not unusual for immunodeficient adults to have chronically red eyes, a condition known as "conjunctivitis." In many patients, if the immunodeficiency can be treated with gammaglobulin, the conjunctivitis often improves although additional antibiotics are sometimes needed.

One of the more common symptoms that antibody deficient patients may experience is diarrhea. This may be caused by a variety of infections or even by an overgrowth of the "normal bacteria" that live in the gastrointestinal tract. Either of the above events result in decreased absorption of important nutrients required for normal body function. Giardia is one of the more common protozoal intestinal infections that can cause diarrhea. Patients with compromised immune systems are uniquely susceptible to Giardia which can be treated easily with oral medication.

Some patients also experience arthritis-like symptoms as well as several other symptoms which are seen in patients with so-called "autoimmune" diseases. These conditions are covered in the chapters in this sourcebook which deal with specific disorders.

It is important that patients be familiar with the common symptoms that accompany their diagnosis, so that appropriate care can be sought. Most doctors who provide care to patients with immunodeficiencies know that these patients may require frequent antibiotics, and that the antibiotics often need to be given earlier in the course of an illness than in people with normal immune systems.

General Care

It is important for any immune deficient patient to understand as much as he or she can about the workings of the immune system. The "well informed" consumer is the "smart" consumer, and when medical care is involved that often means staying healthier longer.

There are a few things that patients can do in their everyday life to help maintain good health. In particular, good nutrition is of great importance. A balanced diet is essential for normal growth, development, body repair and maintenance and especially important in preventing and fighting off disease. The general principles of good hygiene are also very important. Simple things like washing hands before meals and after using the restroom go a long way to prevent illness and should become routine habits. Many viruses, including the ones responsible for the common cold, are spread by unwashed hands. Any cuts or scrapes on the skin should be cleansed completely and any unusual redness or drainage should be reported to a physician so further treatment can be initiated promptly. Dental hygiene and regular dental check-ups are important since some patients are more prone to tooth decay and gum diseases. Regular exercise helps to maintain maximal function of the body and is also a good means of stress relief for the mind.

Specific treatment for the immunodeficiency disease should be coordinated between the patient and the health care team members. Each adult should do everything possible to foster good communication between themselves and their health care providers. Often times patients can give their physicians very important information since they are the ones who have experienced which treatments have truly been of benefit and which have not. Intravenous gammaglobulin and other treatments can be administered at home, saving both money and time and giving the patient more control over their health.

Becoming an Adult Patient

Growing up with illness often speeds the development of a mature personality. The ability to understand and become responsible for complicated medical care can begin at a very early age with parental help.

Including even the youngest of children in the discussions and decisions regarding treatment fosters a positive attitude toward good health rather than anger at "having to take medicine." This sense of responsibility will serve them well in later life once they are on their own.

Having young adults leave home is difficult, compounded by the added needs that often accompany any chronic illness. Knowing that a young adult has been able to gradually take care of his/her own medical problems while living at home eases the fears of moving out. It should be expected that not everything will continue smoothly once the new young adult leaves home. A large part of becoming an adult requires taking your own chances and learning from your own experiences. As mature adults, immunodeficient patients should be cautious that these new experiences do not become life threatening events. Feeling "normal" is an important part of adolescence and early adulthood. If normalcy is established early by the parents, the patient might feel less compelled to fit a lifetime of experience into the first few years away from home. On the one hand, accomplishments and compliance to treatment should be recognized and rewarded, while on the other hand problems should be recognized, discussed in a positive way (in regard to prevention of recurrence) and then dropped with no feelings of guilt or punishment remaining. This creates a good line of communication between patients and their parents. Peer pressure can, on occasion, push someone into unwanted situations. Remember anyone worthy of your friendship will accept your limitations and respect your self-control. Mature adults will quickly realize that the time and attention required to maintain good health will eventually allow for more normal lives and social activities and the continued freedom of living outside the parental home.

Another integral part of preparing for adult problems includes the construction of a medical diary that includes a summary of your past medical history, a list of current problems, medications, physician's phone numbers, insurance information, and even the appropriate chapters/diagrams/paragraphs from this sourcebook. A concise diary is useful when moving to a new area or even on vacation or weekend trips should immediate care be required.

Many adult patients and their friends have commented on the growing number of people who believe that traditional medicine is unnecessary or bad. Frequently they believe that if you "think right" or "eat naturally" you can do without medicine. Most of these people know little about medicine and less about immune deficiency disorders but they are often very persuasive in their offers of easy solutions. Remember that many of these people are motivated by profit and not your good health. Discuss **ANY** variation from your prescribed treatment with your doctor before giving it a try.

The Newly Diagnosed Adult Patient

Some people who have been recently diagnosed have felt unwell for years without an answer to their illnesses and problems. In some cases, a diagnosis can actually be a relief by finally providing an answer. However, at the same time, the newly diagnosed adult patient must face questions and problems which have already been faced by children who have grown up with these disorders. Feelings of self-pity and fear are quite normal. However, sections in this chapter, as well as other chapters of the sourcebook, hopefully, will address some of these feelings. Above all, it is important to realize that you are still the same person, but that you have to come to terms with your diagnosis and treatment and live with them as you go about your life.

Self Education

This is the key to caring for one's own health. The more an individual understands about his or her primary immune deficiency disorder, the more comfortable that person will feel. Just as most parents of children with primary immunodeficiency disorders reach out for as much education as possible, the patients themselves, whether they grew up with the disorder or were recently diagnosed as adults, must ask questions, obtain educational materials and understand the realities of their immune deficiency. Most importantly, patients should read about their disorder and become informed "consumers" getting involved with their own care. This can help produce a feeling of independence and control over their own life.

One way to begin this process is to seek out health care professionals who specialize in these disorders. Physicians who have little interaction with patients with primary immunodeficiency diseases may either overestimate the difficulties or underestimate the need for complete evaluation. It is important to ask as many questions as you can of a specialist. No question about your disorder is too trivial. New methods of investigating and treating these illnesses are being developed over time, and it is in the patient's best interest, regardless of age, to find out what these are.

Another way to gather knowledge is through contact with or attendance at a local support group. Talking to other patients and families is often helpful, and any feelings of isolation you may be experiencing can be dispelled.

Advanced Education

Since the goal of adults is to be self-sufficient, the importance of receiving an education is hard to overestimate. It is important for people with a chronic illness or medical condition to obtain a job with good health insurance and a position with enough flexibility to allow appropriate medical attention when necessary. The bottom line is that advanced training and education provide a greater range of choices and flexibility for anyone, and particularly for a person with a preexisting health condition.

For the individual who goes away from home to college or to be on his/her own, the preceding section on becoming an adult patient suggested potential dangers. Another danger is the tendency of many young adults to "downplay their illness" or fail to disclose their medical history to the school. It is hard for a college or school infirmary to care appropriately for a student who has not informed the school of his/her specific diagnosis. An immunodeficient individual may need antibiotics more often, or sooner in an illness, than another student. For a student with a more serious deficiency, school infirmaries may not be an ideal place to receive care. One way to manage this problem is for the parent or student to find out in advance what physician in the area of the school has had experience in treating immunodeficient patients and to transfer medical records before school starts. Then, if more complicated problems arise, appropriate arrangements can be made. A referral from your current physician may help.

Employment

Adult patients, in choosing a job or career, must think in terms of ones that are suitable for their condition. Depending on the nature of your condition, you may or may not be limited physically. But there may be complications that need to be fully considered. Factors like time and stress, and how they interact with your condition and treatment, cannot be ignored.

In seeking employment, be aware that there are laws against discriminating against an applicant based on a chronic health condition. However, that does not mean that the laws are easy to enforce. You may want to familiarize yourself with the wording of the laws. For many patients it is the health insurance coverage associated with employment that is the most problematic. Small employers, for instance, may not be able to cover you. Hence, large corporations and government jobs should be considered in thinking about careers. For patients who are not able to hold down a full-time job, the section in this sourcebook on health insurance, offers advice on disability.

Home Care

Adult patients must learn to fit their treatment into their school and working lives. For intravenous gamma globulin the use of home health care services permits you to be treated in a home environment. This is particularly useful in avoiding missed time from work. You will want to discuss with your physician whether you are a candidate for home health care, and you will also want to make sure that your insurance will cover the home health care. In many cases, your physician can provide you with the names of home health care agencies in your area. Many adult patients who need infusions of intravenous gamma globulin can learn to give their own infusions. This can be less expensive and more convenient for the working person. In other cases, all of the homecare can be delivered by a nurse who is employed by a home health care company. Discuss with your physician what options are available to ensure that you receive the treatment prescribed for you.

Health Insurance

This is an issue which all people with a primary immune deficiency disorder must face in any decisions they make about school and employment. The section on Health Insurance outlines the options and concerns in detail. Suffice it to say here, that it is important in planning for education and employment that the issue of insurance coverage is addressed. This cannot be taken lightly by anyone with a preexisting condition. If you allow your insurance to lapse, or do not look into what options exist before you are no longer covered by your parents' insurance, or choose or change jobs, your ability to afford the treatment you need may be seriously jeopardized.

Dating, Marriage, and Children

Some people may find it difficult to discuss their disorders with their friends, and particularly with girlfriends and boyfriends. It often depends on an individual's own personality as to how much they want to explain, and when they feel comfortable discussing their medical condition. When you do discuss your disorder with a boyfriend or girlfriend, be sure that you make it clear that you have a primary immunodeficiency disease, and that it is not contagious.

Often when a patient becomes seriously involved with a member of the opposite sex, it may be helpful to have that person accompany them on a visit to the immunologist to better understand the disorder. When a couple is considering marriage, it is important for both to understand the genetic implications of the disorder, and whether it could be passed onto children or grandchildren. This is a question about which the immunologist and a genetic counselor can offer guidance. You may wish to refer to the chapter on inheritance. It is important for an engaged or married couple to also face the issue of health insurance realistically, and understand its importance in career decisions.

Emotional Strains

An adult with a primary immune deficiency disease has all of the medical problems that a child would have, and yet by the definition of adulthood, is supposed to be responsible for his or her life, career, financial planning, and the future of his or her children. Obviously, this can bring various degrees of stress into a family.

For the adult who has recently been diagnosed, there may be feelings of confusion, self pity and, above all, fear. These thoughts and feelings are normal. The positive side of having a diagnosis is that the uncertainty is over and you can be on your way to understanding your illness and the emotional difficulties that may arise from it.

It is difficult to have a chronic illness, and to be susceptible to repeated or recurring infections, or other medical ailments. One of the difficulties about primary immunodeficiency disease is the unpredictability of manifestations. This in itself can place pressures on oneself or family and friends. In addition, the possibility of unexpected absences from work, last minute changes of one's social activities, or even hospitalizations may cause added strain. It is important to discuss with your physician these aspects of an illness, just as much as one would discuss a physical problem. Sometimes just airing your fears can have a therapeutic effect.

A problem in families in which the immunodeficiency is genetically determined are feelings of guilt on the part of the parent who has passed the defect on to a child. Again, the best way to deal with these feelings is to discuss them with your spouse, and also your physician. Remember, that is out of your control, and you also have passed on a number of extremely good qualities. Children with an immune deficient parent may themselves have a fear of becoming ill when they are older. In most cases the fear is unfounded and can be dispelled with the proper information and testing.

There are a variety of ways to help keep your frustrations and anxieties to a minimum. You may simply require some time to discuss these feelings with a spouse, understanding friend or health care professional. Many people are helped by meeting with others in a support group setting. For many patients, learning as much as possible about an illness is one very specific way to guard against confusion about the illness itself. As discussed in the section on Self Education, understanding one's own immune deficiency can lead to taking control of one's own life.

Summary

Adults with primary immune deficiency live in the real world. They work, play, marry and have families like other people. There is no reason why their immune deficiency should alter this. However, they must be aware of the condition and use common sense in recognizing symptoms and treating infections. These adult patients must make sure that they have access to trained specialists who understand their disorder and are aware of the most recent developments in treatment. They must be more careful than people without a pre-existing condition in obtaining and keeping their health insurance coverage and in the laws and regulations which govern insurance. Because of their condition and because of the health insurance risks, some choices of employment may not be optimal. Education and awareness are keys to helping immune deficient adults make life's choices and realize their potential. Always remember that you are not alone and support is only a phone call away.

Chapter 36

General Care

This chapter will provide information pertinent to the care of the immune deficient patient in the home environment. While the discussion centers on the child, the basic information is applicable to the adult as well. General health measures, which maximize the body's natural defenses against infection, will be considered. The psychological effect of immune deficiency and chronic illness on the family unit will be discussed. Finally, specific illnesses will be defined in terms of characteristic symptoms and supportive therapies.

Diagnosis

For some patients and families, the time prior to the actual diagnosis of immune deficiency can be stressful. In addition, the actual diagnosis of immune deficiency often becomes a crisis situation for some families. Learning that your child has a disease which may affect the quantity and quality of his or her life can be devastating. If your child is acutely ill at the time of diagnosis, these feelings are often intensified.

Initial reactions are usually those of shock and disbelief. Denial is a psychological term used to describe these reactions. When limited in duration, denial offers protection from the initial impact of diagnosis.

371

Medical explanations of the disease may be heard, but not remembered or understood at this time.

Once the reality of the diagnosis is acknowledged, feelings of anger and depression tend to dominate. Many parents experience guilt, especially when the disease is known to be inherited.

While everyone is unique in how they handle a crisis situation, generally it tends to bring out the best and the worst in us all. One parent may be consumed with worry, while the other needs the distance of work or hobby. Siblings who initially were concerned, supportive and independent, may suddenly become resentful, demanding and dependent. It is not unusual for them to become jealous of the attention centered around the sick child. Siblings need to verbalize their feelings and concerns. Their concerns may not always center on the sick child. Discipline must be maintained, with firm limits placed on unacceptable behavior.

Tolerance of individual coping methods, and communication among family members are very important. This can be a painful time, but with effort, many families emerge as a stronger unit. Some families may find professional counseling beneficial.

General Health Measures

Nutrition

An adequate diet provides nutrients essential for normal growth and development, body repair and maintenance. While good dietary habits are important for everyone, they are extremely important for the immune deficient individual. Children in particular need good nutrition to grow and develop normally. Recommended Daily Allowances (RDAs) are felt to be the minimal amounts of essential nutrients the healthy population needs to consume in order to maintain an adequate diet. Because nutritional needs and requirements change in response to illness, activity, stress, and age, RDA's may need to be adjusted accordingly.

The Basic Four Food Groups have also been developed by governmental nutrition committees and provide practical guides for nutritious meal planning. Table 36.1 presents the Basic Four Food Groups in terms of RDA's, nutrients supplied, and function. Table 36.2 discusses key nutrients in terms of food sources and basic function. A diet which includes adequate intake of these food sources will provide other essential vitamins and minerals not presented in this table.

BASIC FOOD GROUPS*

TABLE

MINIMUM RECOMMENDED NUMBER OF SERVINGS

FOOD GROUP	SERVING SIZE	CHILDREN	TEENAGERS	ADULTS	SUPPLIED	FUNCTION
MILK GROUP	1 CUP MILK 1 CUP YOGURT *SUBSTITUTE:* 1½ OZ. CHEESE** 1 CUP PUDDING 2 CUPS COTTAGE CHEESE 1¾ CUPS ICE CREAM	3	4	2	CALCIUM RIBOFLAVIN PROTEIN VITAMINS MINERALS CARBOHY-DRATES FATS	NECESSARY FOR STRONG BONES, TEETH, HEALTHY SKIN AND GOOD VISION
MEAT GROUP	2 OZ. COOKED, LEAN MEAT, FISH, POULTRY *SUBSTITUTE:* 2 EGGS 2 OZ. CHEESE* 1 CUP DRIED PEAS OR BEANS 4 TBSP. PEANUT BUTTER	2	2	2	PROTEIN NIACIN IRON THIAMIN RIBOFLAVIN VITAMIN B6 VITAMIN B12 MINERALS	NECESSARY FOR MUSCLE, BONE, BLOOD CELLS AND HEALTHY SKIN AND NERVES
FRUIT AND VEGETABLE GROUP	½ CUP VEGE-TABLES OR FRUIT	4	4	4	VITAMIN A VITAMIN C FIBER MINERALS FOLIC ACID	NECESSARY FOR NIGHT VISION, RESISTING INFECTIONS AND HEALING WOUNDS
BREAD GROUP	1 SLICE WHOLE GRAIN OR ENRICHED BREAD 1 CUP DRY CEREAL ½ CUP COOKED CEREAL, PASTA OR GRITS	4	4	4	CARBOHY-DRATE THIAMIN IRON NIACIN	NECESSARY FOR ENERGY AND A HEALTHY NERVOUS SYSTEM

*This table is adapted in part from information published by the National Dairy Council.
**Count cheese as a serving of milk or meat, not both simultaneously.

Table 36.1.

KEY NUTRIENTS*

TABLE

NUTRIENTS	PLANT SOURCE	ANIMAL SOURCE	BASIC FUNCTION
PROTEIN	LEGUMES (DRIED BEANS, PEAS, ETC.) NUTS	MEAT, FISH, POULTRY, EGGS, MILK AND MILK PRODUCTS	MOST ABUNDANT SUBSTANCE IN THE BODY AFTER WATER. NECESSARY FOR BODY GROWTH AND REPAIR. USED IN THE FORMATION OF ENZYMES, ANTIBODIES, AND SOME HORMONES.
CARBO-HYDRATE	GRAIN PRODUCTS FRUIT STARCHY VEGETABLES SUGAR		PROVIDES THE PRIMARY SOURCE OF ENERGY FOR THE WORK OF THE BODY. SOLE FORM OF ENERGY FOR THE BRAIN AND NERVOUS SYSTEM.
FAT	VEGETABLE OIL PRODUCTS —SALAD DRESSINGS, MARGARINE, ETC.	BUTTER, LARD, FAT MEATS	CONCENTRATED SOURCE OF ENERGY. ACTS AS A TRANSPORT SYSTEM FOR CERTAIN VITAMINS. STORED BODY FAT INSULATES YOU AND PROVIDES A PROTECTIVE CUSHION AROUND VITAL BODY ORGANS.
VITAMIN A	YELLOW VEGE-TABLES AND FRUITS DARK GREEN & LEAFY VEGE-TABLES MARGARINE	LIVER BUTTER EGG YOLK WHOLE MILK	NEEDED FOR HEALTHY MUCOUS MEMBRANES AND SKIN. NEEDED FOR NORMAL VISION, GENERAL EYE HEALTH AND FUNCTIONS.
VITAMIN C	CITRUS FRUITS DARK GREEN & LEAFY VEGE-TABLES POTATOES BROCCOLI CABBAGE CAULIFLOWER TOMATOES		NEEDED FOR HEALTHY BONES, TEETH AND GUMS, TISSUE GROWTH AND HEALING; ELASTICITY AND STRENGTH OF BLOOD VESSELS.
THIAMINE (VITAMIN B1)	NUTS FORTIFIED GRAIN PRODUCTS	LEAN PORK, FISH, POULTRY	NEEDED IN THE DIGESTION OF CARBOHYDRATES. INDIRECTLY PROMOTES GOOD APPETITE AND A HEALTHY NERVOUS SYSTEM.
RIBOFLAVIN (VITAMIN B2)	FORTIFIED GRAIN PRODUCTS GREEN LEAFY VEGETABLES	POULTRY, MILK AND MILK PROD-UCTS, LIVER, EGGS	NEEDED IN THE DIGESTION OF CARBOHYDRATES, FATS AND PROTEINS. ESSENTIAL FOR HEALTHY SKIN AND VISION.
NIACIN	PEANUTS, FORTI-FIED GRAIN PRODUCTS.	LIVER, MEAT, POULTRY, FISH	INVOLVED IN THE ENERGY PRODUCTION WITHIN THE CELLS.
CALCIUM	COLLARD, KALE, MUSTARD AND TURNIP GREENS	MILK AND MILK PRODUCTS BONE MEAL	NEEDED FOR THE FORMATION OF BONES AND TEETH, INVOLVED IN MUSCLE GROWTH AND FUNCTION, BLOOD CLOTTING.
IRON	FORTIFIED CEREAL, LEGUMES, PRUNE JUICE	LIVER, RED MEATS (BEEF, PORK & LAMB)	ESSENTIAL TO THE NORMAL FUNCTION OF HEMOGLOBIN WHICH CARRIES OXYGEN FROM THE LUNGS TO THE REST OF THE BODY. INVOLVED IN STRESS AND DISEASE RESISTANCE.

*Developed in part from information published by the National Dairy Council.

Table 36.2.

Special Diets

In times of infection, illness, or food intolerance, the normal diet may need to be modified. You may want to talk to your doctor in order to understand when these diets are indicated.

Clear Liquid Diet. A clear liquid diet may be used when there is a severe intolerance to food during infection or illness, or when nausea, vomiting and diarrhea are present. Because it is nutritiously inadequate, a clear liquid diet is usually only used for 1 to 2 days. The main purpose of a liquid diet is to replace lost fluids and prevent dehydration. Suggested fluids include: tea, fat-free broth, flattened soda drinks, strained vegetable broth, strained citrus juices, plain jello, fruit ices, and Gatorade.

Full Liquid Diet. A full liquid diet may be ordered when there is difficulty in chewing or swallowing solid foods, as in pharyngitis, or when advancing from clear liquids. When properly planned, this diet can be nutritious and used for extended periods of time. The protein and iron content can be increased by adding eggs and non-fat milk to beverages and soup. A full liquid diet includes all foods which are liquid at room and body temperatures. Eggs (soft-cooked), strained meats, fruits and vegetables, ice cream, milkshakes and creamed soups are examples of food which can be added to the diet.

Soft Diet. A soft or bland diet is the transitional step between a liquid and regular diet. Suggested foods include those which are easily chewed, swallowed and digested. Those foods to be avoided include those which have high fiber content, are rich and highly flavored, or are fried and greasy.

Special Dietary Procedures. *Parenteral and Enteral Nutrition.*

- **Total Parenteral Nutrition (TPN) or Intravenous Hyperalimentation (IVH)** is used to maintain the nutritional status for an individual who is very ill, malnourished, or whose gastrointestinal function is inadequate. The TPN solution contains protein, carbohydrates, electrolytes, vitamins, water and trace minerals. Fats are usually supplied in a separate solution. Various types of intravenous catheters are used to administer the solutions through a large vein, usually located in the neck. Nutrients

375

are introduced directly into the blood stream bypassing the stomach and intestinal tract.

- **Enteral Nutrition.** Enteral nutrition is a term usually used to describe various methods of tube feedings. Enteral nutrition is used when an individual with a normally functioning gastrointestinal system is unable, or refuses, to eat sufficient foods to meet energy needs. The most usual type of tube feeding is the nasogastric which involves placement of a small flexible plastic tube through the nose, into the esophagus and then to the stomach. A prescribed amount of liquid feeding (containing essential nutrients) is poured into the tube continuously, or at regular intervals.

Other methods of tube feedings involve the surgical insertion of a feeding tube into either the esophagus, stomach or small intestine.

Hygiene

General principles of good hygiene are especially important for the immune deficient patient and his/her family. Hand washing before meals, after outings, and after using the toilet should become routine. Individually wrapped and disposable hand wipes are excellent for school lunches and for outings. For younger children, periodic washing of toys may be of some benefit.

Cuts and scrapes should be cleansed, and a first-aid cream applied. Any unusual redness or drainage should be reported to the physician.

Some immune deficient individuals are prone to dental decay. Regular visits to the dentist and proper teeth-brushing technique are to be encouraged.

Immune deficient individuals should avoid exposure to people who are known to be ill. During periods of influenza outbreaks, crowded areas, such as shopping centers and movie theaters, should be avoided.

Hobbies

While it is important to safeguard health, participation in age appropriate activities should be encouraged by parents. Hobbies and sports promote physical fitness and provide an excellent outlet for energy and stress. Swimming, biking, track, and walking may promote optimal lung function, muscle development, strength and endurance.

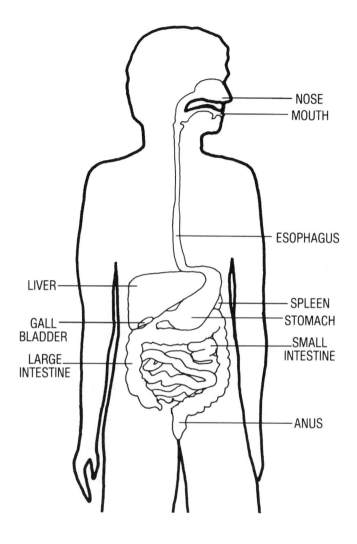

Figure 36.1. *Gastrointestinal System*

Some immune deficient patients may have problems controlling bleeding. In their cases, the types of exercises in which the patients can safely participate should be discussed with their physician. Sedentary hobbies such as reading, puzzles, and model building are useful during periods of illness or confinement.

School Attendance

A major concern for the school-age child is the effect of absentee-ism on academic performance. With the cooperative effort of the school, parents and student, harmful effects can be minimized. At the start of the school year, inform your child's teacher(s) and school nurse of his/her medical condition. The possibility of illness and/or doctor appointments causing absenteeism should be discussed.

If your child is absent from school, ask that a classmate be assigned to take notes, and to record class and homework assignments. Notify the school if a prolonged absence is expected. Arrange to have missed assignments and books sent home with a sibling or friend. These as-signments can be done when your child is feeling better, but not quite ready to return to school.

Encourage your child to complete long-term assignments early. If tests or special assignments are due the day of a scheduled doctor's appointment, help your child to be prepared to take the tests, and to turn in the assignments early.

In some immune deficiencies your child may be too ill to attend school for extended periods of time. In these situations, home tutor-ing may be required.

The Psychological Effect of Illness on the Family Unit

Phases of Illness

The duration of an illness can be divided into various phases, with each phase affecting the family unit differently.

Acute Phase. When a family member becomes ill, there is often an increased awareness of the implications of immune deficiency. When symptoms of an infection are acute, fears and concerns experi-enced at the time of the initial diagnosis often resurface. Your energy needs to be redirected and conserved to meet the needs of your child, your family, and yourself. This phase of illness usually affects the entire family. One parent may assume the care of the ill child, while the other may attempt to maintain his/her job. Siblings may become solicitous. Even the family pet tends to stay with the sick child.

Intermediate Phase. This phase is characterized by the gradual reduction in the severity of symptoms. The patient begins to show some interest in television, reading, and food. Supportive care is still important at this time to prevent complications. This is a good time for the family to spend some quiet moments together.

Recovery Phase. This phase occurs in the immune deficient patient who experiences periods of wellness between infections.

For many families, the resumption of sibling fighting heralds the onset of this phase. The "sick bed" often becomes an arena of twisted sheets, blankets and pillows. It is not unusual to find your child and family pet in the middle of the debris.

This is the appropriate time to begin the completion of missed school assignments. Special attention and treatment should be gradually withdrawn. You may find it necessary to establish definite periods of rest that alternate with periods of activity. Try to spend some separate time with your other children, your spouse, and yourself. This is a time to enjoy and to refuel your energy.

Chronic Phase. Immune deficiency is usually a chronic condition. Many of the infections associated with this disease can become chronic. Coping with chronic illness is comparable to running a marathon race. The key to completion is related to the amount of stamina developed, and the ability to believe in the existence of an unseen finish line.

Frequent periods of illness and hospitalization can strain even the strongest family structure. For the family unit to survive, the needs of all its members must collectively and individually be recognized, met, and balanced with the needs of the immune deficient child or adult. Many times this is a difficult juggling act to master.

Your Child's Reaction to Immune Deficiency

You react to immune deficiency as a parent. As your child grows older and his level of understanding increases, he or she will need to react and accept immune deficiency as the individual who has it. Some children express curiosity at a young age. Other children do not appear interested until they are much older.

Adolescence can be a stormy, rebellious period for many children. Your child may view immune deficiency as something that makes him different from, instead of conforming to, his peer group. It is not unusual for the immune deficient child to balk, or even refuse medical treatment during this time. As with any child, firm limits on unacceptable behavior must be maintained.

379

During the teenage years, your child will need to gradually assume responsibility for his own health care. Parenting includes teaching your children the skills and knowledge necessary for an independent adulthood. Educating your child about his illness, its significance, and treatment is an important facet of this process.

Encouraging your child to develop healthy methods of coping and stress reduction is important. If you have found comfort and strength in a spiritual belief, your child may find the same solace. Listening to your child is probably the most effective parenting tool available. Hopefully, as your child enters young adulthood, he or she will have mastered the skills necessary to deal with the implications of immune deficiency, yet not let it be the primary focus of his or her life.

General Care During Illness: Specific Illnesses

This portion of the General Care chapter provides basic information about some of the illnesses your child may experience which, when uncomplicated, may not require hospitalization. An attempt has been made to define the medical terms often used in association with these illnesses, and to describe their characteristic symptoms. General supportive measures designed to provide relief of symptoms and prevention of complications have also been suggested.

For the sake of organization, these illnesses are grouped according to the body "system" involved. These systems include the visual (eyes), the auditory (ears), the respiratory (nose, throat, lungs) and the gastrointestinal (stomach, intestines).

It is important to stress the need for physician communication and supervision during any illness of an immune deficient individual. The frequency of even "minor" illnesses should be reported, because they can influence the preventive therapy your physician feels necessary for your child (i.e. gammaglobulin, antibiotics). Medical treatment and supportive care of any immune deficient individual seeks to accomplish:

- a reduction in the frequency of infections
- the prevention of complications
- the prevention of an acute infection from becoming chronic

The patient, family, and physician must work together as a unit, if these goals are to be accomplished.

Visual System

Conjunctivitis. Conjunctivitis (pink eye) is an inflammation of the lining of the eyelid and of the membrane covering the outer layer of the eyeball (conjunctiva). It can be caused by bacteria, viruses or chemical irritants such as smoke or soap. Conjunctivitis may occur by itself, or appear in association with other illnesses, such as the common cold.

The symptoms commonly associated with conjunctivitis are redness and swelling of the eyelids, tearing, and discharge of pus. These symptoms are usually accompanied by itching, burning, and discomfort from light. In the morning, it is not unusual to find the child's eyelids "stuck" together from the discharge that has dried during the night. These secretions are best loosened by placing a wash cloth soaked in warm water on each eye. After a few minutes, gently clean each eye, working from the inner corner to the outer corner of the eye. Meticulous hand washing is necessary for anyone coming in contact with the eye discharge in order to prevent the spread of the infection. It may be necessary for your child to be seen by a physician in order to determine the type of conjunctivitis involved, and the type of treatment necessary.

Auditory System

Otitis Media. Otitis Media is an infection of the middle ear, which is usually caused by bacteria or viruses. A small tube called the eustachian tube connects the middle ear with the throat and nose. In the infant and small child the tube is shorter and straighter than in the adult, providing a ready path for bacteria and viruses to gain entrance into the middle ear. In some infections and allergies, this tube may actually swell and become shut, preventing drainage from the middle ear.

The characteristic symptom associated with otitis media is pain, which is caused by irritation of the nerve endings in the inflamed ear. Your baby or young child may indicate pain by crying, head rolling, or pulling at the infected ear(s). The older child or adult may describe the pain as being sharp and piercing. Restlessness, irritability, fever, chills, nausea, and vomiting may also be present. Pressure in the infected ear drum tends to increase when the child is in a flat position. This explains why pain is often more severe at night, causing your child to awaken frequently. As fluid pressure increases within the ear

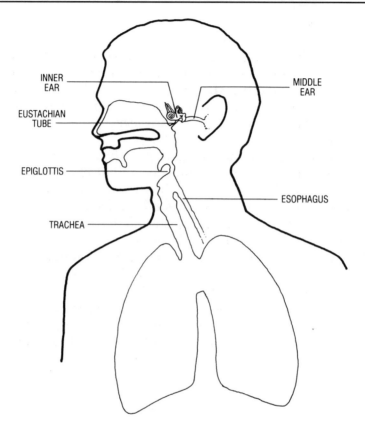

Figure 36.2. *The connection between the nose, throat, and the ear by the Eustachian tube.*

drum, pain becomes more severe and the ear drum may actually rupture. The appearance of pus or bloody drainage in the ear canal is an indication of possible ear drum rupture. Although pain is usually relieved at this time, the infection still exists. Whenever an ear infection is suspected, your child must be seen by a physician for proper diagnosis. Treatment is instituted in order to prevent further infection and hearing impairment. Antibiotic therapy may be initiated. Decongestants may also be prescribed to shrink mucous membranes, promoting better drainage from the middle ear. A follow-up examination may be done in approximately 10 days to be certain that the infection has cleared and that no residual fluid remains in the ear drum.

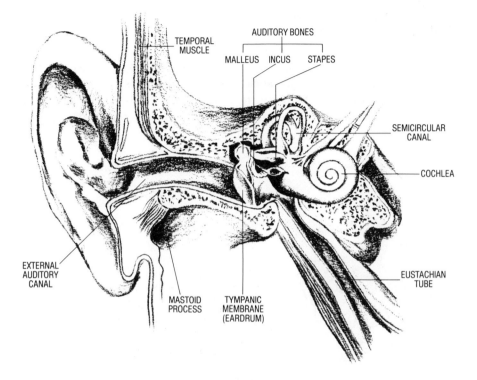

Figure 36.3. *Frontal Section of the Ear*

Respiratory System

The following respiratory illnesses will be discussed in terms of definitions and symptoms. Because the general care of your child during these illnesses is similar, it will be handled as a single discussion at the end of the section.

Rhinitis. Rhinitis is a term used to describe an inflammation of the nose. It is usually caused by bacteria, viruses and/or allergens. Symptoms may include sneezing, difficulty in breathing through the nose, and nasal discharge. The nasal discharge may be thin and watery, to thick, yellow or green.

Pharyngitis. Pharyngitis is a term used to describe an inflammation of the throat (sore throat). It is usually caused by a bacterial or viral infection. Symptoms include a raw or tickling sensation in the back of the throat and difficulty swallowing. Temperature may be normal or elevated. Sore throats caused by streptococcus (strep throat) can, in rare incidences, cause serious complications, such as rheumatic fever or inflammation of the kidneys (nephritis). Whenever your child complains of a sore throat your doctor should be contacted.

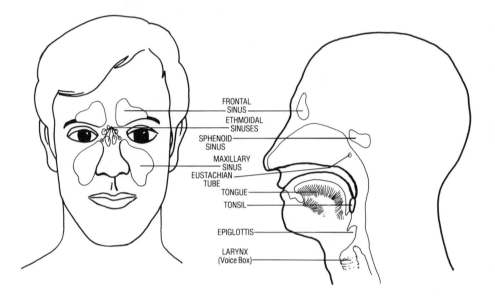

Figure 36.4. Sinus Locations.

Acute Sinusitis. Sinusitis is a term used to describe an inflammation of one or more of the sinuses (see drawing). The sinuses are small cavities, lined with mucous membranes, located in the facial bones surrounding the nasal cavities. The primary purpose of the sinuses is to decrease the weight of the skull and to give resonance and timbre to the voice. The basic causes of sinusitis are the blockage of normal routes of sinus drainage and the spread of infections from the nasal passages. Some of the same bacteria and viruses that cause common colds and respiratory infections can cause sinusitis.

Sneezing, air flow obstruction and nasal discharge are the main symptoms of the early stages of sinusitis. Headache in the area of one or more of the sinuses is also a characteristic symptom. The headache associated with sinusitis is typically more pronounced in the morning (due to accumulated secretions in the sinuses during sleep). Being in the upright position during the day facilitates sinus drainage providing temporary headache relief. Depending on the amount of post-nasal drainage, cough, throat irritation, bad breath and decreased appetite may also be present. Temperature may be within normal limits or slightly elevated. Repeated or prolonged cases of acute sinusitis may cause the condition to become chronic.

Croup. Croup is a general term used to describe the inflammation and narrowing of the air passages leading to the lungs such as the larynx, trachea and bronchi. Croup can be caused by viruses or bacteria. Your child's temperature may be normal or slightly elevated. The onset of croup may be sudden or occur gradually. In some instances the onset occurs at night. The child may awaken with a tight "barking" cough; breathing is difficult due to the narrowing of the trachea (windpipe). The child's voice is hoarse because of inflammation of the larynx. Croup can be a frightening experience for both the parents and child. Unfortunately your child's anxiety may increase the severity of the symptoms. It is important that you stay as calm and as reassuring as possible. High humidity is essential in reducing the respiratory distress (labored, difficult breathing) associated with croup. In the home, the bathroom can provide the best source of a high-humidity environment. Keeping the door closed, run hot water in the shower or tub (allowing the water to continuously drain). The room should be "steamed" in approximately 5-10 minutes. To avoid accidental burning, never leave your child unattended at this time. As your child breathes in the moist air, there should be significant improvement in his breathing.

ALWAYS NOTIFY YOUR PHYSICIAN WHEN YOU SUSPECT YOUR CHILD HAS CROUP.

If the croup is severe, and steaming only partially relieves the child's respiratory distress, or if the child's temperature is markedly elevated, a more serious type of croup, caused by bacteria, may be involved. The child needs to be under the immediate care of a physician. If you are unable to contact a doctor, take your child to the nearest hospital immediately.

Acute Coryza (Common Cold). Acute coryza (common cold) is an acute inflammation of the upper respiratory tract (nose and throat or nasopharynx). Early symptoms include a dry tickling sensation in the throat, followed by sneezing, coughing and increased amounts of nasal discharge. There may also be symptoms of fatigue, chills, fever and general achiness.

Influenza (Flu). Influenza (flu) is a term used to describe a highly contagious respiratory infection which is caused by three closely related viruses. Influenza may occur sporadically or in epidemics. Usually epidemics occur every 2-4 years and develop rapidly because of the short incubation period. The incubation period includes the time a person is exposed to an infecting agent to the time symptoms of the illness appear.

Symptoms of the flu include sudden onset of high fever, chills, headache, weakness, fatigue, rhinitis, and muscular soreness. Vomiting and diarrhea may also be present with one type of influenza.

Acute Bronchitis. Acute Bronchitis is an inflammation of the bronchi (the major branches off the trachea or windpipe). It often accompanies or follows an upper respiratory tract infection, such as the common cold. Symptoms include fever and cough. At the onset, the cough is dry, but gradually becomes productive (producing mucus).

Bronchiectasis. Bronchiectasis is a term used to describe dilation (widening) of the bronchial air passages (bronchi and bronchioles). Please refer to lung illustration. Secretions normally cleared from the lungs by these structures tend to collect in the dilated passages, enhancing the development of infection. Bronchiectasis can develop from frequent pulmonary infections or from obstruction of the bronchi by mucus, pus or foreign bodies.

The main symptom of bronchiectasis is frequent and severe coughing. The cough characteristically produces large amounts of thick, foul smelling sputum. The sputum may also be bloody on occasion.

Pneumonia. Pneumonia is an acute infection of the lungs and can be caused by bacteria, viruses, and fungi. Symptoms include chills, high fever, cough, and chest pain associated with breathing and coughing. In some cases nausea, vomiting, and diarrhea may also occur.

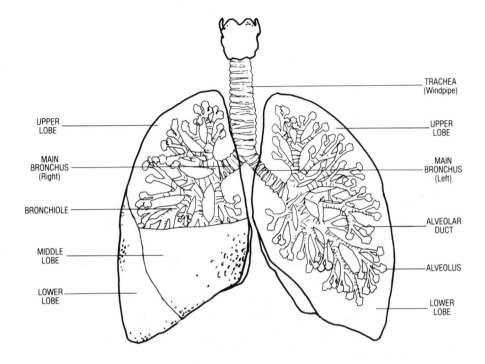

UPPER LOBE

MAIN BRONCHUS (Right)

BRONCHIOLE

MIDDLE LOBE

LOWER LOBE

TRACHEA (Windpipe)

UPPER LOBE

MAIN BRONCHUS (Left)

ALVEOLAR DUCT

ALVEOLUS

LOWER LOBE

Figure 36.5. *The Lungs*

Gastrointestinal System

Diarrhea. Diarrhea is characterized by frequent, loose, watery bowel movements (stools). Diarrhea may be caused by viral or bacterial infections, or be symptomatic of a food allergy or food intolerance. Contaminated foods, drugs and anxiety may also cause diarrhea.

Diarrhea may be mild to severe in nature. Whether it is mild or severe depends on the frequency of stools, their volume, how loose they are, the presence or absence of fever, and how much fluid the child can take by mouth and retain.

The significance of diarrhea is related to the amount of body fluids lost, and the severity of dehydration which develops. Infants and young children, because their body fluid volume is larger and their nutritional reserves smaller, are at a greater risk for dehydration than older children and adults.

Symptoms of dehydration include:

- poor skin turgor (loss of elasticity)
- dry, parched lips, mouth and tongue
- thirst
- decreased urinary output
- in infants, depressed (sunken) fontanelles (soft spots)
- eyes appear sunken
- behavioral changes ranging from increased restlessness to extreme weakness

If your child has diarrhea, a physician should be notified.

General Care of the Individual with Respiratory Illness

The treatment of respiratory infections is directed toward the relief of symptoms and the prevention of complications. Your doctor may prescribe a medication to relieve fever and general body aches. Antibiotics may be prescribed to control infections of bacterial origin and/or to prevent complications. Expectorants may be prescribed to liquify (water down) mucus secretions. Decongestants to shrink swollen mucous membranes may also be ordered.

Fluids should be encouraged, and offering your child a variety of beverages is important. Beverages served with crushed ice can be soothing to a sore throat. Warm beverages, such as tea, may promote nasal drainage and relieve chest tightness.

During the acute phase of any illness, there may be an initial loss of appetite. Your child should not be forced to eat, nor should large meals be offered. It is often better to offer small frequent feedings of liquid and soft foods. Once your child's appetite returns, a high-caloric, high protein diet, to replace the proteins lost during the acute phase of the illness, should be offered. (See section on Nutrition)

General comfort measures also include encouraging your child to rinse his mouth with plain water at regular intervals. This will relieve the dryness and "bad taste" that often accompanies illness and mouth breathing. A vaporizer is helpful in increasing room humidity. If you use a vaporizer, it must be kept clean, to prevent contamination with molds and bacteria. A petroleum jelly coating can provide relief and protection to irritated lips and nose. Body temperature fluctuations may be associated with periods of perspiration. Bed linens and clothing should be changed as often as necessary, and your child should be protected from drafts and chills.

Adequate rest is important. If persistent coughing or post nasal drip interfere with rest, elevation of the head and shoulders with extra pillows during periods of sleep should be attempted.

The individual should be encouraged to cover the mouth and nose when sneezing and coughing. Soiled tissue should be promptly discarded. Frequent hand washing is essential to prevent the spread of the infection.

In some cases of bronchitis and pneumonia (depending on the age and level of understanding) encourage your child to cough and breath deeply at regular intervals. Coughing protects the lungs by removing mucus and foreign particles from the air passages. Deep breathing promotes full expansion of the lungs, reducing the risk of further complications.

In some situations a physician may order chest postural drainage, chest physiotherapy, or sinus postural drainage. Please refer to the special procedures section located at the end of this chapter for a detailed description of these measures.

General Care of the Individual with Gastrointestinal Illness

The general care of diarrhea centers around the replacement of lost body fluids and the prevention of dehydration.

When diarrhea is mild, changes in the diet and increased fluid intake may compensate for fluid losses. The doctor may suggest giving your infant or young child clear liquids. If clear liquids are tolerated (frequency and volume of stools decrease), you may be instructed to offer diluted formula or milk. An infant may find comfort in a pacifier. Sucking may help relieve abdominal cramping. Burping is still necessary to expel any swallowed air. The older child and adult may be encouraged to drink fluids such as weak tea, Gatorade, bouillon and "flattened" soft drinks. If nausea and vomiting are present, offer the older child and adult ice chips and popsicles. Fluids taken too quickly, or in too large of an amount, may precipitate vomiting. If these fluids are tolerated, gradually offer small sips of other fluids. Bland foods, such as rice cereal, yogurt, and low fat cottage cheese can slowly be added to the diet. (See also the section on Nutrition)

General comfort measures include coating the rectal area with a petroleum jelly preparation. This will help protect the skin and reduce irritation from frequent diarrheal stools. Soiled diapers and clothing should also be changed immediately. The older child and adult may be encouraged to regularly rinse his mouth with water. This helps to relieve mouth dryness and "bad taste" associated with illness, and is especially important after vomiting.

In infectious diarrhea, several measures are necessary to reduce the chances of spreading the illness to other family members. Frequent hand washing is essential for everyone. It may be easier for the infected person to use disposable cups, dishes, and utensils. Soiled diapers, clothing and linens should be kept separate and washed separately from other family laundry. Bathrooms should be cleaned with a disinfectant solution as often as necessary.

Special Procedures

Sinus Postural Drainage

In some cases of acute and chronic sinusitis, your physician may instruct you to do sinus postural drainage. Sinus postural drainage facilitates the instillation of medication or irrigating solution into the sinus cavities, and promotes the drainage of nasal contents by gravity. The information listed below is meant as a reference and is not a substitute for physician instruction.

Procedure:

1. Placing your child on his side, elevate his trunk (upper body) with a firm pad or floor pillow such that his head is positioned downward, in a dependent position (lower than his trunk).

2. Instill the irrigating solution or medication into each nostril at this time. With proper head position, the solution should have contact with the various sinus openings on both sides of the face.

3. Encourage your child to breathe through his mouth to prevent "drawing" the irrigating solution or medication into the back of his throat.

4. This position should be maintained for 5-6 minutes.

5. After the appropriate time interval, your child may sit up and, for a few moments, place his head down between his knees, to allow for the drainage of nasal contents. Encourage gentle nose blowing.

6. Your child should sit upright for a few moments to regain his sense of balance.

7. Soiled tissues should be discarded, and hands washed before usual activity is resumed.

General Consideration and Hints

• To avoid vomiting, sinus drainage should be done before meals or 1 to 2 hours after eating.

• Sinus drainage done upon awakening will clear secretions which have accumulated during sleep.

• A warm cloth placed over the sinus area before each session may facilitate the drainage of secretions and enhance the effectiveness of the procedure.

• Listening to a record, conversation, or watching TV helps the time go faster for the younger child. Using a timer is useful in setting a visual or audible time limit.

• Sinus drainage done after the bath or shower, and before bed time is recommended to remove accumulated secretions, and promote a more restful night.

"The following material on segmental bronchial drainage has been adapted from material supplied by the Cystic Fibrosis Foundation, Bethesda, Maryland, and used with their permission."

Segmental Bronchial Drainage

What Is Bronchial Drainage?

Bronchial drainage uses gravity and physical maneuvers to stimulate movement of secretions in order to relieve airway obstruction due to accumulated mucus or "phlegm." This form of chest physical therapy can be prescribed for the prevention and/or treatment of some respiratory problems due to accumulated secretions.

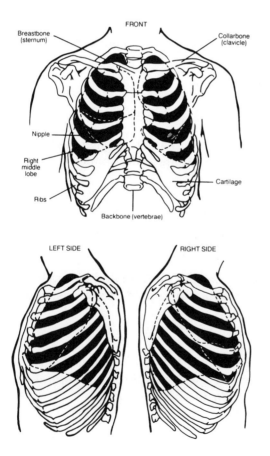

Figure 36.6. *External Anatomy of Chest*

Who Can Benefit from Bronchial Drainage?

As a form of treatment, it helps individuals with respiratory problems caused by:

• increased production of secretions,
• thick or sticky secretions,
• impaired removal of secretions, and
• ineffective cough, or combinations of any of these factors.

As a preventive measure, it benefits those persons with:

• predisposition for increased production or thickness of secretions and/or
• weakness of the breathing muscles.

What Are the Positions for Bronchial Drainage?

Careful positioning helps facilitate gravity in the movement of secretions from small airways into the segmental bronchi and larger airways where the secretions can be coughed up or swallowed. The lung segment to be drained is placed uppermost and the segmental bronchus leading to that segment is placed in as near a straight up-and-down position as possible. This position allows secretions to flow by gravity into larger airways. The positions to be used, as well as the frequency and duration of treatment, should be individually prescribed. To better understand bronchial drainage, please review Figure 36.6, showing the external anatomy of the chest, and Figure 36.7, the bronchopulmonary segments.

The lungs are paired organs of respiration located within the chest. The lungs and other contents of the chest are protected by a firm, but flexible, cage of ribs which are attached to the vertebrae (backbone) and sternum (breastbone) by fibrous tissue (cartilage). During inhalation (breathing in) and exhalation (breathing out), this chest cage changes in size and shape.

The contents of the chest are separated from the contents of the abdomen by a strong dome-shaped muscle, the diaphragm. The diaphragm moves down during inhalation and moves up during exhalation.

The right lung is composed of three lobes: the right upper lobe (RUL), the right middle lobe (RML), and the right lower lobe (RLL).

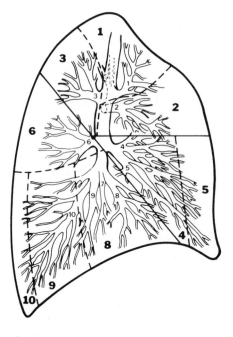

Figure 36.7. Broncho-Pulmonary Segments

The left lung is made up of only two lobes: the left upper lobe (LUL) and the left lower lobe (LLL). The lobes are divided into smaller divisions called segments. In Figure 36.7, each segment is designated by a number corresponding to the positions used for bronchial drainage.

For each position shown in Figure 36.7, the segment and the airway leading to it are identified by the same number. The numbers in Figure 36.7 are also used to show which area of the chest surface should be clapped to assist gravity in the mobilization of the secretions from that segment. The names of the segments and the numbers corresponding to them are shown in Table 36.3. The enclosed pages contain illustrations of the various positions to use for drainage of each bronchopulmonary segment.

Table 36.3.

Name of Segment	No. of Segment
RIGHT UPPER LOBE	
Apical	1
Anterior	2
Posterior	3
RIGHT MIDDLE LOBE	
Lateral	4
Medial	5
RIGHT LOWER LOBE	
Superior	6
Medial	7
Anterior Basal	8
Lateral Basal	9
Posterior Basal	10
LEFT UPPER LOBE	
Apical-Posterior	1-3
Anterior	2
Lingula	
Superior	4
Inferior	5
LEFT LOWER LOBE	
Superior	6
Anteromedial Basal	7-8
Lateral Basal	9
Posterior Basal	10

What Physical Maneuvers Can Assist Gravity in the Removal of Secretions?

Chest physical therapy consists of maneuvers that help remove secretions from the walls of the airways and stimulate coughing. These maneuvers include: clapping with the cupped hand, vibration, deep breathing, and assisted coughing.

Clapping is done with the cupped hand on the chest wall over the segment to be drained. Clapping initiates vibrations which stimulate the movement of secretions and may help remove secretions sticking to the bronchial walls. The hand is cupped by holding the fingers together so that the shape of the cupped hand conforms with the chest wall and tends to trap a cushion of air which softens the blow of clapping.

Clapping should be vigorous, but not painful, and should not be done on bare skin. The therapist should remove rings before clapping.

Clapping is usually performed on the patient by the therapist or a person trained in the technique. Older patients, however, may be taught to self-administer the procedure for some of the segments.

Vibration is also a maneuver which helps to stimulate the flow of secretions. This technique requires that the therapist's hand be pressed firmly over the segment on the chest wall and the muscles of his upper arm and shoulder are tensed (isometric contractions). Vibration is done with the flattened, not the cupped, hand. Vibration is performed during exhalation, with the patient saying "FFF" or "SSS." Exhalation should be as slow and as complete as possible.

Although various mechanical vibrators are available commercially, recommendations differ for their use.

Deep breathing assists in the movement of secretions and may stimulate coughing. An effective cough is an essential part of clearing the airways. A forced but not strained exhalation, following a deep inhalation, may move secretions and may stimulate a productive cough.

Coughing may be assisted by supporting the side of the lower chest with the hands which decreases the strain of coughing and may increase its effectiveness.

Suggestions on the "How" of Bronchial Drainage

It is very important that the individual receiving therapy and the therapist be comfortable during bronchial drainage. A substantial, firm, padded board or table can be inclined to the specific angle or height that is needed for drainage of the right middle lobe (R: 4-5), lingular (L: 4-5), and the basal segments of the lower lobes (R: 8, 9, 10 and L: 8, 9, 10). Tables can be constructed to adjust to various angles or heights or can be obtained commercially. Tilt boards can be elevated at one end by placing blocks on the floor. Infants can be positioned in the therapists lap with or without pillows.

Before beginning bronchial drainage, tight clothing should be removed. Light, soft clothing, such as a "T" shirt, may be worn. Clapping should not be done over clothing seams or buttons. An ample supply of tissues or a receptacle for disposal for expectorated secretions should be readily available.

To minimize the chance of vomiting, bronchial drainage is best done before meals or 1 1/2 to 2 hours after eating. Early morning and bedtime sessions are usually recommended. By helping clear the airways of accumulated secretions, bronchial drainage before bedtime may reduce nighttime coughing.

When used for treatment, bronchial drainage is usually recommended at least twice daily.

Additional bronchial drainage is often advised during acute respiratory infections and in instances where the extent of disease requires it. When drainage is used for prevention, it is usually recommended once or twice daily.

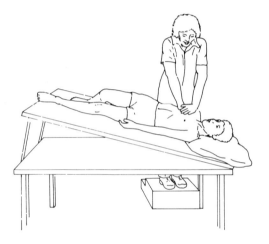

Figure 36.8. *A substantial, firm, padded board or table can be inclined to the specific angle or height that is needed for drainage.*

Chapter 37

Specific Medical Therapy

There are a number of specific medical therapies available to patients with primary immunodeficiency diseases. Only two of the most common of these, gamma globulin therapy and bone marrow transplantation, and two new treatments using gamma interferon and PEG-ADA, will be considered in this chapter. Their specific indications and the disorders for which they may be of benefit should be discussed with your physician.

Gamma Globulin Therapy

Individuals who are unable to produce adequate amounts of immunoglobulins or antibodies may benefit from replacement therapy with gamma globulin. The term, gamma globulin, refers to the chemical fraction of blood that contains immunoglobulins or antibodies. Gamma globulin therapy is used for patients with disorders of humoral immunity, such as X-Linked Agammaglobulinemia and Common Variable Immunodeficiency or hypogammaglobulinemia.

As explained in other chapters of this sourcebook, mature B-lymphocytes (plasma cells), when encountering antigens, manufacture antibodies and release these molecules into the bloodstream. To commercially prepare antibodies that can be given to immunodeficient patients, the antibodies must first be purified (extracted) from the

---

©1987, 1993. Excerpted from *Patient and Family Handbook for the Primary Immune Deficiency Diseases*. Immune Deficiency Foundation. Reprinted with permission.

blood of normal healthy individuals. Blood from each donor is carefully tested for evidence of transmissible diseases, such as AIDS or hepatitis, and any sample that is even suspected of having one of those diseases is discarded. Blood is collected from as many as 2,000-10,000 people, then pooled together. Since different individuals are exposed to different germs, collecting blood from so many different people is the best way to ensure that the final gamma globulin product will contain antibodies to many different types of germs.

The first step in gamma globulin production is to remove all red and white blood cells. Then, the immunoglobulins are chemically purified in a series of steps involving treatment with alcohols. This process results in the purification of antibodies of the Immunoglobulin G (IgG) class, but only trace amounts of IgA and IgM survive.

The purification process removes other blood proteins and is also very effective at killing viruses and other germs that may be in the blood. Purified gamma globulin has been used for approximately 40 years and is extremely safe. No gamma globulin manufactured in the United States has ever transmitted an infectious disease. In addition, the U.S. Food and Drug Administration has tested the manufacturing processes and found that they completely kill the virus that causes AIDS.

There are two forms of gamma globulin that can be given to patients: a form to be injected into muscle (intramuscular, IM) and a form to be injected directly into the bloodstream (intravenous, IV). Gamma globulin products for intramuscular use have been used for decades and continue to be used to give normal individuals a boost of antibodies after exposure to some specific diseases such as hepatitis. The same products were used for many years to treat immunodeficient patients. Unfortunately, immunodeficient patients required frequent injections with much larger doses of gamma globulin than those used in normal individuals. These intramuscular injections were very painful, and only modest amounts of gamma globulin could be given in this way. There simply wasn't enough room inside the muscle for more.

In the early 1980s, new manufacturing processes were developed to make gamma globulin products that could be injected intravenously. There are now many different gamma globulin preparations licensed in the United States for intravenous use. For the most part, the products are equivalent. But, there are some minor differences which may make one particular preparation most suitable for a given individual. Your doctor is your best source of information about which product is best for you.

The new intravenous gamma globulin products are usually very well tolerated by patients. They can be administered either in an outpatient clinic or in the patient's own home. A typical infusion will take two to four hours from start to finish. Use of intravenous products allows physicians to give larger doses of gamma globulin than we could give intramuscularly. Most patients have no side-effects from the IV infusions, but sometimes low grade fever or headache occur. These symptoms can usually be alleviated or eliminated by infusing the gamma globulin at a slower rate.

The dose of gamma globulin varies from patient to patient. In part, the dose is determined by the patient's weight. It is also determined by measuring the blood level of IgG in the patient at some interval after infusion, and by determining how well a given dose of gamma globulin is treating or preventing symptoms in an individual patient. Intravenous infusions of gamma globulin are usually given every three to four weeks, but they may be given more or less frequently depending on the needs of the individual patient.

It is important to remember that although our current gamma globulin products are very good, they do not duplicate exactly what nature normally provides. The manufactured gamma globulin is almost pure IgG, so essentially no IgA or IgM is transferred to the patient. The specific protective functions of these immunoglobulins are therefore not replaced. At least part of the reason that antibody-deficient patients remain somewhat more susceptible to respiratory infections even though they are receiving gamma globulin may be that the IgA on the mucosal surfaces of the respiratory tract is not being replaced.

Bone Marrow Transplantation

Bone marrow transplantation is a highly specialized procedure which can be used to treat some immune deficiency diseases. The immune deficiency diseases for which bone marrow transplantation is performed include those diseases that are characterized by deficient T-lymphocytes or combined deficiencies of T-lymphocytes and B-lymphocytes. Bone marrow transplantation is most often used to treat Severe Combined Immunodeficiency (SCID).

As mentioned in the chapter on the Normal Immune System, the bone marrow is the organ in which the immature cells of the immune system arise and begin their developmental journey on the road to mature T-lymphocytes or B-lymphocytes. Thus, the transplantation of bone marrow from a normal individual to an immunodeficient individual has the potential to replace the deficient immune system of the patient with a normal immune system.

There are two problems in performing a bone marrow transplantation, however. The first is the fact that some patients (or recipient or host) may have enough immune function remaining to cause him/her to recognize the transplanted marrow as foreign, react against it and reject it. In that case, treatment with chemotherapy and/or X-ray therapy may be necessary. This prevents the patient (recipient) from rejecting the transplanted marrow. The second is the fact that the transplanted bone marrow (or graft) carries the immune system of the donor and may therefore recognize the patient (or recipient or host) as foreign, react against the patient and attack the patient. While the first problem is called *graft rejection*, the second problem is called *Graft Versus Host Disease*.

Selection of the Donor: In order to overcome the dual problems of graft rejection by the host and, more importantly, graft versus host disease, "matched" bone marrow is transplanted. A matched marrow is one that is from a donor whose tissue type (or transplantation antigens) is very similar or identical to the recipient. These transplantation antigens are called histocompatibility antigens because they determine whether the transplanted tissue (in this case the bone marrow) is "compatible." Each of us have a collection of these histocompatibility antigens on most of our cells including those of our immune system and our bone marrow. The characteristics of these histocompatibility antigens are determined by a series of genes clustered on one set of our chromosomes, the pair of chromosomes known as the sixth (6th) human chromosomes. Because the genes are closely clustered on the chromosome they are inherited as a single unit called a haplotype. There are so many different forms of these histocompatibility antigens that a person's haplotype (or collection of these genes) is relatively unique. However, because people who are closely related (like brothers and sisters) share some genes they may sometimes share their combinations of genes (their haplotypes) which determine their histocompatibility antigens.

As mentioned in the preceding paragraph, each person's histocompatibility genes are clustered on a single pair of chromosomes and can be divided into four closely linked major groups designated HLA-A, HLA-B, HLA-C and HLA-D. The diagram below shows how they are clustered on the 6th chromosome and how parents would pass them on to their children. Like any other genetic characteristic, the genes that determine our tissue type (or transplantation antigens) are passed on in a random fashion.

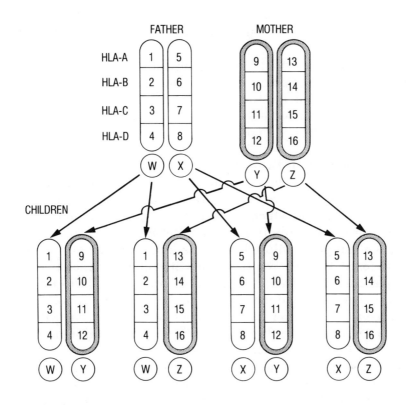

Figure 37.1. Selection of the Donor

There are a number of important points relating to Figure 37.1:

- Each of the transplantation antigens is numbered 1 through 16. Each group of four antigens on each of the chromosomes is called a haplotype and is inherited as a single unit. These haplotypes have been arbitrarily designated W, X, Y and Z in Figure 37.1.

- As with any other genetic characteristic the parents pass on only one chromosome and thus only one set of transplantation genes (haplotype) to each child.

403

- Each child receives one set of transplantation genes (or one haplotype) from each parent.

- There are only four possible combinations of haplotypes in the children. Each of the four combinations is represented in Figure 37.1.

- In the usual situation, a brother or sister of the immunodeficient patient is selected as the donor. Each sibling has a 25 percent chance of having the same transplantation genes as the immunodeficient patient, and therefore being a suitable match, since there are only 4 possible combinations of genes.

The Procedure of Bone Marrow Transplantation: Bone marrow transplantation is accomplished by removing bone marrow from the pelvic bones. Bone marrow is removed by drawing up the marrow through a needle which is about 1/8 of an inch in diameter. Only two teaspoons are taken from each puncture site because, if more is taken, the sample is diluted with the blood which bathes the bone marrow space. Usually two teaspoons are taken for each two pounds of the patient's body weight. The procedure may be performed under general anesthesia or under spinal anesthesia. The discomfort after the procedure varies from donor to donor. Nearly everyone will require some type of pain control medication for 2-3 days, but most are able to return to full activity within a week.

After removal from the donor, the bone marrow is passed through a fine sieve to remove any small particles of bone, placed in a sterile plastic bag and given to the immunodeficient patient through a needle in his/her vein in the same manner as a blood transfusion is given.

Results of Bone Marrow Transplantation: Bone marrow transplantation between "matched" siblings has been successfully employed in the treatment of immunodeficiency since 1968. The first child (a patient with SCID) is still alive and doing well. This case suggests that as best as can be determined the graft is very long lasting and appears to be permanent. In the usual patient with immune deficiency, a bone marrow transplantation involving a "matched" marrow has minimal graft versus host disease and is associated with an overall success rate of approximately 50 percent. A great deal depends on the health of the patient at the time of the transplant. If the patient is in relatively good health and free of infection at the time of the transplantation, the outlook is good.

Newer Methods: Because only 25 percent of the patients have a sibling which is a "match," there has been a major effort to develop alternative methods for transplanting "unmatched" marrows. Using a variety of techniques, it is now possible to remove the mature T-lymphocytes from the bone marrow prior to infusing it into the patient. In this way, the infused marrow is not able to recognize the patient as foreign and the graft versus host reaction is markedly reduced and sometimes eliminated. Although the mature T-lymphocytes have been removed from the grafted marrow, T-lymphocytes of donor origin can still develop from the stem cells and therefore reconstitute T-lymphocyte immunity. The risk of graft versus host disease from these T-lymphocytes is markedly reduced because these cells develop from the immature precursor cells in the grafted marrow, and they have been "educated" during their maturation to not recognize the recipient (host) as foreign. These treated marrows are not grafted as easily as "matched" marrow and occasionally more than one transplant has to be performed. The usual donor for this kind of transplant is a parent since they share one half of the transplantation antigens of their child (see the diagram above).

These kinds of "half-matched" marrow transplants have only been employed since 1980, but they have been quite successful.

Gamma Interferon

Phagocytic cells (neutrophils, monocytes, eosinophils) of patients with Chronic Granulomatous Disease of childhood (CGD) do not kill some types of bacteria and fungi. CGD phagocytic blood cells are unable to produce hydrogen peroxide and other oxygen containing compounds, necessary to kill some microorganisms. Recently, an international study with gamma interferon has shown that CGD patients who are given gamma interferon three times weekly subcutaneously had approximately 70 percent fewer serious infections than those patients not receiving gamma interferon. Also, when those patients taking gamma interferon have infection they require less time in the hospital. Benefit from gamma interferon is most evident in children under 10 years of age, but all age groups benefit.

Interferon is a substance that is found naturally in the body. It is called "interferon" because it was originally discovered to interfere with virus growth. Several different interferons have been identified and it has been shown that they exert numerous effects on the immune system. The interferons are named alpha, beta and gamma interferon.

Gamma interferon is related to alpha and beta interferon for its antiviral activities, but in addition is a potent stimulus of phagocytic cells. Among the phagocytic cell activating properties of gamma interferon is stimulation of hydrogen peroxide production. Increased hydrogen peroxide production improves the bacterial killing by the phagocytic cells.

Gamma interferon (Actimmune, Genentech, Inc.) is supplied in a single-dose vial of 0.5 ml. The dose for each patient is determined by body surface area, which means that both height and weight are considered. For small children, the surface area is not a reliable method, so they are dosed by weight alone. The vials must be kept refrigerated, never frozen, and should not be shaken. There is no preservative in the gamma interferon preparation, so unopened vials should be discarded after 12 hours at room temperature. Expired vials should not be used.

Gamma interferon is given as a subcutaneous injection three times a week (such as Monday, Wednesday, and Friday). The preferred sites for injection are the right and left thigh and arm. Administration is similar to giving insulin to diabetics. Used syringes should be disposed of in an approved needle waste box and the full box returned to the physician or local emergency room for proper incineration. Never discard needles and syringes in your household trash.

Common side effects of gamma interferon therapy include fever, muscle aches, headaches, and occasionally chills. Side effects can be minimized by taking the interferon at bedtime. If headaches persist the next morning, the drug should be given earlier in the evening. If the severity of the side effects are unacceptable, it may be appropriate to reduce the dose. If no side effects are seen but suddenly fevers follow the gamma interferon dose, this should be reported to the physician. In some instances fevers following gamma interferon can be a sign of a subclinical (or hidden) infection. A few patients experience symptoms of depression from interferon gamma and if depression occurs, consult your physician. Patients with a history of seizures should not take gamma interferon.

PEG-ADA

Deficiency of the enzyme adenosine deaminase (ADA) causes a rare, life-threatening form of Severe Combined Immunodeficiency Disease (SCID). About one in a million children are born with ADA deficiency.

The highest levels of ADA occur in cells of the immune system (lymphocytes). When ADA is missing, a substance called deoxyadenosine (dAdo) builds up and is toxic to the developing immune system, while other tissues and organs are resistant to dAdo. Most ADA deficient infants lack both T- and B-lymphocytes and are susceptible soon after birth to repeated, serious infections of the skin, respiratory and digestive tracts. In milder cases, the onset of serious illness may be delayed until 2-3 years of age. The full blown condition is known as Severe Combined Immunodeficiency Disease (SCID). ADA deficiency accounts for a quarter to a fifth of all cases of SCID.

Although antibiotics and regular treatment with intravenous gamma globulin are helpful, SCID is fatal, usually by 2 years of age, if immune function is not restored. Like other forms of SCID, ADA deficiency can be cured by transplanting bone marrow from a donor with the same tissue type as the patient (usually a brother or sister), but in most cases, a "matched" donor is not available. There are three approaches to treating patients who do not have a "matched" donor: transplantation of "partially matched" or haploidentical marrow, enzyme replacement, and gene therapy. The various methods of carrying out bone marrow transplantation, and some experimental approaches to gene therapy are discussed elsewhere in this sourcebook. This section will deal with enzyme replacement therapy.

The rapid elimination of purified enzymes by the body made enzyme replacement for ADA deficiency impractical until it was discovered that linking a polymer called polyethylene glycol, or PEG, to an enzyme could greatly prolong its effectiveness after injection. The New Jersey company that discovered the PEG technique decided to test its clinical application in ADA deficiency, partly in response to the Orphan Drug law enacted in 1983 to promote the development of treatments for rare diseases. A clinical trial of PEG-ADA (Enzon, Inc.), using ADA purified from cows, was begun in April, 1986 in a critically ill child who had failed to benefit from two haploidentical marrow transplants. Based on the results with this patient and others treated subsequently, PEG-ADA was approved for treatment of ADA deficiency by the US Food and Drug Administration in March 1990.

A teaspoon of PEG-ADA has as much ADA activity as almost a gallon of red blood cells or a billion normal T-lymphocytes. Intramuscular injection of this amount or less of PEG-ADA once or twice a week maintains enough ADA activity in the bloodstream of patients to effectively eliminate the toxic effects of dAdo that cause immune deficiency. This gives the immune system a chance to recover over a period of from several weeks to a few months. Continued weekly injections of PEG-ADA are then necessary to maintain a dAdo free environment.

Immune function improves in all patients, but the degree varies, ranging from very little to nearly normal. However, clinical benefit is more uniform and is evident by six months of treatment even in the 20 percent of patients whose lymphocyte counts remain most depressed. Pneumonia, diarrhea and other serious infections present at the start of therapy resolve and growth, which is severely impaired initially, resumes. Over the longer term, treated children have responded well to ordinary childhood infections, allowing them to have normal contact with other children. Older patients are attending school. Thus far IVIG has been discontinued in about half the children receiving PEG-ADA. Those who have caught chicken pox and other viral infections, which can be fatal to untreated patients with SCID, have recovered uneventfully and developed long-lasting, normal levels of antibody to the virus.

Of 30 patients treated with PEG-ADA, there have been two deaths, which were due to infection early in treatment. Aside from the discomfort of an intramuscular injection, PEG-ADA has had no side effects. Initially there was concern that, because a non-human source of ADA was being used, patients might develop antibodies that could neutralize the enzyme or cause allergic reactions. Antibodies to bovine ADA can be detected by sensitive tests in most patients, but there have been no allergic reactions and in only two cases has antibody necessitated an increase in the dose of PEG-ADA.

Because ADA deficiency is so rare it will take much more time to establish the truly long-term benefit of PEG-ADA. For the same reason the cost of producing PEG-ADA is very high and will have to be born by insurance or government. However, in the six years it has been in use, PEG-ADA has proved life-saving and effective in reversing the dire clinical outlook associated with SCID due to ADA deficiency. We anticipate that the children now receiving PEG-ADA will one day be candidates for stem cell gene therapy when that procedure is shown to be safe, reliable and effective.

Chapter 38

Therapies for People with Arthritis

Therapy for arthritis depends on the type of disease being treated, its severity, and patient response. Here are some common forms of treatments being used to treat the major types of arthritis.

Arthritis Medicines

According to research conducted by the Food and Drug Administration, the medicines taken most by people over 45 are those used to relieve the discomfort of arthritis. This is hardly news to older Americans, who know only too well the pain and discomfort caused by this condition.

Of the more than 100 forms of arthritis, osteoarthritis, rheumatoid arthritis, and gout are the most common. According to the Arthritis Foundation, more than 9 million Americans over 65 have some symptoms of osteoarthritis. This condition strikes the joints of the hands, feet, knees, hips, neck, and back. Pain may come and go and can vary from mild to severe. Although rheumatoid arthritis often begins during middle age, it can develop at any age. This type of arthritis, which tends to occur more often in women than men, most commonly affects the joints of the wrists, hands, and feet, but can

NIH Pub No. 1990:241-292/00003, prepared by the National Institute on Aging Food and Drug Administration as part of its series *Age Page. FDA Consumer Reprint DHHS Pub. No 89-1080. For more detailed information on arthritis and rheumatic disorders see Omnigraphics' sourcebook on arthritis.*

affect any movable joint. Gout causes sudden swelling and extreme pain, usually in only one joint, often the big toe.

Most forms of arthritis cannot be prevented or cured, so the goals of treatment are to relieve pain and maintain or restore the function of the arthritic joint. A treatment program may include rest, weight control, heat therapy, exercise, and drug therapy. Appropriate treatment depends on the type of arthritis, the stage of the disease, and the general health of the patient.

Nonsteroidal Anti-Inflammatory Drugs

Nonsteroidal anti-inflammatory drugs (NSAIDs) are commonly used to relieve arthritis pain. These drugs block the production of prostaglandins, chemicals in the body that cause pain and inflammation, which is the stiffness, swelling, and warmth felt by people with arthritis. Although some NSAIDs are available without a prescription, most are prescription drugs. It often takes a few days to a week before NSAIDs start to work and 2 to 3 weeks before the full benefits of treatment are felt.

Some of the most frequently used NSAIDs are listed below. These drugs are divided into two groups: salicylates and nonsalicylates. Although both groups of drugs have similar pain-relieving effects, they may have somewhat different side effects.

Salicylates

Aspirin:

- Bayer,
- Bufferin,
- Easprin,
- Ecotrin, and others

Choline magnesium trisalicylate:

- Trilisate

Choline salicylate:

- Arthropan

Diflunisal:

- Dolobid

Magnesium salicylate:

- Magan

Salicylsalicylic acid:

- Disalcid,
- Mono-Gesic

Nonsalicylates

Diclofenac:

- Voltaren

Fenoprofen:

- Nalfon

Flurbiprofen:

- Ansaid

Ibuprofen:

- Motrin,
- Rufen, and
- over-the-counter brands such as Advil and Nuprin

Indomethacin:

- Indocin

Ketoprofen:

- Orudis

Meclofenamate:

• Meclomen

Mefenamic acid:

• Ponstel

Naproxen:

• Naprosyn

Naproxen sodium:

• Anaprox

Piroxicam:

• Feldene

Sulindac:

• Clinoril

Tolmetin:

• Tolectin

Side Effects of NSAIDs

Along with much-needed pain relief, NSAIDs may cause unwanted side effects in some people. However, side effects do not occur in everyone. They are listed here so that you will know they are possible and so that you can recognize them early and report them to your doctor. In some cases, it may be necessary to adjust treatment to keep side effects to a minimum.

NSAIDs can cause stomach ulcers. Because ulcers sometimes don't cause symptoms, it's important for people taking NSAIDs to see their doctor for regular checkups. Other stomach problems caused by these drugs include heartburn, nausea, stomach pain, vomiting, diarrhea, and occasionally gastro-intestinal (GI) bleeding. GI bleeding, which can be especially serious for older people, is signaled by black or very dark stools or blood in the stool. NSAIDs also can cause headaches, dizziness, and blurred vision.

Coated aspirin tablets and long-acting aspirin products may lessen stomach irritation. NSAIDs should be taken with a full glass of water (or milk), food, or antacids to reduce stomach upset. In addition, an antiulcer drug—misoprostol (brand name Cytotec)—is approved for preventing stomach ulcers which can be brought on by NSAIDs in people at high risk of ulcer complications (for example, older people or those who have had ulcers in the past). Ulcers and other serious stomach problems are more common in smokers and people who drink alcohol while taking these drugs. People who have stomach problems should see their doctor as soon as possible.

Corticosteroids

Corticosteroids also may reduce arthritis inflammation. These drugs closely resemble cortisone, a natural hormone produced by the body. They can be taken by mouth or by injection directly into a stiff, swollen joint.

Although corticosteroids rapidly relieve the pain, swelling, and redness caused by arthritis, these powerful drugs have serious side effects. Lowered resistance to infection, indigestion, weight gain, loss of muscle mass and strength, mood changes, blurred vision, cataracts, diabetes, thinning of bones (osteoporosis), and increased blood pressure can be caused by this treatment. Other side effects may develop and should be discussed with your doctor. Also, serious stomach problems may occur in people who take corticosteroids along with NSAIDs.

Commonly Prescribed Corticosteroids

Betamethasone:

- Celestone

Cortisone:

- Cortone

Dexamethasone:

- Decadron

Hydrocortisone:

• Hydrocortone

Methylprednisolone:

• Medrol

Prednisolone:

• Hydeltrasol

Prednisone:

• Deltasone

Triamcinolone:

• Aristocort

Disease-Modifying Drugs

Researchers believe that disease-modifying, antirheumatic agents slow the progress of rheumatoid arthritis, but these drugs are not used for osteoarthritis. These prescription drugs include gold compounds, D-penicillamine, and antimalarial medications.

Gold compounds. Gold compounds can help people with mild to moderate rheumatoid arthritis. Auranofin (Ridaura) is taken by mouth. Aurothioglucose (Solganol) and gold sodium thiomalate (Myochrysine) are available in injection form. It may be 2 to 6 months before relief is felt. Possible side effects are blood in the urine, easy bruising, sores in the mouth, skin rash, and numbness in the hands and feet. Diarrhea often occurs in those who take gold by mouth, and many people receiving injectable gold notice a metallic taste.

Penicillamine. Penicillamine (Depen and Cuprimine) is also used to treat rheumatoid arthritis. This drug may take 2 to 6 months to work. Side effects include blood in the urine, fever, joint pain, skin rash, sores in the mouth, easy bruising, weight gain, and, in rare cases, muscle weakness. People taking gold compounds or penicillamine should be checked regularly by their doctor.

Hydroxychloroquine. Hydroxychloroquine (Plaquenil) and other drugs originally developed to treat malaria can be used to relieve swelling, stiffness, and joint pain caused by rheumatoid arthritis. People taking these drugs should have regular eye exams because these medicines can permanently damage the retina (the light-sensitive tissue at the back of the eye). Diarrhea, headaches, loss of appetite, skin rash, and stomach pain are other possible side effects. Liver problems may develop in people who drink alcohol while taking antimalarial drugs.

Immunosuppressants

The immune system normally protects the body against foreign invaders such as viruses. Some researchers believe that rheumatoid arthritis is an autoimmune disease, a disease in which the immune system reacts against the body's own tissues. Immunosuppressants, drugs that suppress the immune system, can ease the symptoms of rheumatoid arthritis. Azathioprine (Imuran) and methotrexate are immunosuppressants used to treat this form of arthritis. Side effects, which include mouth sores, infection, fever, chills, sore throat, nausea, diarrhea, and unusual tiredness, should be reported to your doctor.

Gout Medications

Uric acid is a normal waste product found in the body. When uric acid levels become extremely high, crystals form in and around joints causing gout. The pain and swelling caused by this form of arthritis are treated with two types of drugs: one to reduce inflammation and the other to lower uric acid levels. For example, colchicine blocks inflammation. Allopurinol (Zyloprim and Lopurin) reduces uric acid production. Sulfinpyrazone (Anturane) and probenecid (Benemid) increase uric acid elimination. Allopurinol, sulfinpyrazone, and probenecid can help prevent gout attacks, but they must be taken for several months to work effectively. (In fact, allopurinol can actually make gout worse if this drug is started during an attack.) Common side effects may include diarrhea, nausea, vomiting, stomach pain, and a rash.

Over-the-Counter Drugs

Over-the-counter (OTC) products such as aspirin and low-dose forms of acetaminophen (e.g., Tylenol) and ibuprofen (e.g., Advil and Nuprin) temporarily relieve minor arthritis pain. "Extra strength" and "arthritis formula" aspirin products contain more aspirin in each tablet than regular aspirin. As with prescription drugs, these drugs can cause side effects, particularly when directions are not followed carefully. For example, long-term, high-dose use of acetaminophen, ibuprofen, or aspirin may cause liver or kidney damage. Do not take OTC products for long periods without consulting a doctor. Combinations of OTC products, or OTC products and prescription drugs, should not be taken without checking with your doctor first.

In addition, some OTC ointments offer short-term relief of minor arthritis pain. However, these ointments, which are rubbed over painful joints, do not reduce swelling and should not be used for long periods of time.

Taking Arthritis Drugs Safely

Because arthritis drugs may interact with other types of medicine, it is important to let your doctor know if you are taking any other prescription or over-the-counter medications. Be sure to follow your doctor's instructions exactly when taking your medicine—take only the amount specified, ask what to do if you miss a dose, and do not suddenly stop taking your medicine without consulting your doctor. It is also important to keep all appointments with your doctor so that your progress can be checked regularly.

Beware of Unproven Remedies

Americans spend over a billion dollars each year on useless pills, gadgets, and diets hoping to find a cure for arthritis. Because arthritis pain can come and go, many people believe that these phony "cures" really work. Beware of any pill or device that promises miracles. Don't be misled by products that are supposed to cure many different diseases. If you have questions about the safety and usefulness of a treatment, ask your doctor.

Treatment Without Drugs

Medication at times is not the best or only choice of treatment for arthritis. Physical therapy or surgery may be indicated, or prescribed in combination with drugs. A decision should be made by the patient, physician, and any other members of the treatment team.

- **Physical therapy** can be performed at home or with professional supervision.

- **Rest** is important in treatment of painful, inflamed and fatigued joints, but it can lead to temporary stiffening of diseased joints.

- **Moist heat or cold** often reduces pain and increases the range of motion. A shower, a bath, heat packs, hydrotherapy, and paraffin treatments are examples. Occasionally, for acutely inflamed joints, ice packs are an initial treatment.

- **Exercise** helps maintain range of motion in affected joints. Special daily exercises also can strengthen the muscles that surround an arthritic joint.

- **Devices** like splints, braces and crutches may give relief by resting or supporting painful joints. Aids for daily activity can help by supporting a joint that is painful, weak or impaired.

Surgery

Sometimes orthopedic surgery is indicated. Surgeons can correct some deformities, remove inflamed tissue, repair ligament damage associated with arthritis, or replace a diseased joint.

For More Information

Learning about arthritis and arthritis medicines will help you make informed decisions about your health care. The Arthritis Foundation has free booklets on many forms of arthritis and most arthritis medications. This material is available from local chapters, which are listed in the telephone directory, or from the national headquarters at P.O. Box 19000, Atlanta, Georgia 30326; telephone (404) 872-7100.

Free information about arthritis is also available from the National Institute of Arthritis and Musculoskeletal and Skin Diseases, Building 31, Room 4C05, 9000 Rockville Pike, Bethesda, Maryland 20892; telephone (301) 496-8188.

To learn more about drugs and their side effects, contact the Food and Drug Administration, HFD-365, 5600 Fishers Lane, Rockville, Maryland 20857; telephone (301) 295-8012.

The National Institute on Aging (NIA) distributes a number of free Age Pages, including:

- *Arthritis Advice,*
- *Safe Use of Medicines by Older People,*
- *Finding Good Medical Care for Older Americans,*
- *Who's Who in Health Care*, and
- *Health Quackery.*

To receive these publications and other material on health and aging, contact the NIA Information Center, P.O. Box 8057, Gaithersburg, Maryland 20898-8057.

Chapter 39

Intravenous Immunoglobulin: Prevention and Treatment of Disease

Abstract

The National Institutes of Health Consensus Development Conference on Intravenous Immunoglobulin: Prevention and Treatment of Disease brought together biomedical scientists in immunology, infectious disease, and pediatrics, as well as health care providers, patients and their families, and the public to address the safe and effective uses of intravenous immunoglobulin (IVIG) preparations. Following 1 1/2 days of presentations by experts and discussion by the audience, a consensus panel weighed the evidence and prepared a consensus statement.

Among their findings, the panel concluded that all currently available IVIG preparations are safe and effective in treating the conditions for which they have been licensed; however, their efficacy in treating other conditions remains to be established. Effective regimens have been developed for primary immunodeficiencies and secondary immunodeficiencies, idiopathic thrombocytopenic purpura, and Kawasaki syndrome. However, optimal dosages and treatment schedules still need to be established for patients who may benefit from IVIG therapy.

The panel also concluded that the risks of IVIG therapy are minimal, and adverse events, which are rare, can often be alleviated by reducing the rate or volume of infusion. Future research is also important, particularly studies to discern the mechanisms of action of

NIH Consensus Statement, volume 8, number 5, May 21-23, 1990.

IVIG, to compare the effectiveness of IVIG preparations, and to determine their long-term effectiveness and their effect on quality of life for patients receiving IVIG.

The full text of the consensus panel's statement follows.

Introduction

Immunoglobulins are proteins produced by cells of the B lymphocyte lineage that are the major effector molecules of the humoral immune system. Immunoglobulin molecules are antibodies that react with specific antigens, although in many circumstances, the specificity of a given immunoglobulin antibody is unknown. Immunoglobulin preparations from human blood were first used in clinical medicine in 1952 to treat immune deficiency conditions. At that time, the only available preparations required intramuscular administration. In the past decade, several immunoglobulin preparations for intravenous administration have become available. Although initially used for immune deficiency states, intravenous immunoglobulin (IVIG) has also been utilized as a prophylactic and therapeutic reagent in a variety of other conditions. The use of IVIG has undergone tremendous growth in the past several years. This rapid growth in use is the result of improvements in the preparations of IVIG, which have led to reduced morbidity and reports of its benefits in a number of unexpected circumstances. IVIG has been used in such diverse diseases as primary immunodeficiencies, pediatric AIDS, infections in low birth weight infants, bone marrow transplantation, chronic lymphocytic leukemia, idiopathic thrombocytopenic purpura, Kawasaki syndrome, and demyelinating polyneuropathies. However, important questions regarding its use still remain. To assess the usefulness of IVIG in diseases where substantive data existed, the National Institute of Allergy and Infectious Diseases and the Office of Medical Applications of Research of the National Institutes of Health convened a Consensus Development Conference on Intravenous Immunoglobulin: Prevention and Treatment of Disease on May 21-23, 1990. Cosponsors were the National Cancer Institute, National Heart. Lung, and Blood Institute, National Institute of Child Health and Human Development, National Institute of Neurological Disorders and Stroke, and the Food and Drug Administration. In the various disease states in which IVIG has been used, the following questions were considered:

- What are the data to support the efficacy of IVIG in these circumstances?

- What are the appropriate dosage and treatment schedules?
- What are the risks involved in the use of IVIG?
- What are the mechanisms of action?
- Are all IVIG preparations equally efficacious?
- What are the directions for future research?

After a day and a half of presentations by experts in the field and discussion by the audience, a consensus panel drawn from specialists and generalists from the medical profession and related scientific disciplines, clinical investigators, and public representatives considered the evidence and came to the conclusions on the following pages.

What Are the Data to Support the Efficacy of IVIG in These Circumstances?

Primary Immunodeficiencies. The beneficial effects of intramuscular (IM) injection of immune globulin (IG) in the prophylactic treatment of patients with primary immunodeficiency syndromes have been well established. Early studies based on small sample sizes have indicated that almost any desired blood level of IgG can be obtained by use of intravenous immunoglobulin and that infection rates are reduced by use of IVIG as compared with IM IG. IVIG has been shown to ameliorate chronic sinopulmonary disease that developed in patients on long-term IM IG. There is a suggestion that chronic enterovirus meningoencephalitis in patients with X-linked agammaglobulinemia may be less frequent in those receiving prophylactic IVIG as compared with historical data in which IM IG was used. Hence, IVIG has become the current standard in clinical practice for replacement therapy of patients with primary immunodeficiencies (e.g., X-linked agammaglobulinemia and common variable immunodeficiency and immunoglobulin subclass deficiency in which deficiencies of antibody production to common pathogens can be demonstrated). Studies have shown that maintenance of a trough level of 500 mg/dL is beneficial. Dose ranges of 200-800 mg/kg/mo have been shown to be effective, but dose or frequency of infusions must be tailored to the individual patient, because half life of infused IVIG varies widely.

Pediatric AIDS. Because AIDS is an acquired immunodeficiency, it is reasonable to consider the use of IVIG therapy in pediatric patients with HIV infection, given the success of IVIG in primary immunodeficiencies. To date, small, uncontrolled studies have suggested the efficacy of IVIG in pediatric AIDS by decreasing the morbidity from common bacterial pathogens, as well as measles, but no controlled studies have been completed. Currently, the National Institutes of Health (NIH) is sponsoring two large, controlled trials of IVIG with and without zidovudine (AZT) in HIV-infected children. A definitive assessment of the efficacy of IVIG in pediatric HIV infection awaits the results of these trials.

Infections in Low Birth Weight Infants.

- *Prevention of infection in low birth weight infants.* Premature infants have insufficient placental transfer of maternal IgG and have been demonstrated to have low levels of serum IgG. Hence, it is reasonable to consider IVIG prophylaxis in premature infants. Some pilot studies indicated a lower rate of severe infection in IVIG-treated low birth weight infants compared with placebo-treated patients. In a recently completed randomized, double-blind, placebo-controlled trial involving a large number of infants with birth weights of 500-1,500 grams, it was noted that mortality was not significantly reduced among IVIG recipients. However, the number of infections was significantly reduced among IVIG recipients. It should be noted that there was some evidence that beneficial effect may vary by birth weight category, and significantly more placebo patients were small for gestational age. Information about long-term results (greater than 56 days) is not available from this trial. Moreover, preliminary analysis of other trials indicates no significant difference in infection rates between IVIG recipients and placebo recipients. However, differences in study design make direct comparison of the various trials difficult. Further information will become available as a result of the ongoing trial sponsored by the National Institute of Child Health and Human Development Neonatal Research Network. At this time, IVIG cannot be recommended as standard prophylaxis of low birth weight infants.

- *Treatment of presumed neonatal infection.* To date, small trials using primarily historical controls have yielded mixed results. Questions remain concerning dose, schedule, and patient selection. Variability in preparations and lots creates a number of difficulties in predicting results of treatment for specific organisms. There is a potential role for directed preparations containing specific antibodies. Furthermore, studies in neonatal animals have shown that in some situations survival is less with high concentrations of IVIG plus antibiotic compared with antibiotic alone. The routine use of IVIG as adjuvant therapy of neonatal infections cannot be recommended at the present time.

Bone Marrow Transplantation. In a large study of bone marrow transplant recipients, reduced rates of septicemia and local infection were noted for IVIG-treated patients (500 mg/kg weekly) compared with untreated controls. Several studies have shown a decreased rate of acute graft versus host disease (GVHD) in patients receiving IVIG, 500 milligrams to 1 gram per kilogram weekly. Results of limited trials suggest that in pediatric bone marrow recipients, reduction in infection and death but not GVHD has been associated with IVIG administration.

It has been noted that IVIG decreases the incidence of interstitial (presumably CMV) pneumonia but is ineffective in preventing CMV infections. IVIG plus ganciclovir is beneficial in treating CMV pneumonia in patients who are not ventilator dependent.

Chronic Lymphocytic Leukemia. A study in 10 centers in which 57 patients with CLL were followed for one year of observation has been completed. The incidence of major and moderate bacterial infections was significantly reduced in hypogammaglobulinemic CLL patients who received IVIG. The number of trivial infections was unchanged by intravenous immunoglobulin. Maintenance of serum IgG levels greater than 640 mg/dL tended to correlate with fewer infections, especially serious bacterial infections. The data support the conclusion that IVIG may be useful to prevent serious infections in patients with CLL with hypogammaglobulinemia.

Idiopathic Thrombocytopenic Purpura. Among children with ITP, the use of IVIG has been documented to increase platelet counts. This treatment is utilized in the rare pediatric patient with potentially life-threatening bleeding (e.g., 400 mg/kg/d x2-5 or 1 g/kg/d x1 or 2). A number of therapeutic options are available for managing the child with newly diagnosed ITP who does not have serious hemorrhage: IVIG, corticosteroids, or close observation without therapy. IVIG has been used in chronic ITP to postpone the requirement for a splenectomy. There is no firm evidence of curative effects in either acute or chronic ITP. Responses appear to be similar with different manufacturers' products licensed for this purpose. In adult patients with ITP, IVIG, at the doses indicated above, has also been used for the rapid correction of life-threatening thrombocytopenia, with or without corticosteroids. Administration every 10 to 21 days is usually required to maintain adequate platelet counts. Other indications include administration to steroid-refractory patients preoperatively. In addition, IVIG may be employed at the same dosage in patients who cannot use corticosteroids and in patients with immunodeficiency including those with HIV-associated thrombocytopenia. Although IVIG administration before scheduled splenectomy is effective, cost-benefit relationships are unclear because of the low incidence of complications during this procedure, even with extremely low platelet counts.

Kawasaki Syndrome. Studies of IVIG in Kawasaki syndrome using 400 mg/kg daily for 4 days indicate a prompt anti-inflammatory response in the acute phase and a significant decrease in the formation of coronary aneurysms compared with low/moderate aspirin administration regimens. More recently, a dosage schedule of 2 g/kg as a single administration has been shown to be at least as effective as the four-dose schedule. Complications of the larger single-dose administration were few. A smaller study using 1 g/kg as a single dose also seemed to suggest similar efficacy to the four-dose regimen.

IVIG and aspirin administration has become a standard treatment for Kawasaki syndrome. The panel agrees that on the basis of available studies, IVIG administered as a single dose of 2 g/kg is effective therapy for patients who fulfill the diagnostic criteria for Kawasaki syndrome. Treatment of patients recognized after the tenth day of the disease has not been studied systematically.

The advantages of treating patients with Kawasaki syndrome with IVIG as early as possible must be balanced against the probability that children with other inflammatory diseases will also be treated inadvertently. There is no evidence that this latter group of children will be benefitted.

Chronic Inflammatory Demyelinating Polyneuropathies. Several small studies have shown positive responses to IVIG in the majority of treated patients. Treatment needs to be periodically repeated to prevent relapse. When considered in comparison with customary treatments, IVIG may be easier to use and to be associated with fewer complications than repeated therapeutic plasma exchange and long-term glucocorticoids, respectively.

Guillain-Barré Syndrome. In a preliminary analysis of a large, randomized multicenter trial of IVIG compared with therapeutic plasma exchange, there is an indication of improved functional recovery for patients receiving IVIG. Definitive conclusions regarding the efficacy of IVIG in Guillain-Barré syndrome will need to await the final analysis of this study and other confirmatory studies.

Intractable Seizure Disorders. A number of uncontrolled studies and anecdotal reports have indicated benefit of IVIG administration in children with intractable seizures. The absence of randomized, double-blind studies does not allow specific recommendations to be made regarding such treatment. The panel emphasizes the need for controlled human studies in this area.

What Are the Appropriate Dosage and Treatment Schedules?

Effective doses of IVIG have been demonstrated in primary immunodeficiencies, ITP, and Kawasaki syndrome. Whether alterations in amount, frequency, or duration of administration will improve efficacy is not known. Specific details of dosage regimens are discussed in detail in the response to the previous question.

What Are the Risks Involved in the Use of IVIG?

The incidence of adverse events associated with the administration of IVIG is reported by the manufacturers to be in the range of 1 to 15 percent, usually less than 5 percent. Most of these reactions are mild and self-limited. Severe reactions occur very infrequently and usually do not contraindicate further IVIG therapy. Neither HIV nor hepatitis B infection has been transmitted to recipients of products currently licensed in the U.S. The various IVIGs are manufactured from large numbers of donors whose plasma has been tested and found to be negative for hepatitis B surface antigen and HIV antibody. A number of adverse events have been recognized. These include the following:

- pyrogenic reactions marked by high fever and systemic symptoms;

- minor systemic reactions with headache, myalgia, fever, chills, light-headedness, nausea and/or vomiting;

- vasomotor and/or cardiovascular manifestations, marked by changes in blood pressure and tachycardia. These may be related to occasional reports of shortness of breath and chest tightness; and

- hypersensitivity and anaphylactic reactions.

Risk Factors. Patients with primary antibody deficiency syndromes may be at increased risk for reactions. Anaphylactic reactions induced by anti-IgA can occur in individuals who have a total absence of circulating IgA and antibodies to IgA. These are extremely rare in panhypogammaglobulinemic individuals and potentially more frequent in patients with subclass deficiencies. Frequency of reactions may be correlated with volume and/or rate of infusion. Seriously ill patients with compromised cardiac function may be at increased risk of vasomotor or cardiac complications manifested by elevated blood pressure and/or cardiac failure.

Prevention and Management. Adverse reactions often can be alleviated by reducing the rate or the volume of infusion. For patients with repeated severe reactions unresponsive to these measures, hydrocortisone, 1-2 mg/kg, intravenously, can be given 30 minutes before IVIG infusion. In those rare instances when reactions related to anti-IgA antibodies have occurred, use of IgA-depleted preparations will reduce the likelihood of further reactions. Avoidance of anaphylactic reactions may require the use of material completely devoid of IgA. Because the combination of the absence of IgA and the presence of anti-IgA antibodies is infrequent and reactions are rare, screening for IgA-deficiency is not routinely recommended for potential recipients of IVIG.

As with any biologic or pharmacological product, the potential for new or previously unrecognized adverse events should be anticipated. With IVIG these include the following:

- transmission of blood-borne pathogens such as the newly identified hepatitis C virus.

- immunosuppression for example, administration of IVIG has been associated with transient effects on immune response that do not appear to have clinical significance. However, with increased dosage of IVIG or new products for the treatment of specific infections, the possibility of adverse outcomes from immunosuppression should be considered.

• After nearly a decade of experience, the safety of IVIG has been established. For any potential recipient, the small risk of adverse reactions must be weighed against the likelihood of significant benefit. For those patients who require repeated courses of IVIG such as those with a primary humoral immunodeficiency home infusion by the patient or a family member after adequate training has been effectively utilized and is cost effective.

What Are the Mechanisms of Action?

At the present time, we assume that all effects of IVIG are related to the quantity and quality of IgG in the product. Various mechanisms may be important in the different therapeutic uses of IVIG, including:

1. Replacement therapy for primary and secondary immunodeficiencies,

2. Specific passive immunotherapy, and

3. Management of specific inflammatory and/or immunologic disorders.

Efficacy of IVIG infusions in primary immunodeficiency diseases is probably related to replacement of antibodies to environmental pathogens. Despite variations in the titer of specific antibodies, all licensed preparations are apparently efficacious in the treatment of these diseases. In addition, pooled antibodies may have physiologic activities other than pathogen recognition that may contribute to the beneficial effects of replacement therapy.

The effectiveness and the mechanism of action of IVIG in secondary immunodeficiencies such as indolent lymphomas is presumed to be similar to that in primary immunodeficiencies. In these diseases, a reasonable correlation between rates of systemic infection and concentrations of serum immunoglobulins supports this presumption. The benefit of prophylactic replacement of IgG in very low birth weight infants is not established. Attempts to replace antibodies may be rational in this situation. However, it is possible that administration of immunoglobulin from large donor pools could adversely affect the development of the infant's immune system, as there is substantial evidence in mice that anti-idiotypic antibodies may profoundly affect immune responsiveness. For conditions such as bone marrow transplantation and pediatric HIV infection, the complexity of immunologic abnormalities will make determination of mechanisms extremely difficult. IVIG is also being used for specific passive immunotherapy. In these instances, the titers of specific antibodies are of paramount importance. Moreover, consideration must be given to the possibility that large amounts of apparently irrelevant antibodies may block receptors on the surface of phagocytes and thus interfere with effective disposal of microbial pathogens. In the treatment of ITP, there may be multiple mechanisms of IVIG action. The platelet count increase occurring within several days of the initiation of therapy appears to be caused by diminished sequestration of autoantibody-sensitized platelets. This may be caused by interference with Fc receptors on the cells of the monocyte-macrophage system. A similar mechanism may operate in other autoimmune and alloimmune cytopenias. Sustained responses to IVIG may represent spontaneous remissions or may be related to an immunosuppressive effect of IVIG.

There are several possible mechanisms by which the infusion of large concentrations of immunoglobulins may have an immunosuppressive effect. The presence of IgG dimers in immunoglobulin preparations, a result of pooling samples from a large number of individual donors, likely represents the occurrence of idiotype-anti-idiotype complexes. There is evidence that anti-idiotype antibodies in IVIG react with epitopes on the autoantibodies in patients with thyroiditis or spontaneous factor VIII inhibitors. Alterations of T-cell subsets and of in vitro B cell function, both spontaneous and mitogen driven, have been reported in patients treated with IVIG. It is unknown if these observations are related to a mechanism of therapeutic effect.

A striking anti-inflammatory effect of IVIG has been observed. This phenomenon is most apparent in Kawasaki syndrome, where reductions in fever, neutrophil counts, and acute phase reactants regularly occur within a day or so of initiation of treatment. This effect is not unique to Kawasaki syndrome but has been seen in other inflammatory disorders. The mechanisms are unknown but may be distinct from those that mediate immunosuppression. One possible mechanism demonstrated in experimental animals is the inhibition of complement-dependent tissue damage caused by binding of IVIG to active C3 fragments.

There is a great need for an understanding of the mechanisms of IVIG in the various conditions in which it is used. A variety of mechanisms have been suggested but none proven. Mechanistic hypotheses such as the provision of anti-idiotype antibodies, Fc receptor blockade, and alteration of reticuloendothelial cell system function should be rigorously tested. Utilization of appropriate animal models would provide an efficient way to test these hypotheses.

Are All IVIG Preparations Equally Efficacious?

Seven IVIG preparations have been licensed in the U.S.: all seven for use in primary immunodeficiencies, five for idiopathic thrombocytopenia, and one for chronic lymphocytic leukemia. For these disease groups, the limited comparative data available reveal no differences in efficacy among the licensed preparations. For the other uses of IVIG, there is insufficient information to choose one product over another or to know whether each has comparable activity. Given the large number of conditions for which IVIG may have potential value, the prescribing physician should be aware of the demonstrated efficacy of each IVIG preparation to treat a specific disorder. The products and their quality are under the control of commercial firms who must meet general regulatory guidelines of the Center for Biologics Evaluation and Research of the Food and Drug Administration. These include tests for sterility, pyrogenicity, purity, and safety. It is required also to measure antibody levels against polio, measles, hepatitis B, and diphtheria. At the present time, there is no requirement to identify hepatitis C virus in IVIG preparations. Epidemiologic data support the quality and safety of current products. However, guidelines and monitoring methods must be developed as information about transmission of hepatitis C virus and other infectious diseases becomes better defined. Consideration should be given to screening donors for hepatitis C.

Confidence in the capacity of a given preparation to accomplish the desired end result would be enhanced if a more rigorous procedure were established for using IVIG to prevent or treat infections caused by specific microorganisms. The availability of antibody titers to a wider range of pathogens would permit a more rational basis for the choice of a specific product in situations where immunotherapy is directed to a restricted number of infectious agents. Because the factor essential for the effectiveness of IVIG in a number of disorders, such as ITP and Kawasaki syndrome, is unknown, it is not possible to predict efficacy of a given preparation of IVIG for any of these disease processes.

What Are the Directions for Future Research?

The effects of IVIG in the various disease states can probably be accounted for by the presence of one or more specific antibodies. These may be directed against microbial pathogens or their toxins, common idiotypes, cellular components, receptors, or regulatory proteins. The need for massive doses of IVIG to achieve therapeutic effects suggests that many of these antibodies are present at very small concentrations in immunoglobulin pools. One of the major directions of future research therefore should be to identify and isolate these particular antibodies or prepare supplementary monoclonal antibodies so that more specific therapeutic interventions can be designed.

- There is a great need for an understanding of the mechanisms of action of IVIG in the various conditions in which it is employed. Without knowledge of specific mechanisms, progress in this area will be slow. This should be a major focus of future efforts

- Appropriate objective outcome measures, including long-term outcome measures, should be established that can be applied in clinical trials. Cost-effectiveness and objective measures of quality of life should be included in this analysis. Without such outcome measures, results of additional clinical trials will be difficult to interpret.

- Controlled clinical trials in pediatric intractable recurrent seizures, chronic inflammatory demyelinating polyneuropathies, and Guillain-Barré syndrome are warranted in the U.S. In addition, consideration should be given to clinical trials in areas where compelling biologic reasons or experimental data suggest potential efficacy. There is no justification for clinical trials in areas without strong biologic rationales.

- Serious neonatal infections continue to be a major problem. Development of appropriate hyperimmune preparations of IVIG should be undertaken for this purpose.

- Comparative efficacy of various preparations of IVIG should be established, if possible.

- Surveillance for long-term positive and adverse effects should be carried out.

Conclusions

In answer to the question, "What are the data to support the efficacy of IVIG in various clinical circumstances?" the consensus panel concludes the following:

- IVIG is a safe and effective means of replacement therapy in patients with primary humoral immunodeficiency syndromes in which deficiencies of antibody production to common pathogens can be demonstrated. The ideal dosage of IVIG has not been established, although the monthly administration of 200-800 mg/kg appears to be adequate to maintain trough Ig levels at approximately 500 mg/dL in most patients.

- The usefulness of IVIG in pediatric AIDS has not been documented. Results are not yet available from two ongoing NIH-supported multicenter placebo-controlled double-blind trials being carried out to evaluate this issue in more detail.

- The use of IVIG in the prevention of late onset infections in preterm neonates has a rational basis. However, the data indicate that this is of no value in neonates of birth weight of more than 1,500 grams in neonates under 1,500 grams, the results are conflicting. Thus, the currently available data do not support the routine use of IVIG in this group either. Although there may be an impact of IVIG on the rate of bacterial infections in this group and the length of hospitalization, there is no effect on mortality. The use of IVIG as adjuvant therapy in neonates with infections is not supported by the current data. Additional clinical trials, especially involving the use of hyperimmune preparations, would be useful to delineate this issue.

- In immunosuppressed bone marrow transplant recipients, IVIG is useful to treat interstitial (CMV) pneumonia, in combination with ganciclovir. IVIG may be protective against gram-negative septicemia and development of local infections in these patients. In addition. IVIG may suppress GVHD in some patient groups.

- In hypogammaglobulinemia associated with chronic lympho-cytic leukemia, IVIG can decrease the number of infections sig-nificantly. Although it has no effect on mortality, there is a decrease in the number of days per year spent in a hospital or convalescing.

- The comparative efficacy of IVIG versus corticosteroids or other approaches has not been clearly delineated in either adults or children with ITP. IVIG is useful in the treatment of pediatric acute ITP where it usually increases the platelet count rapidly. In adult ITP, it can also induce increases in the platelets. In adults, it is most useful in special circumstances requiring acute increases in the platelet count such as immediately before surgery.

- IVIG in conjunction with aspirin is the current standard of care for children during the first 10 days of Kawasaki syndrome to prevent the development of coronary aneurysms.

- IVIG shows some promise in the treatment of chronic inflamma-tory demyelinating polyneuropathies, and Guillain Barré syn-drome, and therefore additional clinical trials are warranted.

- There is the preliminary suggestion that IVIG might be useful in certain childhood intractable seizure disorders. Therefore, clinical trials are warranted.

In response to the question, "What are the appropriate dosage and treatment schedules?" the consensus panel concludes that in most circumstances this has not been established. For primary and second-ary immunodeficiencies, ITP, and Kawasaki syndrome, effective regi-mens have been developed, but there is no evidence about whether these schedules are optimal.

In response to the question, "Are all IVIG preparations equally efficacious?" the consensus panel concludes that the preparations are efficacious for the indications for which each has been licensed. Al-though it is possible that they can be used for other conditions inter-changeably, the comparability of the various preparations of IVIG for these purposes has not been documented.

In response to the question, "What are the risks involved in the use of IVIG?" the consensus panel concludes that they are minimal. However, appropriate means to monitor IVIG for contamination with potential pathogens should be developed.

In response to the question, "What are the mechanisms of action of IVIG?" the panel concludes that in most circumstances present hypotheses are speculative and not proven.

In response to the question, "What are the directions of future research?" the panel concludes information concerning mechanism of action is critically needed. Deriving information concerning mechanisms of action or other potential uses of IVIG from clinical experiments and trials is costly and inefficient. Without knowledge concerning anticipated objective physiologic end points, trials to establish effective therapeutic regimens are empiric and new initiatives largely exercises in serendipity.

Chapter 40

Drug Therapies for Lupus and Associated Immune Disorders

Nonsteroidal Anti-Inflammatory Drugs (NSAIDS)

Pain and inflammation are common findings in patients with systemic lupus erythematosus. Sometimes these symptoms indicate serious organ involvement which may require potent anti-inflammatory and immunosuppressive drugs, such as steroids (Cortisone, Prednisone). At other times the inflammation is not as severe or does not affect major organs and a less potent drug is indicated. In these cases, other milder anti-inflammatory and analgesic drugs can be used, especially a group of drugs called the nonsteroidal anti-inflammatory drugs (NSAIDS). While NSAIDS are not approved specifically for SLE by the Food and Drug Administration, they are approved for use in many musculoskeletal pain conditions such as arthritis and tendinitis, which also afflict lupus patients.

Types of NSAIDS

There are many different types of NSAIDS, including aspirin and other salicylates. Examples include; ibuprofen (Motrin, Advil), naproxen (Naprosyn), sulindac (Clinoril), diclofenac (Voltaren),

Joint and Muscle Pain in Lupus © 1995, *Steroids in the Treatment of Lupus* © 1994, *Nonsteroidal Anti-inflammatory Drugs (NSAIDS)* © 1993, *Anti-Malarials in the Treatment of Lupus* ©1994, *Imuran, Cytoxan and Related Drugs* © 1993. © Lupus Foundation of America, Inc. Reprinted with permission.

piroxicam (Feldene), ketoprofen (Orudis), diflunisal (Dolobid), nabumetone (Relafen), etodolac (Lodine), oxaprozin (Daypro), indomethacin (Indocin), and newer ones which will be marketed over the next few years. Aspirin is an anti-inflammatory when given in high doses, otherwise it is just a pain killer like acetaminophen (Tylenol).

Mechanism of Action and Use

The body produces substances called prostaglandins which play a role in causing inflammation and pain. NSAIDS work mainly by preventing the formation of prostaglandins which decreases the pain and inflammation.

Although all NSAIDS appear to work in the same way, there are differences between them. The beneficial effects and side effects of individual NSAIDS can vary from patient to patient. Side effects experienced by one patient may not be noted by someone else taking the same drug. Likewise, benefits experienced by one person may not be experienced by another.

As a general rule, NSAIDS are most useful in treating joint pain, muscle pain and joint swelling experienced by individuals with lupus. Occasionally, they can be used to treat the chest pain caused by pleurisy. When used for treatment of a mild flare, a NSAID may be the only drug needed. More active disease may require additional medications. Although there is no absolute reason not to use NSAIDS during pregnancy, it is best to avoid using these medications in the first few months after conception and before delivery.

Side Effects

There are two major drawbacks to NSAID therapy in people with lupus;

1. They do not help serious organ inflammation (e.g. kidney or brain involvement) and

2. They may be associated with troublesome, irritating or even serious side effects. As with all medications, if you experience any adverse reaction when taking one of these medications, you should consult your physician.

Common Side Effects

Common side effects include stomach upset, headache, drowsiness, easy bruising, high blood pressure and/or fluid retention.

NSAIDS commonly cause dyspepsia, a burning, bloated feeling in the pit of the stomach. In some patients, stomach inflammation (gastritis) or gastric ulcers may occur. This can cause bleeding, either obvious and painful or hidden and painless. This loss of blood may lead to anemia. To help protect the stomach, NSAIDS should always be taken with food or directly after a meal. Some patients may need additional medications to control their stomach symptoms. Some may tolerate one kind of NSAID, but have gastric irritation with others. A person on long term NSAID therapy should have a blood count periodically to insure that anemia from gastric bleeding is not occurring. Patients with a history of gastric (stomach) or duodenal (intestinal) ulcers should tell their physician before starting on NSAIDS. Furthermore, any individual who will not accept blood products for religious or other reasons, should inform their doctor of this prior to starting therapy with NSAIDS.

Symptoms of headache or drowsiness are usually mild, but if severe, the medicine may have to be stopped.

NSAIDS affect the function of platelets, a type of blood cell important in normal blood clotting. Although aspirin has the greatest effect, all NSAIDS have some effect on platelet function. If the function of these cells is impaired, it will take longer for blood to clot and bruising can occur more readily. Some patients are very susceptible and experience easy bruising. If severe, the medication should be discontinued.

In older patients or in lupus patients who already have kidney or blood pressure problems, commonly seen side effects include:

- fluid retention,
- high blood pressure and
- reduced kidney function.

In young, otherwise healthy people, these side effects are not common. Patients with lupus nephritis often have some reduction in kidney function. Therefore, NSAID use in this type of SLE may cause further deterioration in kidney function and should be closely supervised.

Uncommon Side Effects

Other rarer, but important side effects include abnormal liver tests, asthma, severe headache with neck stiffness and skin rashes.

Aspirin and other NSAIDS occasionally cause elevations in liver enzyme blood tests, suggesting mild liver inflammation (hepatitis). Patients with active lupus appear to be especially susceptible to this side effect. This usually does not mean that the NSAID should be stopped, but the liver tests may have to be monitored on a regular basis.

Patients with asthma may notice a worsening of their asthmatic symptoms when they use aspirin or other NSAIDS. If this occurs, these drugs should not be used.

Severe headache with neck stiffness is a rare side effect seen almost exclusively in people with lupus. It is important because it mimics meningitis. Hives and other skin rashes, although uncommon, occur with these medications and may require the discontinuation of the NSAID.

Photosensitive skin rashes, which could mimic a flare of SLE, also occur rarely with some NSAIDS.

While NSAIDS are widely used with good results and without problems, individuals with lupus and their prescribing doctors need to pay special attention to the potential side effects. Since drug side effects and symptoms of increased lupus activity may be identical, it is important to alert a physician if any of these symptoms occur. For example: fluid retention headache or rash may be side effects, but they also may occur when the disease activity increases. In any case, notify your doctor when any side effect occurs so therapy can be adjusted. The majority of NSAID-related side effects are reversible once the drug is stopped. Some side effects are seen initially or only in the blood. Therefore, with continued NSAID use regular blood counts, including tests of liver and kidney function, should be monitored every 34 months.

Summary

NSAIDS are often used to treat the musculoskeletal pain and inflammation which may accompany active lupus. If well tolerated, they can be effective as the only treatment for people with mild flares. They can also be used in combination with stronger medications to treat greater disease activity. These medications are not immunosuppressive and, therefore, it is inappropriate to use them alone for the treatment of severe lupus. NSAIDS may have either irritating or serious side effects. People with SLE taking NSAIDS require clinical and laboratory monitoring by their physicians.

Anti-Malarials in the Treatment of Lupus

Anti-malarials were first developed during World War II to treat parasitic infections like malaria. As early as the 1960s it was found that these medications could also be used to treat the joint pain that occurs with rheumatoid arthritis. Soon thereafter, anti-malarials were found to have similar beneficial effects in the treatment of joint pain associated with systemic lupus erythematosus (SLE) and some physicians use it for the treatment of Sjogren's syndrome.

Anti-malarials are particularly effective in treating skin and joint symptoms that may occur in SLE. They have been demonstrated to improve muscle and joint pain, inflammation of the lining of the heart (pericarditis) and lung (pleuritis), and other symptoms of lupus such as fatigue and fever. However, anti-malarials alone are not appropriate treatment for more severe manifestations of systemic lupus such as kidney disease.

Anti-malarials are very effective in the treatment of discoid lupus erythematosus (DLE): 60-90 percent of patients with DLE went into remission or showed major improvement after being treated with anti-malarials. Skin lesions of DLE which have not responded to treatment with topical therapy (e.g., creams, ointments) may improve with the use of antimalarial drugs.

Anti-malarials are useful in subacute cutaneous lupus, and in overlap syndromes in which patients have acute symptoms of lupus and other autoimmune disorders.

The anti-malarials which are utilized in North America for the management of systemic lupus include hydroxychloroquine (Plaquenil), and chloroquine (Aralen). These medications are not equivalent in their side effects. In the United States, hydroxychloroquine (Plaquenil) is the most popular because it is felt to be less likely to cause eye side effects. Quinacrine (Atabrine) is available from compounding pharmacists and will be available again in 1994.

How Do Anti-Malarials Control Systemic Lupus Erythematosus?

The specific mechanisms by which anti-malarials control systemic lupus are unclear. It is known that anti-malarials protect against the damaging effects of ultraviolet light and improve skin lesions. Some researchers suggest that they combine with certain chemicals or groups of proteins and interfere with enzyme groups that play a role in inflammation. Other researchers believe that more complex mechanisms are involved, such as the inhibition of antibody response or the direct inhibition of the lupus erythematosus (LE) cell reaction.

Can Anti-Malarials Be Taken with Other Medications?

Anti-malarials can be taken with other medications used for the treatment of systemic lupus such as corticosteroids (Prednisone), cytotoxics and anti-inflammatory medications including aspirin. In fact, anti-malarials are sometimes given in combination with Prednisone to reduce the amount of steroid that is needed to improve symptoms. Obviously, any combination of medications should always be prescribed by a physician.

Is It Safe to Take Antimalarials During Pregnancy?

The manufacturer recommends that anti-malarials not be given during pregnancy because of the potential for congenital malformations in the baby. However, anti-malarials are apparently safe when used to prevent malaria in pregnant women (lower doses than this are used in the treatment of SLE). Dr. Ann Parke of the University of Connecticut has treated 11 lupus patients who were pregnant with anti-malarials without adverse effects on the fetus. Clearly, more research is needed on this topic. Patients should discuss the pros and cons of continuing treatment with anti-malarials during pregnancy if they are planning to become pregnant.

What Are the Side Effects of Anti-Malarials?

The side effects of anti-malarials include skin rashes and pigmentary changes. Atabrine specifically, can cause yellow pigmentation of the skin. Hair loss and dryness of the skin have also been described. Stomach upset, loss of appetite, abdominal bloating, cramps, nausea, vomiting and diarrhea may also occur with the use of anti-malarials. These side effects usually go away after the patient adjusts to the medication. However, if they continue, a physician should be consulted.

Some patients may experience headaches, muscle aching, and weakness as a result of taking antimalarials. Nervousness, irritability or dizziness can occur, but these side effects are uncommon. Major neurological side effects such as confusion or seizures are quite rare. However, if any of these side effects occur, they should be reported immediately to a physician.

A major potential side effect of anti-malarial use is the possible damage to the retina (back of the eye) that these medications can produce. It is important to note that retinal damage due to the use of antimalarials is dose-related, and that the low doses currently used in the treatment of lupus are rarely associated with retinal damage. Most cases of eye disease occur in patients receiving more than 400 mg of Plaquenil or more than 250 mg of Aralen daily. Atabrine is not known to cause retinal damage.

Retinal damage due to the use of Plaquenil is sometimes reversible, if it is treated early. However, damage due to the use of chloroquine (Aralen) is irreversible. Thus, it is necessary to have the patient see an eye doctor or ophthalmologist prior to beginning treatment with anti-malarials for a baseline examination and to receive follow-up eye examinations every three to six months thereafter. On many occasions, an ophthalmologist can see mild changes in the retinal pigment that indicate early damage due to the use of anti-malarials. In addition to the regular eye check-ups which test visual acuity and eye pressure, tests for color vision and visual field might be necessary. New computer assisted machines for testing the visual field for anti-malarial effects are very sensitive to small changes. Patients can also monitor themselves between visits by the use of an Amsler grid, which can be requested from an ophthalmologist. If visual symptoms do occur (blurred vision or any other changes in vision), these should be reported immediately to a doctor.

In summary, anti-malarials can contribute substantially to the relief of some of the symptoms associated with lupus, especially those of the skin and joints. Other potential benefits of Plaquenil have included decreased levels of cholesterol in some patients who are steroid dependent and decreased thrombosis in some patients with positive cardiolipin antibodies. Plaquenil has also been used by some physicians for the management of Sjogren's syndrome. All of the side effects mentioned are not common and anti-malarials are generally regarded as safe to use in the treatment of lupus.

Imuran, Cytoxan and Related Drugs

Why would anyone take a medicine that might cause their white blood cell count or platelet count to fall abruptly, leading to increased susceptibility to infections or a tendency to bleed? Why would any one take a medicine that might, to a small extent, predispose them to develop certain cancers? People with lupus take them because these medications can be very helpful, especially in cases where the kidneys or other major organs are involved.

While some of the side effects of Imuran (azathioprine), Cytoxan (cyclophosphamide) and other immunosuppressive and cytotoxic drugs are noted above, they are generally reversible by either reducing the dosage or stopping the medication. Although immunosuppressive drugs can have serious side effects, they can be of great value in the treatment of lupus. They can help to prolong life, preserve kidney function, reduce symptoms, and sometimes may serve to put the disease into remission. These drugs help to reduce symptoms and damage to vital organs, such as the kidney, until a natural remission occurs. They sometimes help to achieve a remission earlier.

Immunosuppressive and cytotoxic drugs are sometimes used in the treatment of systemic lupus erythematosus (SLE) for two major reasons. First, they are potent drugs which help to reduce disease activity in major organs such as the kidney. Second, they may reduce or sometimes eliminate the need for steroids (cortisone derivatives such as prednisone). Steroids used alone to treat major organ involvement must sometimes be given in high doses. This increases the risk of both short-term and long-term side effects, which may sometimes be worse than the disease itself. Immunosuppressive drugs can be used either in addition to, or instead of, steroids or to lower the amount of steroid needed and often spare the patient the undesirable side effects of steroid therapy.

How Do They Work?

Cells in the body divide and grow at varying rates. Examples of rapidly dividing cells include the antibody producing cells of the immune system, blood cells, hair cells, gonadal cells and malignant cells. Cytotoxic (cyto=cell, toxic=damage) drugs work by targeting and damaging cells which grow at a rapid rate. In lupus, the immune system is hyperactive and produces auto-antibodies at a rapid rate of growth. Cytotoxic medicines have their greatest effect against rapidly dividing cells and, therefore, can be beneficial in the treatment of lupus by suppressing the cells involved in the hyperactive immune response. The effect is a reduction in disease activity. There are risks associated with the use of cytotoxic drugs. The immune system may be suppressed too much and cause an increased susceptibility to infections such as shingles and pneumonia. The bone marrow may be suppressed and result in reductions in red blood cells, white blood cells and platelets. Suppression of hair cell growth may lead to a net loss of hair. The cytotoxic effects on gonadal cells may lead to sterility.

Imuran

Imuran is less potent and less effective than Cytoxan, but it has far fewer side effects. Its use may cause the white blood cell count, platelet count, or red blood cell count to decrease, and it might increase the risk of developing lymphoma (a cancer involving the lymph glands, liver and spleen). However, it is well tolerated in most cases. Blood tests to determine the white blood cell, platelet and red blood cell count should be taken regularly in patients receiving Imuran. Adjustments in dosage are made if the tests indicate a serious decrease in the blood-count.

Imuran is also used to treat lupoid hepatitis, rheumatoid arthritis and other autoimmune disorders, and to reduce the amount of steroids given.

Cytoxan

Cytoxan may cause many side effects, but it is well tolerated by most patients. Like Imuran, it may cause an upset stomach and its use may cause the white blood cell count, platelet count, or red blood cell count to decrease. Blood tests to determine the white blood cell, platelet and red blood cell count should be taken each month in patients receiving Cytoxan. If the blood count is seriously decreased, the dosage is adjusted and the blood counts will generally return toward normal.

Patients receiving treatment with Cytoxan have an increased risk of developing malignancies including leukemia, bladder cancer and other tumors. Cytoxan may also cause temporary or permanent sterility in both women and men, preventing them from having children.

It may also cause damage to a developing fetus if a woman gets pregnant unintentionally while being treated with the drug. Use of Cytoxan may cause bleeding from the bladder, but this usually can be prevented by drinking large amounts of water. Cytoxan also predisposes a patient to develop shingles, which is a painful, blistering skin condition. It can cause hair loss. Like Imuran, the use of Cytoxan may predispose a patient to develop unusual infections, particularly when it is used in combination with high doses of steroids.

A typical daily dose of Imuran or Cytoxan is 125 to 150 milligrams (mg) a day given orally. A low dose is 75 mg or less. Cytoxan should be taken in the morning with fluid and should not be taken at night, when fluid intake is low. Cytoxan and Imuran are not used together except in certain experimental conditions. Cytoxan (but not Imuran) can be given at a much higher dose intravenously on a monthly basis. This may be quite effective for severe kidney disease and may help to avoid some of the side effects that occur with daily oral dosages of this drug.

Related Drugs

Other cytotoxic drugs related to cyclophosphamide (Cytoxan) are chlorambucil (Leukeran) and nitrogen mustard (Mustargen). Leukeran has similar side effects to Cytoxan. As previously stated, lupus patients taking cyclophosphomide (Cytoxan), azathioprine (Imuran), chlorambucil (Leukeran) or nitrogen mustard (Mustargen) need to have their blood counts monitored each month. In response to the lab tests and side effects, drug dosage is adjusted to prevent or reverse any serious toxicity.

Methotrexate is usually given orally once a week, although it may also be given by injection. The dosage is generally 7.5 to 20 milligrams per week. Methotrexate is well tolerated by most patients. Its use in lupus has not been thoroughly tested, but it is given quite commonly for rheumatoid arthritis and has been shown to produce improvement of joint pain and stiffness. It does not predispose a patient to develop malignancies. However, liver disease and lung reactions can occasionally occur with the use of methotrexate and it can be sun sensitizing. Dosage may need to be decreased if kidney disease is present. Blood counts should also be taken each month in patients receiving this drug and dosage modified if side effects are detected.

Conclusion

While cytotoxic medications are not needed and should not be used in cases of mild lupus, these medications can be very helpful in cases where the kidneys or other major organs are involved, or in cases where the lupus is quite active and symptomatic. Sometimes a kidney biopsy or other tissue biopsy is necessary before deciding whether to use these medications. Even in more serious cases of major organ involvement, they should not be used indefinitely without good reason.

Therefore, it is important to assess the beneficial effects as well as the risks involved in cytotoxic drug therapy. Doctors use the term "risk-benefit ratio" to describe the comparison of side effects to beneficial effects of medications. While these drugs are not FDA-approved, they are commonly used and accepted as standard practice. People with lupus should discuss the risk-benefit ratio of using these medications with their physician.

Steroids Used in the Treatment of Lupus

Many of the symptoms of lupus result from inflammation in various tissues of the body. Cortisone, manufactured naturally by the body's adrenal glands and also made synthetically, has been found to have a marked anti-inflammatory effect.

Cortisone and its derivatives are steroids, the most effective anti-inflammatory drugs known. Their use can substantially reduce the swelling, warmth, tenderness and pain that is associated with inflammation.

While steroid dosage should be kept at the lowest effective level, steroids must not be stopped suddenly if they have been taken for more than four weeks. After that time, some shrinking of the adrenal glands will occur, and they may not produce enough cortisone if the synthetic steroids are discontinued abruptly. A slow reduction in the dosage of steroids allows the adrenal glands to regain their ability to manufacture natural cortisone.

Prednisone

Steroids produced by the outer part (cortex) of the adrenal gland are called "corticosteroids." Prednisone is the synthetic corticosteroid preparation most often used in the treatment of lupus. It comes in tablets of 1, 5, 10, and 20 milligrams (mg). It may be given as often as four times each day, as infrequently as once every other day, or at any frequency in between. Less than 10 mg per day is generally considered a low dose; 11 to 40 mg daily is a moderate dose; and 41 to 100 mg daily is a high dose.

Steroids may also be given by intra-muscular (IM) injection or may be injected directly into a joint. Occasionally, very large doses of steroids may be given for a short period of time. This treatment, referred to as "pulse steroid treatment," involves giving 1000 mg of methyl-prednisone intravenously each day for three days.

Prednisone is an extremely effective drug and may be necessary to control active lupus. Although many lupus patients do not need to stay on steroids continuously, those with severe disease or active and serious kidney lupus may require long-term steroid treatment.

There is usually prompt relief of most symptoms after initiation of treatment with corticosteroids. When pleurisy or pericarditis occur, small or moderate doses of steroids are helpful. Steroids can often be avoided completely in mild cases of lupus (i.e., those involving only the joints and skin).

In addition to prednisone, some other cortisone derivatives include hydrocortisone, methylprednisolone (Medrol) and dexamethasone (Decadron).

Prednisone and other steroids should not be stopped suddenly. Lupus patients should discuss the reasons for using steroids and other treatment alternatives which may be available with their physician.

Side Effects

Some of the more common side effects of steroids include changes in appearance, such as acne, development of a round or moon-shaped face, and an increased appetite leading to weight gain. Steroids may also cause a redistribution of fat, leading to a swollen face and abdomen, but thin arms and legs. In some cases, the skin becomes more fragile, which leads to easy bruising.

Psychological side effects of steroids include irritability, agitation, euphoria or depression. Insomnia can also be a side effect. These changes in appearance and mood are often more apparent with high doses of steroids.

An increase in susceptibility to infections may occur with high doses of steroids. Prednisone may also aggravate diabetes, glaucoma, and high blood pressure, and often increases cholesterol and triglyceride levels in the blood. In children, steroids can suppress growth.

Side Effects from Long-Term Use of Steroids

Side effects that may be caused by the long-term use of steroids include cataracts, muscle weakness, avascular necrosis of bone and osteoporosis.

Avascular necrosis of bone, usually associated with high doses of prednisone over long periods of time, produces pain, an abnormal bone scan, and an atypical X-ray appearance. It occurs most often in the hip, but it can also affect the shoulders, knees and other joints. Avascular necrosis of bone is quite painful and often requires either a core bone biopsy, electrical stimulation, or total surgical joint replacement for pain relief.

Steroids reduce calcium absorption through the gastrointestinal tract which may result in osteoporosis, or thinning of the bones. Osteoporosis can lead to bone fractures, especially compression fractures of the vertebrae, causing severe back pain. Giving calcium and other medications may help to prevent osteoporosis.

There is also a relationship between steroids and premature arteriosclerosis, which is a narrowing of the blood vessels by fat (cholesterol) deposits.

In general, there is a close relationship between the side effects of steroids and the dose and duration of their use. Thus, a high dose of steroids given over a long period of time is more likely to cause side effects than a lower dosage given over a shorter period of time.

Conclusion

Corticosteroids are extremely effective anti-inflammatory agents and can be very helpful in treating active lupus, despite their significant side effects. Treatment with steroids should always be kept at the lowest possible effective dose and should never be stopped suddenly. Hopefully, we will soon develop effective alternative therapies which will not be as toxic as steroids. The history of most therapies shows, however, that those which are extremely effective often are associated with side effects. This is certainly the case with steroids.

Part Six

Manipulating the Immune System

Chapter 41

Immunosuppression and Transplantation

Transplantation of healthy organs and tissue is a powerful and curative therapy for kidney failure, liver failure, leukemias, aplastic anemia, certain immunodeficiency diseases, and heart disease. Since the first unsuccessful attempts tn transplant kidneys in the 1950s, the prognosis for kidney transplantation has improved to an 85 percent success rate, which allows recipients to lead near-normal lives. Although the kidney remains the organ that is most successfully transplanted, procedures involving other organs and tissues also have improved significantly. Advances in three areas of immunology have contributed to the enhanced success of transplantation:

- an increased understanding of human immunogenetics;

- elucidation of the immunology of the events associated with graft rejection and acceptance; and

- the discovery of highly effective immunosuppressive drugs.

The surface of our cells carries proteins known as major histocompatibility complex (MHC) antigens. These proteins act as signals that identify what is uniquely self to our immune system. Although all humans possess variations of the MHC antigens, it is the precise combination of these proteins that constitutes our "immunologic fingerprint." The importance of matching MHC antigens for transplanted

NIH Pub No. 91-2414.

451

organs is similar to the need to match blood types for blood transfusions. However, MHC matches are more complex, and excessive differences between a donor and a recipient will cause the latter's immune system to attack and reject the transplanted organ. Scientists continue to devote considerable effort to improving methods for MHC-typing as well as to conducting basic research in understanding the structure and function of the MHC.

Nevertheless, rejection can occur even when organs are matched for MHC antigens. The discovery of special drugs that suppress the immune system has helped prevent this response. Within the last decade, the introduction of the highly effective immunosuppressive drug CyA (cyclosporin A) has made renal, cardiac, and liver transplantation procedures viable therapeutic options. However, side effects of immunosuppressive drugs demonstrate the need to develop alternative immunosuppressive approaches.

The ultimate goal of transplantation therapy is to induce a state of graft acceptance, or immune tolerance of the transplanted organ or tissue, without compromising the immune system or general well-being of the recipient. Recently, a small number of patients received a form of irradiation prior to renal transplantation that appeared to have induced a degree of "tolerance" such that these patients have retained their kidney grafts without the use of immunosuppressive drugs. This promising result needs to be developed and refined for routine clinical application.

Overview

Clinical transplantation began in the 1950s with unsuccessful attempts to graft kidneys from cadaveric donors. The first successful grafts occurred between identical twins who presented no tissue antigen difference. The modern era of transplantation began in 1962 with the first trials of the immunosuppressive drug azathioprine (Imuran). At that time, there were no concrete data on the nature of the tissue antigens that provoked rejection, and little information was available on the nature of the immune responses.

In the first two decades after the introduction of azathioprine, improved methods of tissue typing established the genetics of the human leukocyte antigen (HLA) system. During the same period, antilymphocyte antibody therapy demonstrated the power of destroying or interfering with lymphocyte function in animal and clinical experiments. However, the most dramatic developments in transplantation have occurred in the past decade.

During the 1980s, scientists made the empiric discovery of cyclosporine, developed detailed knowledge of the molecular biology of HLA, and discovered and developed research applications of monoclonal antibodies (MoAbs). These antibodies now are used both as tools to define various subsets of cells and functional molecules and as selective therapeutic agents to prevent or treat graft rejection. The use of cyclosporine has led to improved kidney graft survival and has allowed the extensive application of transplantation to heart, liver, and pancreas. However, despite these advances, specific tolerance without continuing administration of immunosuppressive drugs has not been achieved.

Immunogenetics and Transplantation

The MHC antigens are cell surface molecules that present foreign antigens to T cells of the immune system. These T cells, in turn, mount a response against the foreign antigens. Curiously, the MHC antigens are themselves very immunogenic, or recognizable, when presented to the immune system of another individual. Thus, they become the principal target for rejection following an organ graft or the transplant of tissue. The structure of HLA molecules differs subtly from individual to individual, producing so-called polymorphisms that are recognized as foreign. In humans, the MHC antigens are encoded by a set of linked genes, which are located on chromosome 6 and designated as HLA. Every individual has 12 HLAs with 6 inherited from each parent. Although more than 120 distinct HLA types are known within the human population, their distribution shows marked racial and ethnic patterns.

Compatibility for HLA yields superior results in clinical tissue transplantation. Other determinants, known as "minor histocompatibility antigens," also play a part in graft rejection. Although these minor antigens are still poorly characterized, they apparently elicit low primary, but strong secondary, immune responses.

Detailed structural information now is available for both the MHC receptor antigen and the T cell receptor complex. MHC molecules on the membrane of an antigen-presenting cell carry a biochemically processed peptide antigen. This MHC/peptide complex interacts with antigen-specific receptors on the T cell membrane, resulting in activation of the T cell. During T cell maturation, T cell selection occurs with specificity for foreign antigens in the context of self-MHC. However, T cell clones with high affinity for self-MHC markers apparently are programmed for destruction in the thymus. This process normally would prevent the immune system from destroying self components.

Many autoimmune diseases occur at a greater than normal frequency among individuals with particular HLA alleles, whose population distributions are not random. Most of these disease associations involve MHC class II antigens rather than class I antigens.

More basic information is needed on the structure of HLA molecules and of the T cell receptors that interact with them. This information will aid in the development of novel approaches for the induction of transplantation tolerance and the prevention of graft rejection. It also may be useful in the diagnosis and prevention of autoimmune diseases.

Research Opportunity

- Elucidate the structure of HLA molecules and T cell receptors, and apply this knowledge to the development of approaches to preventing graft rejection and autoimmune diseases.

Transplantation Tolerance

The conventional definition of immune tolerance entails the acceptance of an organ or tissue graft from another individual, as opposed to the usual rejection of such grafts. Transplantation tolerance is mediated in three ways:

- through clonal deletion of T cells that would have responded to the foreign antigen;

- through clonal inactivation of these cells; and

- through active suppression of T cells.

Chimerism is one approach to effecting transplantation tolerance. A chimera is an organism or individual in which reside cells of different origins. In this procedure, the T cells of a recipient are eliminated to ensure the survival of donor cells. Donor cells are then infused into the recipient. The recipient thus becomes a chimera, whose immune status is dominated by the donor cells. Several other clinical and experimental procedures have been developed to achieve tolerance. These approaches include injecting soluble transplantation antigens, using cyclosporine and other immunosuppressive drugs, destroying host lymph node cells by irradiation, using MoAbs to deplete T cell subsets, matching MHC markers between donor and host, and performing autologous bone marrow transplantation using cells removed from an individual before irradiation. In addition, placing donor tissues in tissue culture or treating them with MoAbs before transplantation sometimes makes them acceptable to the host immune system.

Very few patients have met the criteria for full transplantation tolerance, which entails the acceptance of the donor organ or tissue without the continuing use of immunosuppressive drugs. In these cases, success has been achieved following total lymphoid irradiation before renal transplantation.

Research Opportunity

- Refine clinical criteria for inducing transplantation tolerance, particularly where it involves manipulating the tissues and cells of the donor but not of the host.

Transgenic Mice and Transplant Tolerance

Scientists have learned that transplants from one mouse to another within an inbred strain are accepted, whereas transplants between individuals of different genetic strains are rejected. Experiments show that both positive and negative selection of the T cell repertoire occurs in transgenic mice that contain donor mouse T cell receptor genes. Other experiments using transgenic mice have shown not only negative selection within the thymus but also transplant tolerance involving a poorly understood but apparently novel mechanism in the peripheral lymphoid system.

Research Opportunity

Study the transplant tolerance mechanism that operates in the peripheral lymphoid system of transgenic mice, and explore clinical applications of this mechanism.

Bone Marrow Transplantation

Bone marrow transplantation (BMT) is the preferred treatment in cases of aplastic anemia, severe combined immunodeficiency, and leukemia in patients who have had irradiation to destroy malignant cells. Despite an increasing success rate, BMT can fail for several reasons. For example, the bone marrow graft may be rejected by the recipient or the recipient may develop graft-versus-host disease (GVHD) or infections resulting from the reduced function of the immune system. GVHD is a complication following BMT where the donor cells attack the recipient. HLA matching in industrialized countries often is impeded by the likelihood of only small families being available to study. When possible, autologous transplants, or the use of an individual's own marrow, help reduce tissue rejection. Depleting the donor marrow of mature T cells helps reduce GVHD. However, this procedure also leads to higher rates of engraftment failure and relapse in patients with leukemia. Thus, there is considerable debate concerning the relative value of using T cell depletion or immunosuppressive drugs to control GVHD.

Several approaches to improving the outcome of BMT are being developed based on experiments in mice. For example, treating recipients with monoclonal antibodies that are specific for natural killer (NK) cells and T cells reduces the likelihood of graft rejection. Synthetic compounds also are being tested for their ability to destroy specific T cells *in vitro*, thus reducing GVHD when these cells are reintroduced into mice that have received BMT.

In other studies, the inclusion of host T cells with donor cells dramatically prevents GVHD. Moreover, high doses of donor CD4+ lymphocytes apparently minimize rejection and GVHD.

Research Opportunities

- Elucidate the role of minor histocompatibility antigens and NK cells in BMT.
- Use mouse models to develop new techniques for increasing the success rate of BMT.

Xenogeneic Transplantation

Despite serious efforts in the 1960s, the use of organs from subhuman primates as xenografts in clinical trials has failed to produce long-term successes. However, the current shortage of organs from human donors has sparked renewed interest in xenogeneic transplantation. Several factors complicate the choice of donor species, including the shortage of primates, the need to reasonably match the size of transplanted organs, and the risks associated with endogenous pathogens in the donor species.

Experiments to prevent or inhibit natural antibody formation against xenografts have prolonged survival but have failed to achieve long-term survival of grafts. Although cellular immunity to xenograft antigens often is lower than expected, other mechanisms of graft destruction may be at work. BMT that employs marrow from the same as well as different species may enhance the tolerance of xenografts. However, scientists have not determined if this procedure will lead to long-term survival of the grafts. Neither clinically approved nor experimental immunosuppressive drugs have yet shown any special properties that would improve the success of xenogeneic transplantation.

Research Opportunity

- Encourage efforts to increase our knowledge of xenogeneic transplantation by identifying natural antibody targets and ways to reduce their expression, understanding cell-mediated immunity, understanding tolerance, conducting preclinical testing, and breeding appropriate animal donors.

Nonspecific Immunosuppressive Drugs: Cyclosporin A and FK-506

The modern era of transplantation began a decade ago with the introduction of the immunosuppressive drug cyclosporin A. The more recent discovery of another immunosuppressant, known as FK-506, raises hope that additional drugs will continue to enhance clinical transplantation procedures. However, the rational design of new agents is still lagging.

CyA makes renal, cardiac, and liver transplantation procedures viable therapeutic options, achieving 1-year graft survivals of 85, 80, and 65 percent, respectively. The drug also may be useful in therapy for a variety of autoimmune diseases. However, side effects, particularly damage to kidneys, continue to pose important problems.

FK-506 was identified by a Japanese pharmaceutical company in 1985 and is 10 times more potent *in vivo* than CyA. The two immunosuppressive drugs may act synergistically and generally do not have overlapping side effects.

Both CyA and FK-506 appear to inhibit T cell activation by blocking T cell production of cytokines, such as IL-2 and INF-γ. Both drugs seem to interfere with early signaling of these genes; however, each drug acts on distinct target molecules within the cell.

Research Opportunity

• Continue the search for immunosuppressive drugs with selective activity and reduced side effects, with emphasis on developing drugs that block selective steps in immune activation.

Bibliography

Bach, J.F. Cyclosporine in autoimmune diseases. *Transplantation Proceedings* 21: 97, 1989.

Bjorkman, P.J.; Saper, M.A.; Samraoui, B.; Bennett, W.S.; Strominger, J.L.; Wiley, D.C. The foreign antigen binding site and T cell recognition regions of class I histocompatibility antigens. *Nature* 329: 512-518, 1987.

Cobbold, S.P.; Martin, G.; Qin, S.; Waldmann, H. Monoclonal antibodies to promote marrow engraftment and tissue graft tolerance. *Nature* 323: 164, 1986.

Handschumacher, R.E.; Harding, M.W.; Rice, J.; Druggs, R.J.; Speicher, D.W. Cyclophilin: a specific cytosolic binding protein for cyclosporin A. *Science* 226: 544, 1984.

Kisielow, P.; Bluthmann, H.; Staerz, U.D.; Steinmetz, M.; von Boehmer, H. Tolerance in T-cell receptor transgenic mice involves deletion of nonmature CD4+8+ thymocytes. *Nature* 333: 742-746, 1988.

Korngold, R.; Sprent, J. Lethal GVHD across minor histocompatibility barriers: nature of the effector cells and role of the H-2 complex. *Immunological Reviews* 71: 5, 1983.

Martin, P.J.; Hansen, J.A.; Storb, R.; Thomas. E.D. Human marrow transplantation: an immunological perspective. *Advances in Immunology* 40: 379, 1987.

Mazerolles, F.; Durandy, A.; Platier-Tonneau, D.; Charron, D.; Montagnier, L.; Auffray, C.; Fisher, A. Immunosuppressive properties of synthetic peptides derived from CD4 and HLA-DR antigens. *Cell* 55: 497, 1988.

Sha, W.C.; Nelson, C.A.; Newberry, R.D.; Kranz, D.M.; Russell, J.H.; Loh, D. Positive and negative selection of an antigen receptor on T cells in transgenic mice. *Nature* 336: 73-76, 1988.

Thomson, A.W. FK-506—how much potential. *Immunology Today* 10: 6, 1989.

Chapter 42

Heart and Heart/Lung Transplants

In the two decades since the performance of the first human heart transplant in December 1967, the procedure has changed from an experimental operation to an established treatment for advanced heart disease. Approximately 1,600 heart transplants are performed each year in the United States.

Since 1981, combined heart and lung transplants have been used to treat patients with conditions that severely damage both these organs. As of 1990, about 800 people worldwide have received heart/lung transplants.

In 1983, a major barrier to the success of transplantation—rejection of the donor organ by the patient—was overcome. The drug cyclosporine was introduced to suppress rejection of a donor heart or heart/lung by the patient's body. Cyclosporine and other medications to control rejection have significantly improved the survival of transplant patients. About 80 percent of heart transplant patients survive one year or more. About 60 percent of heart/lung transplants live at least one year after surgery. Research is under way to develop even better ways to control transplant rejection and improve survival.

Organ availability is the second barrier to increasing the number of successful transplantations. Efforts by hospitals and organizations nationwide aim to increase public awareness of this problem and improve organ distribution.

NIH Pub No. 90-2990.

What happens during a heart or heart/lung transplant?

A transplant is the replacement of a patient's diseased heart or heart and lungs with a normal organ(s) from someone who has died, called a donor. The donor's organ(s) is completely removed and quickly transported to the patient, who may be located across the country. Organs are cooled and kept in a special solution while being taken to the patient.

During the operation, the patient is placed on a heart/lung machine. This machine allows surgeons to bypass the blood flow to the heart and lungs. The machine pumps the blood throughout the rest of the body, removing carbon dioxide (a waste product) and replacing it with oxygen needed by body tissues. Doctors remove the patient's heart except for the back walls of the atria, the heart's upper chambers. The backs of the atria on the new heart are opened and the heart is sewn into place. A similar process is followed in heart/lung transplants, except doctors remove the heart and lungs as a unit from the donor; the new lungs are attached first, followed by the heart.

Surgeons then connect the blood vessels and allow blood to flow through the heart and lungs. As the heart warms up, it begins beating. Sometimes, surgeons must start the heart with an electrical shock. Surgeons check all the connected blood vessels and heart chambers for leaks before removing the patient from the heart/lung machine.

Patients are usually up and around a few days after surgery, and if there are no signs of the body immediately rejecting the organ(s), patients are allowed to go home within two weeks.

Why are transplants done?

A transplant is considered when the heart is failing and does not respond to all other therapies, but health is otherwise good. The leading reasons why people receive heart transplants are:

- Cardiomyopathy, a weakening of the heart muscle.
- Severe coronary artery disease, in which the heart's blood vessels become blocked and the heart muscle is damaged.
- Birth defects of the heart.

Heart/lung transplants are performed on patients who will die from end-stage lung disease that also involves the heart. Alternative therapies for these patients have been tried or considered. Leading reasons people receive heart/lung transplants are:

- **Severe pulmonary hypertension:** a large increase in blood pressure in the vessels of the lungs that limits blood flow and delivery of oxygen to the rest of the body.

- **Acquired pulmonary hypertension:** A birth defect of the heart that results in Eisenmenger's complex, which is acquired pulmonary hypertension.

Who can have a transplant?

Patients under age 60 are the most likely heart transplant candidates. Patients under age 45 are generally accepted for heart/lung transplants. In both cases, patients must be suffering from end-stage disease and be in good health otherwise. The doctor, patient, and family must address the following four basic questions to determine whether a transplant should be considered:

1. Have all other therapies been tried or excluded?

2. Is the patient likely to die without the transplant?

3. Is the person in generally good health other than the heart or heart and lung disease?

4. Can the patient adhere to the lifestyle changes including complex drug treatments and frequent examinations required after a transplant?

Patients who do not meet the above considerations or who have additional problems, other severe diseases, active infections, or severe obesity are not good candidates for a transplant.

How are donors found?

Donors are individuals who are brain dead, meaning that the brain shows no signs of life while the person's body is being kept alive by a machine. Donors have often died as a result of an automobile accident, a stroke, a gunshot wound, suicide, or a severe head injury. Most hearts come from those who died under the age of 45. Donor organs are located through the United Network for Organ Sharing (UNOS).

Not enough organs are available for transplant. At any given time, almost 2,000 patients are waiting for a heart or heart/lung transplant. Patients may wait months for a transplant. More than 25 percent do not live long enough. Yet, only a fraction of those who could donate organs actually do.

Does a person lead a normal life after a transplant?

After a heart or heart/lung transplant, patients must take several medications. The most important are those to keep the body from rejecting the transplant. These medications, which must be taken for life, can cause significant side effects, including hypertension, fluid retention, tremors, excessive hair growth, and possible kidney damage. To combat these problems, additional drugs are often prescribed.

A transplanted heart functions differently from the old one. Because the nerves leading to the heart are cut during the operation, the transplanted heart beats faster (about 100 to 110 beats per minute) than the normal heart (70 beats per minute). The new heart also responds more slowly to exercise and doesn't increase its rate as quickly as before.

A patient's outlook depends on many factors, including age, general health, and response to the transplant. Recent figures show that 73 percent of heart transplant patients live at least 4 years after surgery. Nearly 85 percent of patients return to work or other activities they like. Many patients enjoy swimming, cycling, running, or other sports.

About 60 percent of patients who receive combined heart/lung transplants survive at least one year, and 50 percent live at least five years.

What are the risks from transplants?

The most common causes of death following a transplant are infection or rejection of the heart. Patients on drugs to prevent transplant rejection are at risk for developing kidney damage, high blood pressure, osteoporosis (weakness of the major bones such as the hips and spine), and lymphoma (a type of cancer that affects cells of the immune system).

Coronary artery disease is a problem that develops in almost half the patients who receive transplants. Normally, patients with this disease experience chest pain and/or other symptoms when their hearts are under stress. This is called angina and is an early warning sign of a blocked heart artery. However, transplant patients may have no early pain symptoms of a blockage building up because they have no sensations in their new hearts.

Thirty to fifty percent of patients who receive a heart/lung transplant develop destructive changes in the lung tissue, bronchiolitis obliterans.

What does rejection mean?

The body's immune system protects the body from infection. Cells of the immune system move throughout the body, checking for anything that looks foreign or different from the body's own cells. Immune cells recognize the transplanted organ(s) as different from the rest of the body and attempt to destroy it; this is called rejection. If left alone, the immune system would damage the cells of a new heart and eventually destroy it. In a heart/lung transplant, immune cells may also destroy healthy lung tissue.

To prevent rejection, patients receive immunosuppressants, drugs that suppress the immune system so that the new organ(s) is not damaged. Because rejection can occur anytime after a transplant, immunosuppressive drugs are given to patients the day before their transplants and thereafter for the rest of their lives. To avoid complications, patients must strictly adhere to their drug regimen. The three main drugs now being used are cyclosporine, azathioprine, and prednisone. Researchers are working on safer, more effective immunosuppressants for future testing.

Doctors must balance the dose of immunosuppressive drugs so that a patient's transplanted organ(s) is protected, but his or her immune system is not completely shut down. Without an active enough immune system, a patient can easily develop severe infections. For this reason, medications are also prescribed to fight any infections.

To carefully monitor transplant patients for signs of heart rejection, small pieces of the transplanted organ are removed for inspection under a microscope. Called a biopsy, this procedure involves advancing a thin tube called a catheter through a vein to the heart. At the end of the catheter is a bioptome, a tiny instrument used to snip off a piece of tissue. If the biopsy shows damaged cells, the dose and kind of immunosuppressive drug may be changed. Biopsies of the heart muscle are usually performed weekly for the first three to six weeks, every three months for the first year, and yearly thereafter.

How much do transplants cost?

According to the Health Resources and Services Administration, the average cost of a heart transplant ranges from $57,000 to $110,000. In most cases these costs are paid by private insurance companies. More than 80 percent of commercial insurers and 97 percent of Blue Cross/Blue Shield plans offer coverage for heart transplants. Medicaid programs in 33 states and the District of Columbia also reimburse for transplants. Heart transplants are covered by Medicare for Medicare-eligible patients if the operation is performed at approved centers.

Approximately 70 percent of commercial insurance companies and 92 percent of Blue Cross/Blue Shield plans cover heart/lung transplants. Medicaid coverage for heart/lung transplants is available in 20 states.

What will transplants be like in 5 to 10 years?

Hospitals nationwide are trying to set up a better system for distributing organs to patients in need. Researchers are looking for easier methods to monitor rejection to replace the regular biopsies that are needed now. Work is progressing to make immunosuppressive drugs with fewer long-term side effects so that coronary artery disease development and lung destruction may be prevented.

Where can I get more information on transplants?

Information is available 24 hours a day, 7 days a week from the United Network for Organ Sharing at 1-800-24-DONOR. This hotline provides general information on transplants, current statistics, and listings of transplant centers.

Information on organ donation can be obtained from the American Council on Transplantation at 1-800-ACT-GIVE. The address is P.O. Box 1709, Alexandria, VA 22313.

Additional information is available from the Division of Organ Transplantation, Health Resources and Services Administration, Room 11A22, 5600 Fishers Lane, Rockville, MD 20857.

Chapter 43

Transplantation Therapy in an Animal Model for Krabbe's Disease

Administration of high doses of a drug that destroys bone marrow cells may be as effective as total body irradiation in preparing a patient for autologous bone marrow transplantation, according to scientists at the Johns Hopkins University School of Medicine in Baltimore, Maryland. Twitcher mice, an animal model for an inherited demyelinating human lipid storage disease called Krabbe's disease, did not develop hind limb paralysis—as they usually would—when treated with a conditioning regimen of high-dose busulfan (BU) prior to transplantation of normal bone marrow and spleen cells. In Krabbe's disease deficiency of the enzyme galactosylceramidase causes incomplete buildup of the insulating myelin sheath around nerve cells and accumulation of a particular type of lipid in the brain. The scientists suggest that in Krabbe's disease gene replacement therapy with infusion of an individual's own bone marrow cells, into which a cloned enzyme gene has been inserted, may be possible following conditioning only with BU. The drug destroys bone marrow without causing immunosuppression.

"Up to this point all studies on gene insertion in hematopoietic, or blood-forming, cells and reconstitution of recipient animal cells used total body irradiation before transplantation. Because genetically identical transplants may not require immunosuppression, busulfan seems to be an alterative conditioning regimen," says Dr. Andrew Yeager, associate professor of oncology, pediatrics and neurology at the

Research Resources Reporter. July/August 1992.

Johns Hopkins University School of Medicine and pediatrician-in-charge of the university's bone marrow transplantation program.

According to Dr. Yeager, the possibility of using only BU as a conditioning regimen, without exposing the patient to irradiation, is significant because it reduces not only the risk of opportunistic infections associated with immunodeficiency but also other toxic side effects commonly associated with irradiation. He explains that BU has "space-making" properties but causes no immunosuppression. By killing old, inefficient cells the drug creates space for proliferation of new hematopoietic cells and helps achieve a full and rapid engraftment of normal donor cells. In previous marrow transplantation studies between different strains of mice, in which BU was combined with the immunosuppressive agent cyclophosphamide, higher doses of BU were associated with more rapid engraftment.

The Johns Hopkins scientists are especially interested in studying the treatment of Krabbe's disease, a relatively rare disorder, because of the availability of an excellent animal model. "The Krabbe model, the twitcher mouse, is the first murine model for a known neurodegenerative disease associated with a lysosomal hydrolase [galactosylceramidase] deficiency," says Dr. Yeager. Unlike other murine models, the twitcher resembles the human condition—neurodegeneration plus deficiency of galactosylceramidase. Also, there are similarities between Krabbe's disease and other lipid storage diseases such as metachromatic leukodystrophy, in which there are both neurodegenerative processes and enzyme deficiencies. The study of Krabbe's disease therefore has potential implications for the treatment of such analogous disorders.

To test the effects of BU and hematopoietic cell transplantation (HCT), the scientists gave 9-day-old twitcher mice and control littermates single intraperitoneal injections of BU. Bone marrow and spleen donor cells were derived from normal 6- to 8-week-old mice that had the same genetic background as the twitcher mice and then administered by intraperitoneal injection 24 hours after BU conditioning. At selected times following HCT samples of blood, bone marrow, spleen, and lymph node tissues were obtained from recipient mice and analyzed for repopulation by blood-forming and lymphoid donor cells and for galactosylceramidase activity.

The 17 twitcher mice that received high-dose BU followed by HCT at 10 days of age survived a median of 94 days. They had improved gait and did not develop the hind limb paralysis usually seen in untreated twitchers.

At 90 days after HCT the treated animals' blood, bone marrow, spleen, and lymph nodes showed evidence of repopulation with donor-derived lymphoid and blood-forming cells, and this engraftment was sustained without any attrition of donor cells. Galactosylceramidase activity in livers and spleens of treated twitcher mice reached 45 and 80 percent of control values, respectively: a sevenfold to ninefold elevation of enzyme activity compared to that seen in untreated twitchers. Three months after transplantation enzyme activity also rose in the animals' brains to 20 percent of control values, approximately five times the value noted in untreated twitchers. The enzyme level in the sciatic nerves of HCT-treated twitcher mice exceeded normal values, rising to 30 times the level of untreated mice, and damaged nerve sheaths showed repair.

In contrast, after the first three weeks of life the 51 untreated twitcher mice developed body tremor, hind-limb paralysis, impairment of gait, and changes in foraging and grooming behavior. They failed to thrive and had extensive sciatic nerve sheath demyelination. They died when they were approximately 40 days old.

Because there appears to be a barrier between the blood and brain and nervous tissue that prevents entry of large molecules into those tissues, the appearance of the missing enzyme in the neural tissues and brains of treated twitcher mice was significant, according to Dr. Yeager.

"One of the concerns in clinical transplantation for genetic diseases involving deficiency of lysosomal hydrolase enzymes, in which there also may be central nervous system abnormalities, is whether one can get adequate levels of the missing enzyme into neural tissues," Dr. Yeager explains. The Johns Hopkins researchers are now tracking the appearance of donor-derived mononuclear cells in nervous system tissue, especially the brain. Dr. Yeager theorizes that total body irradiation or BU may disturb the blood-brain and blood-nerve barriers and thus make them permeable to either the enzyme or the cells that make or contain the enzyme. In ongoing work Dr. Yeager and his colleagues quantitate both lymphoid and hematopoietic repopulation in twitcher mice and normal mice following a BU preparatory regimen.

"We are looking at whether lower doses of BU might provide the same disease-free survival as the higher doses," Dr. Yeager says. He notes that this would be encouraging because in normal mice high doses of BU are associated with growth retardation and loss of hair pigmentation. Long-term follow-up of normal mice treated with BU has led him to believe that a dose that is about one-third of the dose he used in the study will achieve sustained, complete engraftment. At doses lower than this, engraftment is only transient.

Looking toward the future, Dr. Yeager says, "Our results suggest that when gene replacement therapies using the patient's own bone marrow are moved into clinical trials, it might be valid to use busulfan alone as conditioning. It might be used not only for lysosomal storage diseases but also potentially for other conditions of ineffective marrow function, for example, sickle cell anemia. In a situation where immune suppression is not needed but engraftment of modified cells is needed, busulfan may be very attractive."

Additional Reading

Yeager, A. M., Hematopoietic cell transplantation after administration of high-dose busulfan in murine globoid cell leukodystrophy (the twitcher mouse). *Pediatric Research* 29:302-305, 1991.

Shull, R. M., Brieder, M. A., and Constantopoulos, G. C., Long-term neurological effects of bone marrow transplantation in a canine lysosomal storage disease. *Pediatric Research* 24:347-352, 1988.

Yeager, A. M., Brennan, S., Tiffany, C., et al., Prolonged survival and remyelination after hematopoietic cell transplantation in the twitcher mouse. *Science* 225:1052-1054, 1984.

Tutschka, P. J. and Santos, G. W., Bone marrow transplantation in the busulfan-treated rat. *Transplantation* 24:52-62, 1977.

The research described in this article was supported by a Biomedical Research Support Grant from the NIH National Center for Research Resources, the National Institute of Neurological Disorders and Stroke, the National Institute of Child Health and Human Development, the March of Dimes Birth Defects Foundation, the Children's Cancer Foundation, the National Children's Cancer Society, and the United Leukodystrophy Foundation.

—by L. Anne Hirschel, D.D.S.

Chapter 44

Transgenic Animal Model for Human Inflammatory Disease

By transplanting a pair of human genes into rats, a team of Texas researchers has developed the first animal model for a family of human inflammatory diseases. Their work has confirmed the long-suspected genetic basis of these diseases, known as spondyloarthropathies. In the rat model the scientists will study development of the illnesses and potential treatments.

"We can use these rats to study how each of the diseases is triggered and progresses," says Dr. Robert E. Hammer, assistant professor of biochemistry at the University of Texas Southwestern Medical Center at Dallas. According to the investigators, more than 200,000 Americans have spondyloarthropathy, the most common form of which is ankylosing spondylitis, an arthritis involving inflammation of the spine that in severe cases leads to fusing of the vertebrae and bent posture. In addition to arthritis, patients with these illnesses can develop inflammatory diseases of the gastrointestinal tract, genitourinary tract, skin, eye, and heart.

Disease in the genetically engineered rats seems to mimic these human diseases. "The constellation of involved organ systems, the types of disease, and their sequence of appearance parallel what happens in people," says Dr. Joel D. Taurog, associate professor of internal medicine at the University of Texas and co-principal investigator with Dr. Hammer. "At about 2 months of age the rats develop gut inflammation and diarrhea. Arthritis occurs by 4 months, and some rats later develop a skin disease."

Research Resources Reporter. April 1992.

471

Affected male rats develop arthritis much more often than do female rats, a characteristic that is also seen in the human disease. However, the rats in one of the affected lines also often develop a mild neurologic disease, which is a divergence of the model that has no counterpart in humans with spondyloarthropathy, Dr. Taurog explains.

Human leukocyte antigen (HLA)B27, a protein that is found in about 7 percent of Caucasians, appears to cause these diseases. HLA proteins, which are associated with the outer surface of an individual's cells, are important participants in immune reactions and help the immune system distinguish an individual's own cells and tissues from foreign materials. In some people the presence of certain HLA proteins appears to be linked to immunological diseases. For example, some types of HLA-DR or HLA-DQ proteins are associated with rheumatoid arthritis and insulin-dependent diabetes. By the mid-1970s, researchers had epidemiologic evidence that the HLA-B27 gene was linked to the spondyloarthropathies, the investigators say.

Drs. Taurog and Hammer, as well as other teams of investigators, hoped to get firmer evidence of HLA-B27's involvement in these disorders by transferring the gene into unaffected rats. Dr. Hammer microinjected copies of the B27 gene into fertilized, one-cell rat eggs together with the gene for human beta-2-microglobulin (ß2m), another cell surface protein. "On cell surfaces, the B27 protein binds to the B27 protein," explains Dr. Taurog. "If human ß2m were not available, B27 would bind to the rat form of the protein, which differs from human ß2m. We wanted an authentic model," he notes.

The researchers placed the injected eggs into pseudopregnant female rats. After gestation and delivery, cells in five of the newborn animals produced both of the human proteins encoded by the transferred genes, and these five animals produced offspring that continued to make the human proteins. Two of the rat lines yielded animals with overt spondyloarthropathy-like disease. (For more information about production of transgenic animals, see the Research Resources Reporter, January 1991).

Drs. Hammer and Taurog note that it is not clear why only some of the rats that make human B27 and ß2m develop the disease. "One possibility is that the B27 protein causes disease by being involved in an immune response that gets out of hand," says Dr. Taurog. This immune response might be triggered by another tissue protein, a foreign protein from an infecting pathogen, or by a reaction to B27 itself. "Our goal is to try to understand the molecular mechanism that is the basis for the genetic predisposition to these diseases," he adds.

The Dallas scientists have already uncovered one disease correlate. "The amount of the B27 protein on the cell surface goes way up as the animals become sick," says Dr. Taurog. "The B27 expression does not increase as much in animals that do not get sick, but it is still unclear what role the B27 increase plays in causing the disease."

"We assume that it is probably the level of B27 expression that controls whether the disease appears, but we are not sure," says Dr. Hammer. "The gut is the main site we are studying now because human B27 disease starts there. So far, we know that B27-containing immune cells are in the rat's gut when there is overt disease, but it is difficult to determine whether there is B27 expression in the gut prior to the onset of disease. We are now trying to determine when the first B27-containing cells appear in the gastrointestinal tract."

To further prove that the disease in the rats is caused by B27, Drs. Taurog and Hammer engineered additional rat lines that contain different HLA genes. One line carries an HLA-A2 gene, another an HLA-B7 gene. Both lines also produce the human ß2m proteins, but no rat from either line has shown signs of an inflammatory disease.

"Because the gut seems to be the place where disease begins, we think it may start with a gut peptide [a short chain of linked amino acids] that associates with B27," says Dr. Hammer. "We hope to get a better understanding of the disease-triggering process by raising B27 rats in a germ-free environment and then seeing whether they still get sick. If they don't, we can then introduce a defined gut flora to them to see whether that triggers the disease."

The rat B27 lines also provide a means to study drugs that might block the progression of spondyloarthropathy or alleviate its symptoms.

"We will soon make B27 animals available to drug companies for drug screening studies," says Dr. Hammer.

The Dallas group has faced an unexpected bottleneck in breeding sufficient numbers of B27 rats for all the experiments they and others want to do. Unlike affected humans, B27 male rats often become sterile from their disease. This has forced Drs. Taurog and Hammer and their colleagues to breed animals of the two diseased rat lines through females, which limits them to producing single litters at a time. An additional complication is that the females are often sick by the time their litters are born, which has forced researchers to use surrogate rat mothers to nurse the newborns. "This is expensive and time-consuming," says Dr. Taurog.

Despite this limitation, Drs. Taurog and Hammer, and many other researchers who study HLA-linked diseases, are hopeful that the B27 rats will yield new insights into human spondyloarthropathies as well as other human inflammatory diseases. "Scientists are now trying to make transgenic rats for every type of HLA-associated disease," says Dr. Hammer. "It's nice to think that the system will be useful for other diseases, but we don't know that yet."

Additional Reading

Arnold, B. and Hammerling, G. J., MHC class-I transgenic mice. In *Annual Review of Immunology*, (Paul, W. E., Fathman, C. G., and Metzger, H., eds.), Palo Alto, California: Annual Reviews Inc., 1991, pp. 297-322.

Hammer, R. E., Maika, S. D. Richardson, J. A., Tang J.-P., and Taurog, J. D., Spontaneous inflammatory disease in transgenic rats expressing HLA-B27 and human ß2m: An animal model of HLA-B27-associated human disorders. *Cell* 63:1099-1112, 1990.

David-Watine, B., Israel, A., and Kourilsky, P., The regulation and expression of MHC class I genes. *Immunology Today* 11:286-292,1990.

Taurog, J. D., Lowen, L., Forman, J., and Hammer, R. E., HLA-B27 in inbred and non-inbred transgenic mice: Cell surface expression and recognition as an alloantigen in the absence of human beta2-microglobulin. *Journal of Immunology* 141:4020-4023, 1988.

Bergfeldt, L., Insulander, P., Lindblom, D., Moller, E., and Edhag, O., HLA-B27: An important genetic risk factor for lone aortic regurgitation and severe conduction system abnormalities. *American Journal of Medicine* 85:1218, 1988.

The research described in this article was supported by the Comparative Medicine Program of the National Center for Research Resources, the National Institute of Arthritis and Musculoskeletal and Skin Diseases, the Howard Hughes Medical Institute, the Harold C. Simmons Arthritis Research Center, and the North Texas Chapter of the Arthritis Foundation.

—by Mitchel Zoler, Ph.D.

Chapter 45

Immunotoxicology

From an immunologic perspective, our environment can be viewed as hostile. We are constantly bombarded by "natural" immunotoxicants such as pollens, molds, animal proteins, food, natural radioisotopes, and a variety of organic dusts. In addition, people have polluted the environment with threatening agents such as pesticides, heavy metals, radioactive waste, and drug and chemical metabolites. Scientists have learned that certain substances hyperstimulate the immune system and actuate allergic responses as well as autoimmune-like disorders. Other substances cause a depression of the immune response, which renders us vulnerable to infections and cancers.

Although scientists recognize the significant threat of environmental toxins, they have not yet determined the links between certain agents and specific diseases. Researchers need to elucidate the mechanisms whereby certain classes of toxicants produce deviations in the immune system, and the consequences thereof, and to quantitate aspects of their toxicity in terms of dose and duration of exposure.

Overview

The developing field of immunotoxicology addresses two broad types of adverse effects that can occur when chemicals or their metabolic products interact with biological systems (table 45.1). The first

NIH Pub No. 91-2414.

type occurs when the immune system recognizes the chemical or its metabolites as foreign or nonself, producing immune responses that may lead to immunopathologic changes that are recognized as hypersensitivity or autoimmune-like disorders. A second type of adverse effect is evident when a chemical or its metabolites injure the immune system in any of its broad capabilities. When this injury occurs, the affected individual risks succumbing to diseases such as serious infections and neoplasia.

Class	Example
Polyhalogenated aromatic hydrocarbons	TCDD, PBB, PCB[a]
Metals	Lead, cadmium, arsenic, methyl mercury
Aromatic hydrocarbons (solvents)	Benzene, toluene
Polycyclic aromatic hydrocarbons	DMBA, BaP, MCA[b]
Pesticides	Trimethyl phosporothioate, carbofuran, chlordane
Organotins	TBTO[c]
Aromatic amines	Benzidine, acetyl aminofluorene
Oxidant gases	NO_2, O_3, SO_2
Particles	Silica, asbestos
Natural products	Selected vitamins, antibiotics, fungal products, vinca alkaloids, estrogen, plant alkaloids
Abused drugs	Ethanol, cannabinoids, cocaine, opioids
Therapeutics	Diphenylhydantoin, lithium
Others	Nitrosamine, BHA[d]

[a] TCDD = 2,3,7,8-tetrachlorodibenzo-p-dioxin; PBB = polybrominated biphenyls; PCB = polychlorinated biphenyls.
[b] DMBA = dimethylbenzanthracene; BaP = benzo(a)pyrene; MCA = methylcholanthrene.
[c] TBTO = bis(tri-n-butylene)oxide.
[d] BHA = butylated hydroxyanisole.

Table 45.1. Examples of toxins that can induce immunologic changes.

Immunostimulants and Immunodepressants

The most easily recognized adverse effects of certain chemicals or their metabolites are those that manifest as allergic or autoimmune diseases. It is estimated that more than 40 million Americans have allergic disorders, such as rhinitis, conjunctivitis, and asthma, that result from immunostimulation by natural pollens and molds. "Natural" chemical agents, such as cotton dust, animal proteins, grain dust, and a variety of other organic dusts and occupational environmental antigens, may trigger brisk immune responses that can lead to asthma or hypersensitivity pneumonitis. Conversely, abundant evidence from animal model studies indicates that exposures to various chemicals may seriously depress immune responses. Evidence for similar immunodepression in humans currently is limited by the confines of study methodology. Data to verify the accuracy of results extrapolated to humans from animal study findings also are inadequate. Nevertheless, it appears likely that chemicals that depress immunity in animals also will depress immunity in humans. If this hypothesis is correct, human exposures to chemical agents—especially prolonged, chronic exposures—may lead to pathological conditions such as serious infections or cancers. Individuals who have fragile immune systems, such as infants and the elderly, are the most likely to be affected by this exposure.

Research Opportunity

- Identify the agents that affect the immune system; quantitate their toxicity in terms of dose and duration of exposure; and determine the manner in which they affect the immune system. Emphasize efforts to understand the mechanisms whereby classes of toxic substances produce deviations in immune reactivity.

Model Systems for Immunotoxicologic Research

Several manifestations of immune system toxicity may follow exposure to toxins and chemicals. In experimental animals, these manifestations include effects on organ weights, functions, and histology; qualitative or quantitative changes in the cellular composition of lymphoid tissues, peripheral blood, and bone marrow; impaired cell function at the effector or regulatory levels: and increased susceptibility to infectious organisms or tumors. Although immune functions can be monitored to help detect subclinical toxic injury, no single function can demonstrate conclusively the deleterious effects of a chemical, drug, or natural agent on the immune system. Thus, research and testing must involve a combination of animal models and *in vitro* cell systems. The latter approach offers the potential to identify adverse actions on the immune system as well as to determine targets of noxious substances and mechanisms of effect.

Research Opportunity

- Develop models of both immunostimulation and immuno-depression, including both animal research and human model systems. This research should attempt to perfect systems for detecting exposures and quantifying levels of exposure to noxious substances. Researchers should stress the understanding of how these substances affect the functions of the immune system.

Chemistry of Immunoreactants

A central feature of the adverse effects of many chemicals and drugs on the immune system is the reactivity of these substances with accessible macromolecular structures at the surface of cells. This reactivity may lead to immune responses directed against self-macromolecules that have been altered by reacting with the chemical agent. A variety of clinical syndromes may result, including occupational asthma, pneumonia, generalized allergic reactions to drugs, and contact dermatitis. Examples of immunoreactive chemicals include the drug penicillin (figure 45.1) as well as anhydrides and isocyanates. The latter substances, used widely in industry, are known to combine readily with tissue proteins.

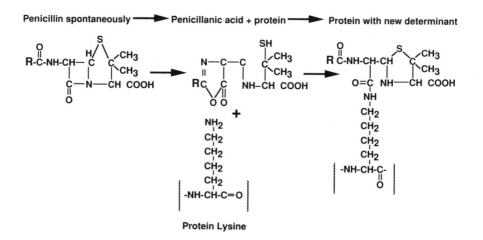

Figure 45.1. Penicillin protein interaction.

Research Opportunities

- Use traditional as well as new methods and techniques to analyze the interactions between noxious or toxic chemicals, drugs, and tissue proteins.

- Conduct systematic studies of the immunogenicity of these immunoreactants, including the induction of autoimmunity.

The Workplace and Other Human Environments Conducive to Exposure As the Clinical Research Laboratory

Even if scientists undertake extensive animal testing to detect noxious substances, humans probably will continue to be exposed to new immunotoxins that have not been defined by animal research. Therefore, to define emerging problems and to guide surveillance and prevention measures, researchers need to develop ways of ensuring early recognition and evaluation of immunotoxins.

Research Opportunities

- Develop standardized immunoassays for measuring antibodies of various immunoglobulin isotypes against immunostimulants.

- Establish standardized reagents and assays for measuring immune status in humans.

- Establish serum banks as reference sources for emerging human immunostimulants and immunosuppressive diseases.

- Establish a relationship between altered immune function and clinical disease to develop guidelines for diagnostic standards that will prevent the misuse of immunodiagnostic technology.

Bibliography

Bekesi, J.G.; Holland, J.F.; Anderson, E.A.; Fischbein, A.S.; Rom, W.; Wolff, M.S.; Selikoff, I.J. Lymphocyte function of Michigan dairy farmers exposed to polybrominated biphenyls. *Science* 199: 1207-1209, 1978.

DeSwarte, R.D. Drug allergy. In: *Allergic Diseases. Diagnosis and Management* (3rd ed.), edited by R. Patterson. Philadelphia: L.B. Lippincott Co., p. 855, 1985.

Johnson, K.W.; Munson, A.E.; Kim, D.H.; Holsapple, H.P. Role of reactive metabolites in suppression of humoral immunity by N-nitrosodimethylamine. *Journal of Pharmacology and Experimental Therapeutics* 240: 847855, 1987.

Law, F.; Tsang, P.; Holland, J.F.; et al. High frequency of immune dysfunctions in asbestos workers and in patients with malignant mesothelioma. *Journal of Clinical Immunology* 6: 225, 1986.

Lee, T.P.; Chang, K.J. Health effects of polychlorinated biphenyls. In: *Immunotoxicology and Immunopharmacology*, edited by J.H. Dean, M.I. Luster, and A.E. Munson. New York: Raven Press, p. 415, 1985.

Luster, M.I.; Munson, A.E.; Thomas, P.T.; Holsapple, M.P.; Fenters, J.D.; White, K.L.; Lauer, L.D.D.; Germolec, D.R.; Rosenthal, G.J.; Dean, J.H. Development of a testing battery to assess chemical-induced immunotoxicity: National Toxicology Program's guidelines for immunotoxicity evaluation in mice. *Fundamental and Applied Toxicology* 10: 2-19, 1988.

McGrath, K.G.; Zeiss, C.R.; Patterson, R. Allergic reactions to industrial chemicals. *Clinical Immunology Review* 2: 1-58, 1983.

Penn, I. Neoplastic consequences of immunosuppression. In: *Immunotoxicology and Immunopharmacology*, edited by J.H. Dean, M.I. Luster, and A.E. Munson. New York: Raven Press, p. 79, 1985.

Salvaggio, J.E.; Butcher, B.T.; O'Neil, C.E. Occupational asthma due to chemical agents. *Journal of Allergy and Clinical Immunology* 18: 1053-1058, 1986.

Uber, C.L.; McReynolds, R.A. Immunotoxicology of silica. *Critical Reviews in Toxicology* 10: 303-319, 1982.

White, K.L., Jr.; Munson, A.E. Suppression of the *in vitro* humoral immune response by chrysotile asbestos. *Toxicology and Applied Pharmacology* 82: 493-504, 1986.

Chapter 46

Biotechnical Applications in Immunology and Allergy

In the past decade, scientists have achieved remarkable technological advances in cell biology that have significantly affected the field of immunology. Researchers now have the ability not only to isolate and characterize cells and important cell surface markers but also to purify, analyze, and trace the proteins produced by these cells. New techniques, collectively known as "recombinant deoxyribonucleic acid (DNA) technology," also allow investigators to examine the structure and function of a cell's DNA. Passive observation of cellular functions has progressed to active intervention through genetic engineering, which alters DNA sequences to make modified versions of genes that are then reinserted into cells and organisms. This procedure enables scientists to produce vitally important substances in quantities that were previously unattainable. For example, by using gene sequencing and cloning, researchers now can produce cytokines, which are the regulatory hormones secreted by cells, in amounts sufficient for therapeutic purposes. Researchers will continue their efforts to perfect molecular techniques and to apply them to our understanding of gene control and resultant protein products.

One important aspect of our immune response is the production of antibodies that target a wide variety of antigens. Researchers have developed procedures for screening and isolating an immune cell that will produce an antigen-specific antibody. In 1975, they devised a way to fuse an immune cell with a tumor cell. The resultant immortal cell line, known as hybridoma, produced large quantities of a monospecific

NIH Pub No. 91-2414.

or monoclonal antibody (MoAb). MoAbs have provided scientists with tools for developing extensive diagnostic reagents. These antibodies have been linked to toxins that target and eliminate specific cells prior to bone marrow transplantation. This system has had limited potential for *in vivo* use in humans because it uses mouse cells whose MoAb would be recognized as foreign and eliminated. However, scientists recently developed a technique that combines the recognition portion of the mouse antibody with a human antibody. This genetically engineered "humanized" MoAb has shown promise for use in humans. Researchers now are focusing concerted efforts on developing a MoAb of human and chimeric monoclonals.

Overview

During the 1980s, much of our progress in understanding both normal and abnormal immune functions has paralleled advances in biotechnology. Three technological advances that have significantly affected both basic and clinical research include:

- methods for preparing MoAbs;
- development of ingenious molecular biological techniques; and
- procedures for acquiring new and deeper insight into peptide and protein structure.

Technologies that were unknown a decade ago are now virtually routine in many immunology laboratories. In addition, many of these new procedures currently are being applied to clinical problems. The new technologies are themselves undergoing change as modifications and improvements are introduced. Thus, these technological advances will continue to play a vital role in future biomedical research.

Protein Structure and Function

X-ray diffraction and two-dimensional nuclear magnetic resonance have allowed scientists to determine an increasing number of three-dimensional structures for proteins and to improve the quality of these structures. The number of proteins for which amino acid sequences are available is growing even more rapidly and will increase exponentially as work progresses on the Human Genome Project, a federally funded effort devoted to elucidating the structure and sequence organization of all human genes. In the last few years, research has generated important information in such areas as the structure of antibody-combining sites and their association with cognate ligands, the structure and binding sites of class I and class II histocompatibility substances, and the nature of enzyme-substrate interactions. New attempts to locate important structural parameters of proteins by statistical and computer modeling have been reasonably successful. Detailed knowledge of protein structure is essential to understanding the functions of antibody-combining sites; the functions of molecules such as cytokines, cytokine receptors, and T cell receptors; and a variety of critical molecules that are known to be associated with lymphocytes and other leukocytes. However, the roles of these sites and molecules remain largely unknown. The most challenging task facing structural biology over the next decade is the development of strategies to predict the folding of protein molecules based on the knowledge of amino acid sequences.

Research Opportunity

- Develop rapid and precise methods to predict secondary and tertiary protein structure from primary amino acid sequences.

Cytokines

The study of cytokines is, perhaps, the aspect of immunology that has benefited most directly from recent technological advances. Progress in this area includes:

- the perfection of specific *in vitro* assays for cytokines, which allowed documentation of cytokine function at the clonal level;

- the development of stable, clonal cell lines as reliable sources of the cytokines, thus providing immunochemists and molecular biologists with the necessary quantities of materials; and

- the application of sophisticated technology for isolating and characterizing individual cytokines as well as identifying and cloning the genes encoding the cytokines.

Advances made in the past decade have furthered the realization that the biological effects of cytokines are varied, complex, and fraught with apparent overlap and redundancy. Scientists now must acquire the knowledge needed to construct a rational view of the cytokine reactive and interactive network.

Cytokine genes are expressed in a variety of heterologous hosts, ranging from bacteria to yeast to insect cells. This expression has led to the production of pure, recombinant cytokines in quantities sufficient for research that addresses their use in the treatment and prevention of human diseases. As a result, a profound increase in the clinical use of cytokines will occur in the next 10 years.

Research Opportunities

- Elucidate the cytokine reactive and interactive network.

- Identify the diseases that can be successfully treated or prevented with a given cytokine, and determine efficacious combinations and dosages that do not have severe side effects.

Monoclonal Antibodies

The ability to routinely produce MoAbs to an almost unlimited array of antigens has given immunologists extraordinary tools for isolating and characterizing the important cell types and molecules that are involved in the immune response. Murine MoAbs have been extremely useful as *in vitro* diagnostic reagents. However, their inherent immunogenicity limits their potential use as long-term therapeutic agents in humans. Recent breakthroughs in molecular biology have permitted the production of genetically engineered antibodies that contain the murine variable region and the human constant region. Because these "humanized" antibodies are not expected to elicit strong immunologic responses in humans, they should prove to be more effective therapeutic agents for treating immunologic and infectious diseases as well as for treating and preventing graft rejection.

Research Opportunity

- Develop more effective and efficient methods for generating MoAbs and appropriate fragments of such antibodies; focus particularly on all-human, humanized, and chimeric monoclonals.

Immunoconjugates

Immunoconjugates contain a cell binding component that is linked to a toxic moiety. They have been developed in recent years for treating a variety of malignant and nonmalignant diseases. Scientists initially chose MoAbs as the cell binding component These antibodies were directed at a specific molecule that is present on the surface of the cell targeted for elimination by the immunoconjugate. However, recent immunoconjugates have linked toxins to growth factors or growth hormones. Bacterial or plant toxins that inhibit protein synthesis have been used as the toxic component of immunoconjugates. Immunoconjugates have been shown to be effective in eliminating tumor cells *in vivo* in several animal models and now have entered clinical trials. However, the initial results of these studies fail to indicate marked antitumor effects. Factors influencing these results may include the inaccessibility of solid tumors to the circulating immunoconjugate and the production of anti-immunoconjugate antibodies after repeated treatment. Other clinical studies show that first generation immunoconjugates are more effective in treating autoimmune diseases and graft-versus-host disease. Scientists now are developing new generations of immunoconjugates that will enhance the antitumor effects in humans.

Research Opportunities

- Develop procedures for optimizing the delivery of immunoconjugates *in vivo*.

- Devise solutions to the problems associated with the development of neutralizing antibodies in recipients of immunoconjugates.

The Polymerase Chain Reaction

The impact of the polymerase chain reaction (PCR) on both basic and diagnostic aspects of molecular biology has been similar to that of recombinant DNA technology. Recombinant DNA techniques create molecular clones by conferring on a specific sequence the ability to replicate after insertion into a vector and the introduction of that vector into a host cell. PCR allows the production of large amounts of a specific DNA fragment from small amounts of a complex template.

Thus, PCR represents a form of *in vitro* cloning that can generate as well as modify DNA fragments of defined length and sequence by using a simple automated reaction. In addition to its many applications in basic molecular biological research, PCR promises to play a critical role in the identification of DNA sequences that are associated with disease as well as in the detection and diagnosis of these diseases.

Research Opportunity

Develop the PCR technique into a routine, quantitative procedure that is suitable for detecting DNA fragments such as aberrant genes, genes encoding cytokines and cytokine receptors, and genes associated with infectious organisms.

Bibliography

Alzari, P.M.; Lascombe, M.B.; Poljak, R.J. Three-dimensional structure of antibodies. *Annual Review of Immunology* 6: 555-580, 1988.

Blakey, D.C.; Wawrzynczak, E.J.; Wallace, P.M.; Thorpe, P.E. Antibody toxin conjugates: a perspective. In: *Progress in Allergy (Monoclonal Antibody Therapy)*, edited by H. Waldmann. Basel. Switzerland: S. Karger. p. 50, 1988.

Lerner, R.A.; Tramontano, A. Catalytic antibodies. *Scientific American* 258: 58-60, 65-70, 1988.

Liberman, T.A.; Nusbaum, H.R.; Razon, N.; Kris, R.; Lax, l.; Soreq, H. Amplification, enhanced expression and possible rearrangement of EGF receptor gene in primary brain tumors of glial origin. *Nature* 313: 144-147, 1985.

Moller, G. Antibody carriers of drugs and toxins in tumor therapy. *Immunological Reviews*: 62, 1982.

Morrison, S.L.; Johnson, M.J.; Herzenberg, L.A.; Oi, V.T. Chimeric human antibody molecules: mouse antigen-binding domains with human constant region domains. *Proceedings of the National Academy of Sciences of the USA* 81: 6851-6855, 1984.

Riechmann, L.; Clark, M.; Waldmann, H.; Winter, G. Reshaping human antibodies for therapy. *Nature* 332: 323-327, 1988.

Vitetta, E.S.; Fulton, R.J.; May, R.D.; Till, M.; Uhr, J.W. Redesigning nature's poisons to create anti-tumor reagents. *Science* 238: 1098-1104, 1987.

White, T.J.; Arnheim, N.; Erlich, H.A. The polymerase chain reaction. *Trends in Genetics* 5: 185-189, 1989.

Chapter 47

Immunology of Infectious Diseases

Infectious disease remains one of the leading challenges to modern science and medicine. Twenty percent of the world's population suffers from disease, malnutrition, or both of these conditions. Furthermore, infectious disease is the leading cause of death among children. Researchers have devised celebrated cures for diseases that have plagued mankind for centuries, including syphilis, polio, and smallpox. However, such victories have eluded investigators who are addressing well-known diseases such as malaria, the common cold, and AIDS. To develop new vaccines and effective therapeutic interventions, scientists must focus on understanding the pathogenesis and escape mechanisms of pathogens. Molecular technology will help delineate the precise genetic basis for susceptibility and resistance to infectious disease, thereby providing fundamental insight about the regulation of immune responses.

Overview

No aspect of immunology has more direct impact on the quality of life for people around the world than the immunology of infectious diseases. The World Health Organization recently reported that 20 percent of the world's population is suffering from disease or malnutrition, and infectious diseases remain the major killer of children worldwide. Furthermore, the AIDS epidemic has demonstrated that no infectious disease remains truly remote. The United States has an

NIH Pub No. 91-2414.

opportunity to improve significantly the world's health by making a relatively small investment in research that is developing new vaccines and diagnostics for infectious diseases. The practical applications of this research have the potential to benefit hundreds of millions of people around the world.

The uniqueness of the immune response is inherent in its elaborate and diverse mechanisms for recognizing myriad foreign antigens. Infectious diseases clearly represent the strongest evolutionary pressure for the development and diversification of the immune system. Understanding of the fundamental biological roles of the immune response and its evolution requires knowledge of the many host defense mechanisms, such as antibodies, cytotoxic and helper T cells, and lymphokines, as well as their roles in resisting infection. The study of diseases such as AIDS, influenza, malaria, and sleeping sickness has shown that immune responses select for the emergence of antigenic variants of pathogens that are capable of escaping immunologic surveillance. Thus, infectious diseases represent a constant challenge to the immune system and to immunologists who strive to engender effective immune responses to infectious pathogens and their genetic mutations.

Vaccines remain the most cost-effective medical intervention for disease prevention in developing as well as industrialized countries. To provide effective and long-lasting immunity to the pathogenic infectious agents in our environment, scientists need to elucidate the nature of protective immune mechanisms and to define the nature of protective antigens. However, the easy vaccines already have been developed new approaches using sophisticated techniques of immunology and molecular biology are needed to understand the basic pathogenic mechanisms of various infectious agents. This understanding entails very specific knowledge of the strategies used by each viral, bacterial, and parasitic pathogen that is associated with human disease. This knowledge, in turn, will allow scientists to identify targets for immunologic attack. Research on the immunology of infectious diseases is providing new approaches to the development of novel vaccines that are capable of immunizing simultaneously against multiple pathogens as well as new adjuvants and delivery systems that will enhance and prolong effective immune responses to a wide variety of antigens. Thus, few areas of research offer comparable opportunities for developing insights into fundamental mechanisms and practical applications concerned with the prevention or cure of disease.

New Molecular and Immunologic Approaches to Understanding Basic Mechanisms of Microbial Pathogenesis

To develop new vaccines and diagnostic tools, scientists need more precise information on how viral, bacterial, and parasitic pathogens attach to, enter, alter, or destroy cells of the host. These defined molecular "virulence factors" become targets for immunologic attack by antigens and vaccines. They also serve as molecular probes for gene amplification techniques that are revolutionizing the diagnosis of infectious diseases.

Research Opportunities

- Define the mechanism whereby the HIV virus inactivates or kills the CD4+ T cells.

- Determine if a vaccine against "invasion molecules" protects colon cells from infection by enteric pathogens such as Salmonella, Shigella, and Yersinia.

Pathways of Antigen Presentation And Immunologic Mechanisms of Resistance to Infectious Pathogens

Increasing evidence from studies with viral and soluble protein antigens indicates that the pathways of antigen processing and presentation to MHC class I and class II restricted T cells are distinct. The paradigm currently confronting scientists is that, whereas antibodies recognize conformational, three-dimensional determinants on antigen molecules, the T lymphocytes recognize linear, nonnative (i.e., processed or fragmented) forms of foreign antigens in association with MHC molecules. Scientists have determined that T helper and cytotoxic T lymphocytes recognize antigen fragments associated with different MHC antigen classes. Moreover, the pathway whereby antigens are processed and presented apparently is critical to determining the type of immune response obtained. Researchers now need to understand the pathways whereby complex antigens of viruses, bacteria, and parasites are handled in antigen-presenting cells. They also need to know which antigens associate with MHC class I and class II molecules and thus can be recognized by cytotoxic and helper T cell subsets.

With this knowledge, scientists will be able to define the immunologic mechanisms that are necessary and sufficient to engender protective immunity.

Research Opportunity

• Elucidate the role played by the internal antigens of viral and other pathogens, which are carried to the cell surface of infected cells by the MHC antigens and thus can be targets of cytotoxic T cells.

Development of a New Generation of Vaccines

Vaccines represent the most cost-effective medical intervention in the world. Molecular biological approaches are revolutionizing concepts for creating new vaccines. For example, by introducing genes encoding protective antigens from a variety of pathogens into one live vaccine vector, a single immunization can generate long-lasting immunity against multiple infectious agents. Examples of potential new recombinant vaccine vectors include vaccinia poliovirus and adenovirus vaccines, Salmonella, and BCG (table 47.1). In each of these vectors, the genes for foreign antigens have already been expressed.

For certain viruses, research studies have documented the ability of short synthetic peptides to mimic the moiety on the antigenic polypeptide that is recognized by T lymphocytes. In some instances, scientists can define the critical residues necessary for peptide recognition by the T cell antigen receptor and for peptide binding to the MHC. Although peptides have been extensively studied as antigens, peptide-based vaccines have not yet been developed. However, synthetic peptides may have great potential as future vaccine candidates because they bypass processing events in antigen-presenting cells that may be limiting in natural infection. Scientists now need to determine whether they can design peptides with the capacity to bind to a range of alleles of human MHC products and whether they can develop specific peptide vaccines with "universal" MHC-binding capacity. Considerable amino acid variation in malaria sporozoite antigens allows these agents to elude specific immune responses. However, researchers have identified several peptides that are likely to be broadly immunogenic because either they are nonvarying or they bind to many different MHC types.

Research Opportunities

- Develop live vaccine vehicles that use genes encoding protective antigens for a variety of pathogens.

- Develop peptide and synthetic vaccines that will offer broad immunogenic protection against a variety of pathogens.

- Develop immunologic adjuvants that will extend the immunizing period and enhance the effectiveness of vaccines, particularly those using synthetic and peptide antigens.

Bacterial	Parasitic	Viral
Bordetella pertussis	Plasmodia	Human immunodeficiency virus
Enterotoxigenic *Escherichia coli*	Schistosoma	Hepatitis A virus
Hemophilus influenzae	Toxoplasma	Hepatitis B virus
Mycobacterium leprae	Trypanosoma	Hepatitis C (non-A, non-B) virus
Mycobacterium tuberculosis	Leishmania	Influenza A and B viruses
Neisseria gonorrhoeae		Parainfluenza virus
Neisseria meningitidis		Rotavirus
Pseudomonads		Varicella virus
Salmonellae		Herpes simplex virus types 1 and 2
Shigellae		Respiratory syncytial virus
Streptococcus pneumoniae		
Streptococcus groups A and B		
Vibrio cholerae		

Table 47.1. *Pathogens targeted by vaccines under development.*

Viruses, Molecular Mimicry, And Autoimmunity

Viruses and bacteria are being implicated increasingly as important environmental stimuli that lead to the induction of autoimmune responses. Scientists urgently need to examine further the existing models of autoimmune diseases and to develop new models based on emerging clinical data. They particularly need to understand the contribution of molecular mimicry of self-constituents by viral gene products. This information is important because the primary, rather than tertiary, structure of an antigen is the focus of the T cell antigen receptor.

Researchers also need to determine the extent to which cross-reactivities between viral and self proteins contribute to the induction of autoimmune disease.

Research Opportunities

- Enhance our understanding of the immunopathogenesis of autoimmune diseases by studying the known antigenic similarities between viruses and host tissues.

- Study the similarities between evolutionarily conserved proteins in bacteria and those in host cells that are known to be active in experimental models of multiple sclerosis, diabetes, and rheumatoid arthritis.

Genetic Basis of Resistance

The precise factors governing resistance and susceptibility to most infectious diseases remain unknown. However, genetically controlled mechanisms that govern host resistance to various infectious agents are known to exist in animals. Strategies to map the human genome offer unprecedented possibilities for defining new genetic factors that affect resistance and susceptibility to infectious disease. The identification of these factors could provide fundamental insights with respect to the regulation of normal immune responses as well as the mechanisms of host resistance.

Research Opportunity

- Clarify the mechanism whereby a single gene on a mouse chromosome plays a major role in resistance to the infecting organisms in salmonella, leishmaniasis, and tuberculosis. Explore the potential applicability to humans, who may have a counterpart gene on chromosome 2.

Clinical Trials in Humans

Many infectious diseases have no appropriate or effective animal model. Moreover, studies using animal models, such as macaque monkeys with simian immunodeficiency viruses (SIV), often cannot obtain enough animals to derive definitive conclusions on the effectiveness and safety of potential vaccine candidates in humans. After conducting appropriate animal and safety testing, researchers need to emphasize human volunteer studies to assess the safety and efficacy of many of the vaccines currently under development.

Research Opportunity

- Explore and prepare appropriate study centers that will focus on vaccine trials in humans. This approach would permit more widespread clinical testing and development of the next generation of vaccines.

Bibliography

DeWolf, F.; Lange, J.M.A.; Houweling, J.T.M.; Coutinho, R.A.; Schellekens, P.T.; Vander Noordaa, J.; Goudsmit, J. *Journal of Infectious Diseases* 158: 615, 1988.

Fauci, A.S. The human immunodeficiency virus: infectivity and mechanisms of pathogenesis. *Science* 239: 617-622, 1988.

Ho, D.D.; Pomerantz, R.J.; Kaplan, J.C. Pathogenesis of infection with human immunodeficiency virus. *New England Journal of Medicine* 317: 278-286, 1987.

Ho, D.D.; Rota, T.R.; Hirsch, M.S. Infection of monocyte/macrophages by human T lymphotropic virus type III. *Journal of Clinical Investigation* 77: 1712-1715, 1986.

Levy, J.A. Mysteries of HIV: challenges for therapy and prevention. *Nature* 333: 519 522, 1988.

Lyerly, H.K.; Matthews, T.J.; Langlois, A.J.; Bolognesi, D.P.; Weinhold, K.J. Human T-cell lymphotropic virus IIIB glycoprotein (gp120) bound to CD4 determinants on normal lymphocytes and expressed by infected cells serves as target for immune attack. *Proceedings of the National Academy of Sciences of the USA* 84: 4601-4605, 1987.

Rusche, J.R.; Javaherian, K.; McDanal, C.; Petro, J.; Lynn, D.L.; Grimaila, R.; Langlois, A.; Gallo, R.C.; Arthur, L.O.; et al. Antibodies that inhibit fusion of human immunodeficiency virus-infected cells bind a 24 amino acid sequence of the viral envelope, gp120. *Proceedings of the National Academy of Sciences of the USA* 85: 3198-3202, 1988.

Seligmann, M.; Pinching, A.J.; Rosen, F.S.; Fahey, J.L.; Khaitov, R.M.; Klatzmann, D.; Koenig, S.; Luo, N.; Ngu,].; Riethmuler, G.; Spira, T.J. Immunology of human immunodeficiency virus infection and the acquired immunodeficiency syndrome. An update. *Annals of Internal Medicine* 107: 234-242, 1987.

Walker, B.D.; Chakrabarti, S.; Moss, B.; Paradis, T.J.; Flynn, T.; Durno, A.G.; Blumberg, R.S.; Kaplan, J.C.; Hirsch, M.S.; Schooley, R.T. HIV-specific cytotoxic T lymphocytes in seropositive individuals. *Nature* 328: 345-348, 1987.

Walker, B.D.; Flexner, C.; Paradis, T.; Fuller, T.C.; Hirsch, M.S.; Moss, B. HIV-1 reverse transcriptase is a target for cytotoxic T lymphocytes in infected individuals. *Science* 240: 64-66, 1988.

Part Seven

Socioeconomic Implications

Chapter 48

The Socioeconomic Impact of Immunologic and Allergic Disease in the United States

Overview

Allergic and immunologic diseases are among the leading causes of illness and disability in the U.S. population. More than one out of every ten persons are reported to have a condition related to immunologic illnesses. Table 48.1 lists more than 30 diseases that demonstrate immunopathology as their underlying mechanism. Several of these, such as asthma or rheumatoid arthritis, affect millions of individuals. Other immunologic conditions, such as scleroderma, combined immunodeficiency syndrome, or Wegener's granulomatosis, occur less frequently. However, when viewed collectively, even these less prevalent immunologic diseases constitute a significant disease burden within the U.S. population.

This chapter reviews how immunologic diseases affect the health of the U.S. population. The first section reviews current knowledge about the overall prevalence, morbidity, disability, and mortality associated with selected immunologic conditions. The second section presents a case study of the economic impact of a specific immunologic disease, asthma. The third section focuses on how immunologic diseases disproportionately affect two vulnerable subsets of the U.S. population: children/young adults and minorities. The final section emphasizes the direct and indirect socioeconomic benefits of the clinical applications of immunologic research.

NIH Pub No. 91-2414. A special report to the NIAID Task Force on Immunology and Allergy.

501

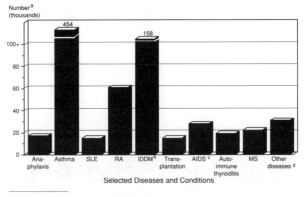

[a] Based on 1987 Hospital Discharge Survey data, first listed diagnosis (10).

[b] Insulin-dependent (type I) diabetes mellitus; see text.

[c] AIDS hospitalization based on 1985 estimate (11).

[d] Selected other diseases, including urticaria from allergies, hemolytic anemia, myasthenia gravis, contact dermatitis and other eczema, and "other diseases of the immune system."

Figure 48.1. *U.S. hospitalizations for selected immunologic diseases and conditions.*

Allergic diseases
    Allergies—insect, food, drug, environmental

Immunologic diseases involving the respiratory system
    Allergic rhinitis/hay fever
    Chronic sinusitis
    Asthma
    Hypersensitivity pneumonitis

Collagen vascular diseases
    Vasculitis syndromes, including Wegener's granulomatosis
    Systemic lupus erythematosus
    Cutaneous lupus
    Scleroderma
    Eosinophilic fascitis
    Panniculitis
    Dermatomyositis/polymyositis

Immune endocrinopathies
    Autoimmune-mediated thyroiditis
    Autoimmune-mediated diabetes mellitus (type I)
    Autoimmune-mediated primary adrenal insufficiency

Immunologic diseases involving the hematopoietic system
    Immunodeficiency diseases
    Acquired immunodeficiency syndrome
    Autoimmune hemolytic anemia
    Idiopathic thrombocytopenic purpura
    Plasma cell disorders
    Amyloidosis

Immunologic diseases involving the nervous system
    Multiple sclerosis
    Guillain-Barré syndrome
    Myasthenia gravis

Immunologic diseases involving the connective tissue
    Rheumatoid arthritis
    Ankylosing spondylitis
    Sjögren's syndrome

Immunologic diseases involving other organ systems
    Eczema/allergic dermatitis
    Immune complex diseases
    Immunologically mediated renal diseases

Table 48.1. *Immunologic diseases, by organ site*

This review is based on readily available data sources. Whenever possible, the information has been extracted from U.S. population-based surveys. Some of the surveys provide information on a variety of immunologic conditions; for example, figure 48.1 summarizes U.S. Hospital Discharge Survey information for several immunologic diseases. However, many of the population-based surveys are not designed to provide comprehensive information on every disease. Therefore, our understanding of the socioeconomic impact of many immunologic diseases is based on fragmented information that has been obtained from smaller, community-based studies. Although substantial information may be gained from this type of review, many critical data on the impact of immunologic diseases are currently unavailable.

Impact of Selected Diseases

Allergic Diseases

The conditions that are often referred to as allergic diseases represent one of the largest causes of illness and disability in this country. The diseases range in severity from allergic rhinitis, with its clinical expression of moderate nasal discomfort, to asthma or anaphylaxis, where death may be sudden and unexpected. The exact number of persons in the United States who are affected by allergic diseases is uncertain; however, a composite of related information suggests the impact of these conditions. Table 48.2 lists the estimated number of people in the United States who are affected by selected allergic conditions.

Data from NHANES II (the second National Health and Nutrition Examination Survey) provide an estimate that more than 40 million Americans—1 out of every 5—are reactive to at least one of eight selected antigens that are known to contribute to allergic illness (1). Immunotherapy—in this context, defined as the use of allergy shots—is a common drug intervention that is used frequently in ambulatory care for allergic diseases. More than 5 million allergy shots are prescribed annually for children with asthma and allergic rhinitis (2).

Allergic rhinitis. Allergic rhinitis, often referred to as hay fever, is a common disorder that affects an estimated 19.6 million individuals in the United States (3). This disorder is the principal reason for more than 8.4 million office visits to ambulatory care physicians.

Allergic Condition	Estimated Number Affected[a]
Allergic rhinitis	19.6 million persons (3)
Chronic sinusitis	32.5 million persons (3)
Contact dermatitis and eczema	5.8 million annual office visits (3)
Allergy immunotherapy	5.4 million administrations to children annually (2)
Skin rashes and allergic skin reactions	12 million annual office visits (4)
Asthma	9 to 12 million persons with active disease (3, 8)
Anaphylaxis and allergic reactions	1 to 2 million episodes annually (6)

[a]*Numbers in parentheses refer to reference list on page 75.*

Table 48.2. *Impact of selected allergic conditions on the U.S. population.*

Approximately two-thirds of such visits are by individuals with chronic allergic rhinitis (4).

Ninety percent of the office visits for allergic rhinitis result in medication therapy, which accounts for more than 10.5 million prescriptions annually. Antihistamines constitute the class of drugs prescribed most frequently for this condition (62 percent of all therapy) (5). However, antihistamines are often purchased without prescription, and therefore the estimated number of prescriptions issued annually for allergic rhinitis is probably a gross underestimate of the total drugs used for this condition (5).

Chronic sinusitis. Chronic sinusitis is the most prevalent allergic disease, with 32.5 million persons reporting this condition (3). Contact dermatitis and other eczemas represent a group of allergic conditions that account for 5.8 million office visits to physicians annually. Concern about skin rashes and allergic skin reactions produces 12 million office visits each year (4).

Anaphylaxis. Anaphylaxis is one of the most dramatic expressions of an allergic disorder—a severe allergic reaction that can lead to the sudden death of an apparently healthy person. An estimated 1 to 2 million people experience severe allergic reactions to insect stings each year (6), and anaphylactic reactions to penicillin are responsible for an estimated 1 to 7.5 deaths per million population (7).

Anaphylactic reactions can occur also from exposure to many other antigens, so the full impact of this condition on the U.S. population is unknown.

Much remains to be learned about the effects of allergic diseases on the U.S. population. In general these conditions are an infrequent cause of hospitalization and mortality; therefore, the national surveillance systems, such as hospitalization and mortality surveys, provide limited insight with respect to the importance of allergic diseases. Furthermore, the economic costs of most of these common illnesses have not been determined. Nevertheless, allergic diseases unquestionably constitute one of the Nation's most common and expensive health problems.

Asthma

Like other allergic diseases, asthma usually is expressed clinically as a chronic illness and is often associated with significant disability. However, unlike other allergic diseases, asthma frequently causes severe morbidity and occasionally causes death. The estimated number of individuals affected with asthma varies according to epidemiologic definition. The information most often used is derived from NHANES II or the National Health Interview Survey (NHIS). On the basis of these two surveys based on 1987 Census data, it is estimated that between 9 million and 12 million persons in the United States have asthma (3,8). There are no national data sources to estimate the incidence of this disease.

Asthma is associated with significant disability. It is responsible for more than 18 million restricted activity days annually, confining individuals to bed for more than 6 million days each year (9). In 1985, asthma was responsible for 6.5 million visits to private physicians and accounted for nearly 1 percent of all office visits to ambulatory care physicians (4). These visits generated 11.5 million prescriptions for drug therapy (5). Additional ambulatory services for asthmatic patients included nearly 5 million visits to hospital outpatient clinics and more than 1.5 million emergency room visits (9).

The clinical expression of asthma can lead to severe morbidity and occasional mortality. In 1987, asthma was the first-listed diagnosis for more than 450,000 hospitalizations (10). Rates for asthma hospitalization in the United States increased 9 percent between 1982 and 1986. Furthermore, in 1981, there were 4,360 deaths from asthma reported in the United States. (Data from 1987 mortality, underlying cause of death, U.S. Vital Records, National Center for Health Statistics.) Although asthma deaths are still infrequent, mortality rates have increased 66 percent since 1980. Non-whites are almost three times as likely as whites to die from asthma (8,12,13).

Unlike the case with most other allergic diseases, detailed information has been compiled on the economic impact of asthma in the United States. Both direct and indirect costs associated with asthma are discussed in a subsequent section of this report.

Rheumatoid Arthritis

Rheumatoid arthritis (RA) is a multi-system, autoimmune disease of unknown origin that characteristically leads to polyarthritis and progressive chronic joint deformities. The risk of developing RA increases with age. According to data from the NHIS, an estimated 2.1 million adults in the United States suffer from RA. Affected persons include approximately 0.6 million males and 1.5 million females aged 18 and older (14).

More than 80 percent of people with RA report some limitation of activity, and more than 10 percent are unable to perform one or more activities of daily living (15). In 1987, RA was responsible for an estimated 2.1 million lost workdays, 12.0 million days in bed, and 27.8 million days of restricted activity. (Figures derived from National Health Interview Survey estimates (15) as applied to 1987 census data.)

As with other immunologic diseases, much of the impact of RA is seen in the ambulatory care setting; but, unfortunately, national surveys do not provide data on ambulatory care visits for this condition. Information about the socioeconomic impact of RA comes primarily from three community-based longitudinal studies. These studies have demonstrated that persons with RA made more than 1.0 visit per month for symptoms related to this condition, in contrast to 1.7 to 3.1 visits per year for symptoms related to other conditions (16). These studies also showed that individuals with RA were hospitalized frequently, with a rate of 0.2 hospital stays per person per year (15).

Although RA is a major cause of morbidity in the United States, it is listed infrequently as the underlying cause of death.

The total economic costs of RA in the United States are unknown, however, in 1980, the economic impact of all rheumatic diseases combined was estimated at $21 billion (15). RA is clearly a major contributor to that sum. Recent advances in surgical science have enabled doctors to replace joints damaged by RA, and these procedures will change the socioeconomic impact of the disease dramatically.

Autoimmune Mediated Diabetes Mellitus

During the past decade, biomedical research has increased significantly our understanding of diabetes mellitus. Researchers have learned that most cases of what historically has been termed type 1, or insulin-dependent, diabetes mellitus (IDDM) are actually cases of an autoimmune disease resulting from an immunologically mediated destruction of the beta islet cells of the pancreas.

It has been estimated that 6.1 million persons in the United States have diabetes mellitus of some type (1985 estimate) (3). The proportion of this condition that is attributable to autoimmune-mediated disease is uncertain. However, some information about the socioeconomic impact of autoimmune-mediated diabetes can be inferred from an examination of childhood IDDM, in which immunopathology is acknowledged to be the primary mechanism of illness.

Approximately 1 child for every 600 in the population under age 16 is affected by diabetes mellitus. Based on this self-reported information, an estimated 118,000 total cases occur among persons under 18 years of age (3). (Figures derived from National Health Interview Survey estimates (15) as applied to 1987 census data.) It is expected that almost all of these cases would be IDDM. Estimates of the incidence of childhood IDDM are derived from community-based studies. These estimates range from 7 to 27 persons per 100,000 population per year for children under age 16 (17), or approximately 3,900 to 14,900 new cases of childhood IDDM diagnosed per year. (Based on 1987 census information.)

Hospitalization and mortality rates for IDDM in the general population are unknown, but hospitalization and mortality rates for children with IDDM can be inferred from hospitalization rates for all types of diabetes mellitus in this age group. During 1987, diabetes mellitus was the first-listed discharge diagnosis for 21,000 hospitalizations among children under 15 years of age. During the same year, diabetes mellitus was reported as the principal discharge diagnosis for 113,000 hospital bed-days for children in that age group. Diabetes mellitus is an infrequent cause of death in children under age 15; however, recent evidence suggests that as many as 9 percent of deaths from diabetes mellitus in this age group may be preventable (18). There is no commonly accepted information regarding other aspects of illness, disability, or costs for this important immunologic disease.

Systemic Lupus Erythematosus

There are no national data on the incidence or prevalence of SLE (systemic lupus erythematosus). The only SLE data available are derived from regional studies of populations that are not representative of the entire United States; therefore, any national estimates based on these studies should be viewed with caution. The National Institutes of Health recently conducted a National Arthritis Data Workshop to review these regional studies. The workshop, sponsored by the National Institute of Allergy and Infectious Diseases and the National Institute of Arthritis and Musculoskeletal and Skin Diseases, recommended a 1985 figure of 131,000 cases of SLE in the United States. SLE is much more prevalent in females than in males and more prevalent in blacks than in other segments of the population. The community studies suggest that 90 percent of the people affected with SLE are women between the ages of 15 and 45 years (14).

SLE often leads to severe morbidity and disability. In 1987, SLE was mentioned as a discharge diagnosis for more than 40,000 hospitalizations (10). In 1986, SLE was identified as the underlying cause for 1,067 deaths and was mentioned as a contributing factor for another nearly 2,000 deaths. (Figures based on 1986 U.S. Vital Records, both underlying cause of death and any-listing on record axis of multiple causes of death, National Center for Health Statistics.) The economic costs of SLE in the U.S. population are unknown.

Multiple Sclerosis

Multiple sclerosis (MS) is a demyelinating disease of the central nervous system in which autoimmunity plays a major pathogenic role. There are no recent population-based estimates of the number of persons who are affected with MS; however, estimates based on regional data indicate that there are more than 150,000 diagnosed cases of MS in the United States (19). The average estimated cost of MS in this country is $1.6 billion. (Figure is a 1985 estimate based on applying a 1984 estimate to 1987 census data. 1984 estimate from the Multiple Sclerosis Society, prepared by Herbert Baum, Director, Data and Research Services, ELM Services, Inc., Rockville, Maryland.)

Ankylosing Spondylitis

Ankylosing spondylitis is a chronic inflammatory disorder involving the spine and adjacent soft tissues. Again, there are no national estimates of the prevalence of this disease. Based on community studies, however, an estimated 318,000 individuals in the United States are affected by ankylosing spondylitis. (Figure is a 1985 estimate derived by applying a prevalence estimate (14) to 1985 census data.)

Transplantations

Transplantation of major organs represents one of the most significant advances in modern medical science. Each year thousands of individuals develop end organ failure that can benefit from organ replacement. Table 48.3 summarizes transplantation activity for 1988. During that year, more than 10,000 persons benefited from organ transplantation. However, demand for transplantation procedures continues to exceed the availability of organs for transplant. As of August 1989, more than 18,000 persons were waiting to receive transplant organs (20).

Kidneys are the most frequently transplanted organ. Chronic dialysis and kidney transplantation are the only two treatment options for end-stage renal disease (ESRD). During 1987, 157,944 patients in the Medicare system had ESRD. Annual Medicare payments for their care averaged more than $28,000 per patient. In 1987, 3.4 percent of the Health Care Financing Administration budget for Medicare and 5.5 percent of the Medicare Part B outpatient budget were used to provide either maintenance dialysis or kidney transplantation to patients with ESRD (21).

The costs of ESRD are enormous, and transplantations represent a large portion of these costs. Improvements in the recognition and treatment of early renal disease will reduce considerably the impact of ESRD; however, improvements in transplantation knowledge also will be required if the morbidity, disability, and costs of ESRD are to be reduced.

Organ	Number of Transplants	Number of Persons Awaiting Transplantation
Kidney	7,278	15,721
Heart	1,647	1,227
Lung	31	77
Heart/Lung	74	231
Liver	1,680	734
Pancreas	243	298
Bone Marrow	2,000[a]	n/a
Cornea	n/a	30

[a] *Data obtained from reports of listed procedures, National Hospital Discharge Survey, 1987. The standard error for this estimate is large, so the figure should be used only with caution.*

SOURCE: **USRDS Annual Report,** 1989.

Table 48.3. Organ transplantation activity, selected organs, United States, 1988.

Acquired Immunodeficiency Syndrome

AIDS is caused by an infection with human immunodeficiency virus, which disrupts the normal function of the immune system. AIDS continues to have a major socioeconomic impact on the U.S. population. The prevalence of HIV infection in the general population is unknown; however, as of October 1989, a total of 109,167 persons had been diagnosed with AIDS, an incidence rate of 13.1 per 100,000 population per year. As of October 1989, 63,836 deaths had been attributed to AIDS (22). More than 1,000 of those who died were children under 13 years of age. The total estimated cost of AIDS in the U.S. population was more than $4 billion in 1988 (23).

Economic Impact of Immunologic Disease: Asthma as a Case Study

The preceding descriptions of immunologic diseases provide a broad understanding of how these conditions affect the U.S. population. However, with few exceptions, documented information concerning the economic costs of these conditions is scarce. Because the most extensive available data are about asthma, this condition is considered in detail here to provide insight regarding the economic costs of immunologic diseases. The estimated costs of asthma can be separated into two broad categories: direct costs and indirect costs. The direct costs for asthma are measured as medical care expenditures. These costs include an estimated $1.3 billion in hospital charges for inpatient, outpatient, and emergency room visits; over $210 million in physician charges for inpatient and private office visits; and $900 million for prescription medications. No available data support estimates of other associated expenditures, such as diagnostic services, nonprescription medications, home health care, or long-term care. The total estimated direct medical expenditures for asthma in 1985 approached $2.5 billion.

	Direct medical expenditures ($ millions)
Hospital charges inpatient, outpatient, and emergency room	$1,295
Physician charges inpatient and private office	271
Medications	905
Diagnostic services	n/a
	Indirect costs ($ millions)
Disability through work and school loss	1,417 [a]
Mortality	676
Total estimated costs	$ 4,564

[a] See text.

[8] Based on analysis by Weiss, Gergen, and Hodgson (unpublished report).

Table 48.4. Economic Impact of Asthma, estimated direct and indirect costs, 1995.

The indirect costs associated with asthma include the loss of income from disability and mortality. Loss-of-income figures are derived from both days away from work, absenteeism caused by the need to care for a sick child, and the imputed value of foregone housekeeping. These costs amount to $1.4 billion. An additional indirect cost of illness is based on the reduction of lifetime earnings because of death, $616 million. For asthma, these indirect costs exceed $2 billion annually. Therefore, as summarized in table 48.4, the total estimated annual costs associated with asthma exceed $4.5 billion (1985 dollars). (Based on analysis by Weis, Gergen, and Hodgson—unpublished report.) The figures in table 48.4 provide a gross estimate of the total economic costs of asthma within the United States. However, they do not give any insight into the economic impact of the disease on affected individuals and their families. A recent study examined the costs associated with the management of childhood asthma, and the results indicate that an average family with a moderately severely asthmatic child will spend 6.4 percent of its yearly income on asthma-related expenses (24).

Immunologic Diseases Affecting Vulnerable Populations

Immunologic Diseases in Children and Young Adults

Immunologic diseases affect persons of all ages and most often are clinically expressed as conditions of chronic morbidity and disability rather than conditions associated with significant mortality. Another important aspect of these diseases is their unique impact on children and young adults. One way to view the impact of immunologic diseases in this younger population is through health care utilization. Table 48.5, for example, shows that in 1980 to 1981, immunologic diseases accounted for 10.5 million, or nearly 1 out of 10, office visits to U.S. pediatricians (2).

Allergic conditions are the immunologic disorders that occur most frequently in childhood. In the United States, there are more than 3 million asthmatic children who are 3 to 11 years old (8), and nearly 40 percent of all physician office visits for asthma are by patients in this age group (2). In addition, more than 5.4 million allergy injections are delivered annually to children by pediatricians (4). In fact, allergy injections are the single most common drug therapy mentioned for pediatrician office visits of all children more than 6 years of age (2). **Juvenile rheumatoid arthritis (JRA)** is a striking expression of an immunopathologic arthritis that affects children and young adults. According to data from community studies, JRA affects 57 children per 100,000 in the population. From this prevalence figure, it is estimated that 71,000 children under the age of 18 years were affected with this condition in 1987 (14).

As described in a preceding section, **autoimmune-mediated diabetes mellitus** is another immunologic disease that affects children disproportionately. Many children with this type of diabetes will eventually become disabled through loss of vision, end-stage renal disease, or other disease complications; and many will die prematurely.

Immunologic Diseases in Minority Populations

Over the past few decades, scientists have achieved unprecedented advances in scientific knowledge about the diagnosis, treatment, and cure of disease. However, individuals of African American, Hispanic, Native American, and Asian and Pacific Islander heritage apparently have not benefited fully or equitably from these advances. According to the 1985 HHS Secretary's Task Force on black and Minority Health, an average of 59,000 excess deaths among blacks under age 70 occurred annually between 1979 and 1981. (Excess deaths are those that would not have occurred if the black population had experienced the same age-sex death rates as whites [25].) The relative risk for death in the Hispanic population was found to be intermediate between blacks and whites. The Secretary's Task Force made many recommendations, including the need to target Federal categorical initiatives to identify large gaps between the health experiences of whites and those of minorities.

However, the report of the Task Force focused entirely on issues relating to mortality. It did not examine the impact of morbidity and disability in our minority populations. As previously noted, immunologic conditions are not common causes of mortality but they have an important socioeconomic impact on U.S. minority health by causing years of chronic illness and disability.

Asthma is more prevalent among black children who are 6 to 11 years old than among white children of the same age (rates of 9.4 and 6.2 percent, respectively) (26). In addition, asthma hospitalization and mortality rates are both higher for blacks than for whites, and for blacks the rates are disproportionately increasing (8, 12, 13, 27). Recent evidence suggests that U.S. asthma mortality rates are highest among urban minorities (13, 28). The levels of morbidity and disability related to asthma within other minority populations are not well known; however, the costs of asthma appear to affect minorities disproportionately because these groups tend to be poor. As previously noted, the average family with a moderately severely asthmatic child will spend 6.4 percent of its yearly income on asthma-related costs; for low-income families, however, these costs amount to nearly 12 percent of yearly income (24).

Systemic lupus erythematosus is another immunologic condition that disproportionately affects minority health. The estimated rate of SLE prevalence per 10,000 population among blacks is 7.5, compared to 4.0 among whites. However, this general figure underestimates the combined sex and racial distribution. Prevalence estimates for black females are greater than 50 times those for white males (38.0 and 0.7 per 10,000 population, respectively, based on 1985 estimated number of cases (14) and 1985 census population estimates. Although evidence suggests the possibility of genetic risk factors, the etiology of the difference in SLE prevalence between blacks and whites is not known. Prevalence rates for SLE among other minority populations also are unknown.

Blacks and other minority populations have not benefited fully or equitably in the area of **organ transplantation**. Rates for kidney transplantation, the most frequent transplant procedure, demonstrate this inequity. In 1987, blacks were more than four times as likely, and Native Americans were approximately three times as likely, as whites to have ESRD, which is the primary reason for kidney transplantation (29). Despite the higher incidence of ESRD among the black population, members of this group receive kidney transplantations at slightly more than half the rate of the white population.

During the past few years, the demographics of **AIDS** in the United States has shifted from populations represented primarily by white males to a population that is represented increasingly by blacks and Hispanics and by women. The prevalence of AIDS in the United States disproportionately affects these minority groups. As of September 1989, 27 percent of all AIDS cases reported to the Centers for Disease Control occurred among blacks (22), who represent only 12 percent of the U.S. population. Similarly, 15 percent of all reported AIDS cases occurred among Hispanics who constitute only 6 percent of the U.S. population.

Socioeconomic Benefits of The Clinical Applications of Immunologic Research

A comprehensive description of the benefits of immunologic research is beyond the scope of this special report. However, research within the discipline of immunology has produced dramatic socioeconomic benefits. Developments in immunologic research result in both expected and unexpected gains. Vaccines are perhaps the most obvious ongoing expected benefit from immunologic research. Investments in this area of immunologic research have high expected rates of return and produce an enormous socioeconomic benefit to society. Future development of vaccines for diseases such as influenza, respiratory syncytial virus, and streptococcus group B may prevent millions of days of morbidity and allow substantial cost savings for the U.S. population (30).

In addition to the expected socioeconomic benefit of certain developments in immunologic research, there are unexpected gains from research in this area. For example, the radioimmunoassay now is used in nearly all facets of clinical and research applications.

Conclusions and Recommendations

Immunologic conditions represent a broad spectrum of diseases that affect many organ systems. When viewed collectively, these diseases affect nearly 10 percent of the U.S. population. Although only a few immunologic conditions are fatal, most of these illnesses are clinically expressed through years of relentless morbidity and disability. Thus, the economic costs of immunologic diseases differ from those of other diseases. For example, a large proportion of costs for diseases such as cancer and heart disease are related to loss of expected years of life. However, as Table 48.4 illustrates, the economic costs of immunologic diseases such as asthma consist primarily of direct medical expenditures and disability. (Indirect costs of income loss due to caring for a sick child not included in the indirect costs of morbidity for neoplasms and circulatory diseases.) Therefore, the socioeconomic impact of these diseases can be quantified best by measuring the use of ambulatory care and disability such as school days or work days lost.

Although information is available on the socioeconomic impact of immunologic diseases and organ transplantation, many large gaps in our knowledge still remain. More information on this impact can provide critical insight about approaches for reducing the burden of immunologic diseases. Thus, it would be useful to establish a long-range plan that addresses these gaps in our knowledge regarding the socioeconomic impact of immunologic disease upon the U.S. population.

References

1. Gergen, P.J.; Turkeltaub, P.C.; Kovar, M.G. The prevalence of allergic skin test reactivity to eight common aero-allergens in the U.S. population: results for the Second National Health and Nutrition Examination Survey. *Journal of Allergy and Clinical Immunology* 80(5): 679-99, 1987.

2. National Center for Health Statistics; Cypress, B.K. Patterns of Ambulatory Care in Pediatrics: The National Ambulatory Medical Care Survey, United States, January 1980-December 1981. *Vital and Health Statistics*, series 13, no. 75. DHHS Pub. no. (PHS)841736. Washington, D.C.: U.S. Government Printing Office, Oct. 1983.

3. National Center for Health Statistics; Moss, A.J., Parsons, V.L. Current Estimates from the National Health Interview Survey, United States, 1985. *Vital and Health Statistics*, series 10, no. 160. DHHS Pub. no. (PHS)861588. Washington, D.C.: U.S. GPO. Oct. 1986.

4. National Center for Health Statistics; Nelson, C., McLemore, T. The National Ambulatory Medical Care Survey, United States, 1975-81 and 1985 Trends. *Vital and Health Statistics,* series 13, no. 93. DHHS Pub. no. (PHS)88-1754. Washington, D.C.: U.S. GPO, Oct. 1988.

5. National Center for Health Statistics; Cypress, B.K. Medication Therapy in Office Visits for Selected Diagnoses: The National Ambulatory Medical Care Survey, United States, 1980. *Vital and Health Statistics*, series 13, no. 71. DHHS Pub. no. (PHS)83-1732. Washington, D.C.: U.S. GPO, Oct. 1983.

6. Reisman, R. Insect sting allergy in children. In: *Current Therapy in Allergy, Immunology and Rheumatology*, edited by L.M. Lichtenstein and A.S. Fauci. Toronto: B.C. Decker, Inc., 1988.

7. Idsoe, O.; Gruthe, T.; Wilcox, R.R.; deWeck, A.L. Nature and extent of penicillin side-reactions with particular reference to fatalities from anaphylactic shock. *Bulletin of the World Health Organization* 38: 159-63, 1968.

8. Evans, R., et al. National trends in the morbidity and mortality of asthma in the U.S. *Chest* 91(6):65s-74s, 1987.

9. National Health Interview Survey, NCHS, 1983-1987 combined (unpublished data).

10. National Center for Health Statistics; Graves, E.J. Detailed Diagnoses and Procedures, National Hospital Discharge Survey: 1987. *Vital and Health Statistics*, series 13, no. 100. DHHS Pub. no. (PHS)89-1761. Washington, D.C.: U.S. GPO, Oct. 1989.

11. Graves, E.J.; Molen, M. Hospitalization for AIDS, United States, 1984-1985. *American Journal of Public Health* 77: 729-30, 1987.

12. Sly, R.M. Mortality from asthma, 1979-1984. *Journal of Allergy and Clinical Immunology* 82: 705-17, 1988.

13. Weiss, K.B.; Wagener, D.K. Changing patterns of U.S. asthma mortality: identifying target populations at high risk. *Journal of the American Medical Association* (in press): 1990.

14. Lawrence, R.C., et al. Estimates of the prevalence of selected arthritic and musculoskeletal diseases in the United States. *Journal of Rheumatology* 16: 427-441, 1989.

15. Felts, W.; Yelin, E. The economic impact of rheumatic diseases in the United States. *Journal of Rheumatology* 16: 867-84, 1989.

16. Yelin, E.; Shearn, M.; Epstein W. Health outcomes for a chronic disease in prepaid group practice and fee for service settings. *Medical Care* 24: 236-247, 1986.

17. Krolewski, A.S.; Rarram, J.H.; Rand L.I.;, Kahn, C.R. Epidemiologic approach to the etiology of type 1 diabetes

mellitus and its complications. *New England Journal of Medicine* 317(22): 1390-1398, 1987.

18. Will, J.C.; Connell, F.A. The preventability of premature mortality: an investigation of early diabetes deaths. *American Journal of Public Health* 78(7): 831-836, 1988.

19. Baum, H.M.; Rothschild B.B. The incidence and prevalence of reported multiple sclerosis. *Annals of Neurology* 10: 420-428, 1981.

20. United Network for Organ Sharing. *Organ Procurement and Transplantation Network Annual Status Report to the Health Resources and Services Administration: January 1, 1988, to December 31. 1988.* Report date: April 21, 1989.

21. USRDS Annual Data Report, 1989.

22. HIV/AIDS surveillance, USPHS, CDC, Division HIV/AIDS, issued October 1989.

23. Winkenwerder, W.; Kessler, A.R; Stolec, R.M. Federal spending for illness caused by the human immunodeficiency virus. *New England Journal of Medicine* 320(24): 1598-1603, 1989.

24. Marion, R.J; Creer, T.L.; Reynolds, R.V.C. Direct and indirect costs associated with the management of childhood asthma. *Annals of Allergy* 54: 31-34, 1985.

25. U.S. DHHS. *Report of the Secretary's Task Force on Black and Minority Health, Volume 1: Executive Summary.* Washington, D.C.: U.S. GPO, 1987.

26. Gergen, P.J., Mullally, D.I.; Evans R. National survey of prevalence of asthma among children in the United States, 967, to 1980. *Pediatrics* 81: 1-7, 1988.

27. Gergen, P.J., Weiss, K.B. Changing patterns of asthma hospitalization among U.S. children 0-17 years of age, 1979-1987. *Journal of the American Medical Association* 1990 (in press).

28. Weiss, K.B., Wagener, D.K. Geographic variations in the U.S. asthma mortality: Small-area analyses of excess mortality 1981-1985. *American Journal of Epidemiology* 1990 (in press).

29. National Kidney and Urologic Disease Advisory Board. 1990 "Long-Range Plan: Window on the 21st Century" (final draft), November 10, 1989.

30. Division of Health Promotion and Disease Prevention, Institute of Medicine. *New Vaccine Development: Establishing Priorities. Vol. 1, Diseases of Importance in the United States.* Washington, D.C.: National Academy Press, 1985.

31. Rice, D.P.; Hodgson, T.A.; Kopstein, A.N. The economic costs of illness: a replication and update. *Health Care Financing Review* 7: 61-80, 1985.

Chapter 49

Health Insurance for Primary Immune Deficiency: Taking Control

As we are all aware, having a chronic condition, like a primary immunodeficiency, can be financially taxing. If therapy is not administered on a regular basis, the cost of complications and subsequent hospitalizations is burdensome. Most individuals with primary immune deficiency rely on private third party payers to assist them with these expenses, but often are frustrated when faced with the overwhelming task of paperwork, phone calls, and other issues, simply to justify the use of a therapy prescribed by their physician. In addition, looking for health insurance and understanding the maze of issues involved can be an overwhelming process that can often lead to feelings of isolation and helplessness.

The purpose of this chapter, while not designed to solve each and every health insurance problem, is to prepare you with some of the information you will need to be your own best advocate. Most of the information that follows is practical. We begin by describing the various payers, what they cover and who they serve. Next, you will learn about what to look for when changing insurance coverage, a very important issue when a chronic condition is involved. You will read about other features that you should have a general working knowledge of, like COBRA, a name for extended benefits.

Other hands-on information follows with how to prepare yourself to face your insurer confidently with questions about your coverage.

And last, but not least, as in every profession these days, health insurance has its own "language." We will arm you with a glossary of terms so that you will feel confidently "bilingual."

When it comes to your health coverage, never hesitate to ask lots of questions and search for as many resources as possible. Your well-being and that of your family relies on it.

Who Are the "Payer Players?"

In order to best prepare for working with your health insurer, you must understand who the various "payer players" are in the scheme of things.

Medicare

Medicare is a federal health insurance program which provides coverage for people age 65 and older or individuals of any age who are on Social Security disability or have end-stage renal disease. Medicare is divided into two parts: Parts A and B. Part A is a basic hospital insurance plan that reimburses for most of the cost of inpatient care (hospital and skilled nursing facility) and some care after you go home. There is an annual deductible to meet, but after that, Medicare will pay for most of your approved costs. Medicare Part B covers physicians services and other medical expenses. Unfortunately, neither prescription drugs nor home infusion of IGIV is covered. Beneficiaries must pay a monthly premium and a small deductible each year for all services covered under Part B. For most of these services, Medicare pays 80 percent of the bill and the beneficiary pays the 20 percent co-payment. You must first have Part A before receiving Part B. If you apply for Social Security disability, you will receive Medicare benefits after being on disability for two years.

Medicaid

Medicaid is a welfare program sponsored by both the federal and state governments which is administered by the individual states. Coverage varies from state to state although each of the state programs adheres to certain federal guidelines. Medicaid enrollment criteria also vary from state to state, but coverage is usually available only to those who are not eligible for any other type of health insurance.

Each state has a predetermined income level that an individual or family must meet in order to qualify for Medicaid benefits. The local office of the State Department of Social Services is responsible for reviewing applications and managing eligibility requirements.

Medicaid programs may require prior authorization for certain forms of treatment or prescription drugs. This means that your physician must contact Medicaid to obtain approval for reimbursement of the treatment before you receive it.

State Assistance Programs

Your state may have a special assistance program for particular chronic conditions. Most of these programs are funded by state and local budgets and are designed to meet the needs of adults and/or children who are not eligible for any other medical coverage. They may also serve as a secondary or supplemental coverage to Medicaid. The level of coverage available will change according to such variables as state needs and available funding. These programs may be identified under such names as Children with Special Health Care Needs, Crippled Children's Services, or Children's Medical Services. Coverage for children with a Primary Immune Deficiency may be severely restricted or not available at all. It is best to check with your local sources of information for eligibility information before considering this as a coverage option.

SSI

SSI or Supplemental Security Income makes monthly payments to aged, disabled, and blind people with limited income and resources. Disabled children as well as adults, may qualify for SSI payments. Eligibility and benefits vary by state, but more information can be obtained by contacting your local Social Security Office listed in the White Pages of the phone book.

Third Party Insurers

Third party insurers offer various types of plans; for example, fee-for-service plans or 80/20 plans are normally obtained through your employer. The services covered by the policy will vary depending on your employer, so read the summary of benefits carefully, **especially the exclusionary language**.

The beneficiary is free to choose his own provider. A premium is paid for coverage by the beneficiary, the employer, or the cost is shared. The beneficiary is usually responsible for an annual deductible before the insurance coverage becomes effective. Once the deductible is met, the plan pays a portion of the bill normally 80 percent. The beneficiary is then responsible for the remaining 20 percent, which is called a co-payment.

Prepaid Managed Care

These plans cover medical services provided by "participating" physicians. Premiums are paid in advance for most covered services, depending on the nature of the problem. Group practice health maintenance organizations or HMOs cover you only if you go to HMO-affiliated health care providers (doctors, labs, hospitals) for all your health needs. You may go to one central facility for your care, or you may visit an HMO-affiliated physician at his or her office. There are also preferred provider organizations or PPOs. These plans are similar to HMOs in that members pay a set amount each month for health care services. A group of physicians or other types of health care providers contract with the PPO, to provide services to members. These plans offer greater flexibility of choice of provider. Under most situations, a PPO offers a financial incentive, in the form of the percentage of co-payment, for the patient to use a participating provider. The co-payment may be set at 90/10, for example. If, however, the patient sees a provider outside the network, the co-payment for the patient may increase to 70/30.

You the Consumer

It is important to consider specific issues when deciding on a health insurance policy. You should compare:

- The lifetime maximum
- Any pre-existing condition waiting period
- Out-of-pocket cost including premium cost sharing, deductible, and co-payment
- inadequate or no coverage

Your lifetime maximum (LTM) will differ according to the health coverage you have. Most LTMs will range from $250,000 to $1 million.

Once you have exhausted your LTM, you no longer have health coverage, so it is wise to keep a running total of the major expenses that affect it: hospitalizations, surgeries, annual cost of drug therapy, etc...

The pre-existing condition waiting period is an amendment to your coverage that states that if you have a chronic condition, or are, for example pregnant, you're subject to a waiting period before your benefits cover you for that "condition." Look for a pre-existing condition waiting period clause in the summary of benefits booklet.

Out-of-pocket costs are those co-payments, deductibles, or premium cost-sharing expenses you may incur to meet your financial obligation under the plan. These were reviewed under the previous payer section.

Language in your health policy can differ. It can be explicit or vague, so knowing what to look for is important. You must always check the exclusionary language in your summary of benefits booklet.

Finally, if you are considering signing up with an HMO, but you are concerned because you may have to change to a different doctor, check with others who are members to ask about their level of satisfaction. Ask such questions as:

- How are chronic conditions like primary immune deficiency covered within the plan?
- What about referrals to specialists?
- What are the procedures?
- Do they have restrictions on prescription drugs?

COBRA

COBRA or the Consolidated Omnibus Budget Reconciliation Act was enacted into Federal law in 1985. Should you leave your job for any reason other than gross misconduct, your employer is required under the law to offer you continuing health benefits for a period of time—the same benefits you were receiving while you were employed. You are responsible for paying the premium, which is usually kept at 102 percent of what your employer was paying on your behalf. (The 2 percent is for administrative fees).

For job termination or a reduction in hours, COBRA's duration is normally 18 months. In the case of a divorce, separation or death of a spouse, COBRA may be available for up to 36 months. When these situations, known as "qualifying events" occur, it is your responsibility, as the employee, to notify the human resources department of your employer (that person or group responsible for medical insurance) within 60 days or you lose the option, For further information on COBRA coverage and your rights under COBRA law, you should contact the human resource department or the benefits manager within your organization or call the COBRA information lines at (202) 523-8776 or (202) 523-8784.

Small employers (less than 20 employees), church groups, and the federal government, are exempt from COBRA legislation. Federal employees, however, are not without help. Those employees should contact the personnel office serving their agency for more information on temporary extensions of health benefits.

High Risk Pools

High risk pools provide coverage for individuals whose medical conditions have prevented them from obtaining private health insurance and those who may not qualify for government or state assistance. At this writing, high risk insurance pools are now available in 26 states. While the operation of plans varies considerably from state to state, there is a basic pattern. The state generally forms an association of all health insurance companies doing business in the state. One organization is selected to administer the plan under the guidelines for benefits, premiums, deductibles, etc., as set forth under state law. Individual policies are available through the risk pool and are subject to the very same restrictions as private, third party insurance. So do not be surprised if you see co-payments, deductibles, lifetime maximums, and pre-existing condition waiting periods. Coverage usually includes physician and in-patient hospital services, home health care, skilled nursing care and prescription drugs.

If high risk insurance is available in your state, be sure to inquire about eligibility requirements and the specific benefits which are covered. There can be waiting lists for enrollment in these programs in some states.

Words to the Wise

As you've repeatedly just read, it is very important for you to be your own best advocate when dealing with your health plan. First, read your policy and then ask your personnel department, and any other resource you can find lots of questions. Try to keep current information concerning the new rules affecting your policy. Review your medical bills to check for mistakes. (Billing errors occur more often than you would think!) Keep important information such as your policy number, your ID number, insurer's address and phone number, and doctor's address and phone number in one place to refer to whenever you communicate with your insurer.

If there's a possibility you might reach your lifetime maximum, please explore the alternatives before your maximum runs out. Many employers offer open enrollment once a year when you may change your coverage to another plan offered by your employer. Ask your employer if and when an open enrollment period is offered. If you have difficulty getting benefits through your employer, consider coverage through associations, schools, professional groups, farm groups, or local chambers of commerce. You may qualify for individual or group benefits.

Document each time you contact your insurer. Get the full name and title of each person you talk with. This information will be important if you experience difficulties with your coverage and need to document your situation in writing.

If your problem becomes more complicated, don't panic. You may appeal to the medical director of the insurance company and may need to work with the provider to submit additional justification of your claim. Often, in the case of primary immune deficiencies, insurers need to be educated as to what the condition is and what the approved forms of treatment are. Most of the manufacturers of intravenous immune globulin (IVIG) offer reimbursement support services for their products and should be an excellent source of information. The Immune Deficiency Foundation can refer you to these sources.

There may come a time when an insurance company terminates your policy. If it does for any other reason than bankruptcy, they are required by state and federal law to find you new coverage. Enforcing this law is up to the State Insurance Commissioner. You should contact them especially if you feel your cancellation is due to a pre-existing condition. Arbitrary cancellation is illegal.

Conclusion

You could spend a major portion of every waking day working on coverage and reimbursement issues for yourself or your family. Some of you are fortunate enough to never experience problems. Others of you are in an endless search for coverage or adequate reimbursement.

While we do not assume to have provided all the answers to your questions in this section, we hope you have picked up a few bits of information. Never hesitate to seek assistance from resources. There is no such thing as a stupid question when it comes to you or your family's well being.

Glossary of Insurance Terms

ASSIGNMENT OF BENEFITS: A written authorization by the patient/insured to make payment to the provider of services (hospital, physician, home care company, etc.) directly.

BALANCE BILLING: If a provider chooses not to accept assignment, he or she can "balance bill" the patient for the portion of the charge not recognized by Medicare.

BASIC BENEFITS: Refers to the portion of the insurance policy which generally provides coverage for inpatient services: room and board, surgery, drug therapy, physician services, etc.

BENEFICIARY: A person entitled to insurance benefits under the insurance plan; a patient.

"CAP": The maximum length of time or dollar amount that a plan will continue to pay benefits; also referred to as **"contract maximum."**

CARRIER: A private insurer that contracts on a regional basis with the Medicare program to process and pay claims. Also a term generally to describe an insurer.

CHARGE-BASED: Reimbursement based upon billed fees for physician's services.

CLAIM FORM: Requests for payment are submitted to insurers on claim forms. Claim forms include spaces for showing the patient's name and address, diagnosis, documentation of medical necessity and kinds of services received.

CODING: Several coding systems are used to describe patients and the services they receive in the health care system. These are used on medical records and billing forms.

CO-PAYMENT: A percentage of medical costs which the patient is required to pay, usually up to a certain limit.

COST-BASED: Reimbursement methodology typically used to pay institutions on the basis of accounting cost audits. The books of the provider are examined in an effort to avoid paying profits and unallowed items.

COVERAGE: The products and services your health plan is willing to pay for.

DEDUCTIBLE: A flat amount that the patient is automatically responsible for paying before the insurance plan begins to pay benefits.

EFFECTIVE DATE: The date that coverage begins for the insured.

ELIGIBILITY: The screening method used by an insurance company or government program to determine whether the patient qualifies for benefits.

EXCLUSIONS: Illnesses, injuries, devices, procedures, or conditions for which the policy will not pay.

EXPLANATION OF MEDICAL BENEFITS: This form is sent to patients to report on the status of their insurance claim. It outlines the services for which a bill was received, describes whether the service is covered and delineates the reimbursement that will be made for the service or product.

FEE-FOR-SERVICE: A predetermined charge for a given medical service.

FEE SCREEN: Many insurers established a price cap, also called a fee screen, on the total they will pay for a service or product.

HEALTH CARE FINANCING ADMINISTRATION: A branch of the federal government's Department of Health and Human Services that administers the Medicare program.

HEALTH MAINTENANCE ORGANIZATION (HMO): A prepaid health plan that provides comprehensive benefits using certain health care professionals, at times in specified locations, generally within certain geographic areas.

INSURED/POLICY HOLDER: The person for whom the insurance policy is registered under.

LIFETIME MAXIMUM: The maximum amount that the insurance company will pay for medical expenses. This amount may be listed as the maximum amount for each illness or condition. Or it may be listed as total costs paid from a portion of a policy; e.g. inpatient expenses vs outpatient.

MAJOR MEDICAL: Refers to the portion of the insurance policy which usually provides coverage for outpatient services: doctor's office visit, outpatient pharmacy services, factor concentrate home therapy, etc.

MEDICAID: A federally and state funded program for low income people. Eligibility criteria will vary by state but are usually tied to income and assets.

MEDICAL NECESSITY: In order to be financed by an insurer, a service must be medically necessary.

MEDICARE: A federally funded medical insurance program for people age 65 and over, individuals with end stage renal disease, or those who qualify for Social Security disability.

OPEN ENROLLMENT: a time period when a person can obtain insurance coverage or change insurance carriers without penalty for a pre-existing condition. This opportunity may be available from some employers on an annual basis.

PRE-EXISTING CONDITION CLAUSE: Any medical, obstetrical or psychiatric condition that the patient had at the time the plan became effective. If your plan contains this clause there is usually a defined waiting period beyond the effective date of the plan before the plan will make payment for treatment of the preexisting medical condition.

PREFERRED PROVIDER ORGANIZATION (PPO): A group of health care providers (physicians, hospitals, and other providers) located within a specific geographical area who have contracted with an entity (a physicians' group or hospital, for example) to provide health care services.

PREMIUM: The payment a subscriber must pay in order to maintain medical benefits.

PRIMARY COVERAGE: The insurance plan that is required to pay benefits first based on state and federal insurance regulations.

PROVIDER: Refers to any party that delivers health care services. For example, can be used to describe doctors, hospitals, or suppliers.

REIMBURSEMENT: The amount the plan pays for a particular product or service. Your plan may reimburse the full amount charged by your doctor, pharmacy, or hospital; or it may reimburse a percentage or set amount.

SECONDARY COVERAGE: An insurance plan that is required to pay benefits after the primary plan has paid or denied payment for medical expenses.

STOPLOSS/OUT-OF-POCKET EXPENSE: The maximum amount of money an insured individual is required to pay (as a deductible or co-pay) before the plan will pay benefits at 100 percent.

UTILIZATION REVIEW: The process of evaluating the appropriateness, necessity and quality of medical care for purposes of insurance coverage.

Appendix

Appendix

Chapter 50

Glossary of Medical Terms

Acquired immunodeficiency syndrome (AIDS): A life-threatening disease caused by a virus and characterized by breakdown of the body's immune defenses. A disorder resulting from infection by the human immunodeficiency virus (HIV), which greatly depletes the helper T cell population, causing various infections and/or tumors.

Active immunity: Immunity produced by the body as a result of previous exposure to an antigen, an allergen, or vaccination.

Acute phase proteins: Serum proteins whose levels increase during infection or inflammatory reactions.

Adjuvant: A substance that non-specifically enhances the immune response to an antigen.

Agammaglobulinemia: An almost total lack of immunoglobulins, or antibodies.

AIDS: See Acquired immunodeficiency syndrome.

Allergen: Any substance that causes an allergic response.

Allergy: An inappropriate and harmful response of the immune system to normally harmless substances. A specific IgE antibody response to a specific antigen.

Altered self: The concept that the combination of antigen and a self-MHC molecule interacts with the immune system in the same way as an allogeneic MHC molecule.

Anaphylactic shock: life-threatening allergic reaction characterized by a swelling of body tissues including the throat, difficulty in breathing, and a sudden fall in blood pressure.

Anaphylatoxin: Complement peptides (C3a and C5a) that cause mast cell degranulation and smooth muscle contraction.

Anaphylaxis: An antigen-specific immune reaction mediated primarily by IgE, which results in vasodilation and constriction of smooth muscles, including those of the bronchus, and which may result in death.

Anergy: A state of unresponsiveness, induced when the T cell's antigen receptor is stimulated, that effectively freezes T cell responses pending a "second signal" from the antigen-presenting cell (see co-stimulation).

Antibody: A soluble protein produced by B cells, which reacts to a specific antigen in some demonstrable way (e.g., binding or coating the antigen).

Antibody-dependent cell-mediated cytotoxicity (ADCC): An immune response in which antibody, by coating target cells, makes them vulnerable to attack by immune cells.

Antigen presentation: The process by which certain cells in the body (antigen-presenting cells) express an antigen on their cell surface in a form recognizable by lymphocytes.

Antigen: Any substance that, when introduced into the body, is recognized and elicits a response by the immune system.

Antigen processing: The actions that a cell makes to convert antigen into a form in which it can be recognized by lymphocytes

Antigen-presenting cells: B cells, cells of the monocyte lineage (including macrophages as well as dendritic cells), and various other body cells that present antigen in a form that T cells can recognize.

Antinuclear antibody (ANA): An autoantibody directed against a substance in the cell's nucleus.

Antiserum: Serum that contains antibodies.

Antitoxins: Antibodies that interlock with and inactivate toxins produced by certain bacteria.

Antiviral proteins: Proteins induced by Interferons that render a cell resistant to viral replication.

Appendix: Lymphoid organ in the intestine.

Asthma: A genetically linked problem, believed to cause airway obstruction, that is associated with narrowing of air passages, airway inflammation, and airway hypersensitivity to multiple stimuli.

Atopic: See atopy.

Atopy: A genetically determined clinical manifestation of type 1 hypersensitivity, which includes reactions such as eczema, asthma, and rhinitis.

Attenuated: Weakened; no longer infectious.

Autoantibody: An antibody that reacts against a person's own tissue.

Autocrine: Acting on self; e.g., describes hormones that are produced and utilized by the same cell or organ.

Autoimmune disease: A disease that results when the immune system mistakenly attacks the body's own tissues. Rheumatoid arthritis and systemic lupus erythematosus are autoimmune diseases.

Autologous: Referring to a graft in which the donor and recipient areas are in the same individual.

B cell growth factor (BCGF): A factor that is involved in B cell proliferation.

B cell differentiation factor (BCDF): A factor that is involved in the induction of antibody secretion by B cells.

B cells: Small white blood cells crucial to the immune defenses. Also known as B lymphocytes, they are derived from bone marrow and develop into plasma cells that are the source of antibodies.

Bacterium: A microscopic organism composed of a single cell; many, but not all, bacteria cause disease.

Basophil: A white blood cell that contributes to inflammatory reactions. Along with mast cells, basophils are responsible for the symptoms of allergy. They contain numerous lysosomes and granules (secretory vesicles), which release histamine and serotonin in certain immune reactions.

Biological response modifiers: Substances, either natural or synthesized, that boost, direct, or restore normal immune defenses. BRMs include interferons, interleukins, thymus hormones, and monoclonal antibodies.

Biotechnology: The use of living organisms or their products to make or modify a substance; biotechnology includes recombinant DNA techniques (genetic engineering) and hybridoma technology.

Bone marrow: Soft tissue located in the cavities of the bones; consists, in varying proportions, of fat cells and maturing blood cells. The bone marrow is the source of all blood cells.

C1-C9 complement: The components of the complement classical and lytic pathways, which are responsible for mediating inflammatory reactions, opsonization of particles, and lysis of cell membranes.

CD markers: Cell surface molecules of lymphocytes, including

- **CD1:** A cortical thymocyte differentiation marker
- **CD2:** A receptor involved in antigen; nonspecific T cell activation (E receptor)
- **CD3:** A constant portion of the T cell antigen receptor
- **CD4:** A marker of T helper cells involved in MHC class II recognition

- **CD5:** A T cell marker also present on a sub-population of B cells
- **CD8:** A marker of T cytotoxic cells involved in MHC class I recognition
- **CD25:** The IL-2 receptor present on activated T cells and on some activated B cells

Cellular immunity: Immune protection provided by the direct action of immune cells (as distinct from soluble molecules such as antibodies).

Chemotaxis: Increased directional migration of cells, particularly in response to concentration gradients of certain chemotactic factors.

Chimera: An organism whose body contains different cell populations of the same or different species.

Chromosomes: Physical structures in the cell's nucleus that house the genes; each human cell has 23 pairs of chromosomes.

Class I, II, and III molecules: Three major classes of molecules coded within the MHC:

- **Class I molecules:** Expressed on virtually all cell types, consisting of a heavy alpha chain associated with a light beta chain (ß2 microglobulin) not encoded by the MHC
- **Class II molecules:** Tend to be expressed on B cells, macrophages, and activated T cells; consisting of two noncovalently linked alpha and beta chains, which are thought also to interact to form a common binding site
- **Class III molecules:** Predominantly plasma proteins that act as complement proteins; thought to involve the induction of the immune response

Class I/II restriction: The observation that immunologically active cells will cooperate effectively only when they share MHC haplotypes at either the class I or class II loci.

Clone: A group of genetically identical cells or organisms descended from a single common ancestor, OR, to reproduce multiple identical copies.

Co-stimulation: The delivery of a second signal from an antigen-presenting cell to a T cell. The second signal rescues the activated T cell from anergy, allowing it to produce the lymphokines necessary for the growth of additional T cells.

Complement cascade: A precise sequence of events usually triggered by an antigen-antibody complex, in which each component of the complement system is activated in turn.

Complement system: See C1-C9.

Complement: A complex series of blood proteins whose action "complements" the work of antibodies. Complement destroys bacteria, produces inflammation, and regulates immune reactions.

Constant region: That part of an antibody's structure that is characteristic for each antibody class.

Cyclosporine (cyclosporin A): A drug derived from fungal extracts; used to suppress immune reactions and to prevent rejection of transplanted organs and tissues.

Cytokines: Powerful chemical substances secreted by cells. Cytokines include lymphokines produced by lymphocytes and monokines produced by monocytes and macrophages.

Cytotoxic T cells: A subset of T lymphocytes that carry the T8 marker and can kill body cells infected by viruses or transformed by cancer.

Cytotoxic: Having the ability to kill cells.

Degranulation: Exocytosis of granules from cells such as mast cells and basophils.

Dendritic cells: White blood cells found in the spleen and other lymphoid organs. Dendritic cells typically use thread-like tentacles to enmesh antigen, which they present to T cells.

DNA (deoxyribonucleic acid): A nucleic acid that is found in the cell nucleus and is the carrier of genetic information.

ECF (eosinophil chemotactic factor): A factor produced at sites of inflammation by T cells that attracts eosinophil; other ECFs are produced by triggered mast cells.

Edema: Swelling of tissue due to injury or disease.

Effector cells: Generally denotes T cells that are capable of suppressing cytotoxicity (helper T cell function).

Endotoxin: Lipopolysaccharide component of the cell wall of several species of gram-negative bacteria; a potent immunostimulant.

Enzyme: A protein, produced by living cells, that promotes the chemical processes of life without itself being altered.

Eosinophil: A white blood cell that contains granules filled with chemicals damaging to parasites and enzymes that damp down inflammatory reactions.

Epitope: A unique shape or marker carried on an antigen's surface, which triggers a corresponding antibody response.

Extrinsic asthma: Asthma caused by external sources, e.g., allergens.

Fc receptor: A protein on the surface of a cell that recognizes and binds Fc portions of antibody molecules.

Fc: The portion of an antibody that is bound by specific receptors on cells and the C1a component of complement.

Fungus: Member of a class of relatively primitive vegetable organisms. Fungi include mushrooms, yeasts, rusts, molds, and smuts.

Gene: A unit of genetic material (DNA) that occupies a definite locus on a chromosome and contains the plan a cell uses to perform a specific function (e.g., making a given protein).

Genetic association: A term used to describe the condition in which particular genotypes are associated with other phenomena such as particular diseases.

Glycoproteins: Proteins combined with a carbohydrate; frequently on cell surfaces.

Graft-versus-host disease (GVHD): A life-threatening reaction in which transplanted immunocompetent cells attack the tissues of the recipient. A condition caused by allogeneic donor lymphocytes reacting against host tissue in an immunologically compromised recipient.

Granulocytes: Phagocytic white blood cells filled with granules containing potent chemicals that allow the cells to digest microorganisms; neutrophils, eosinophils, basophils, and mast cells are examples of granulocytes.

H-2: The mouse major histocompatibility complex.

Haplotype: A set of genetic determinants located on a single chromosome.

Helper T cells: A subset of T cells that typically carry the T4 marker and are essential for turning on antibody production, activating cytotoxic T cells, and initiating many other immune responses.

Helper factors: Molecules that can deliver T cell help to other lymphocytes; the term is usually reserved for antigen-specific interferons and interleukins.

Helper cells: A functional subclass of T cells that can help to generate cytotoxic T cells and cooperate with B cells in the production of an antibody response; helper cells usually recognize antigen in association with class II MHC molecules.

Hematopoiesis: The formation and development of blood cells, usually taking place in the bone marrow.

Heterologous: Refers to interspecies antigenic differences.

Histamine: A major vasoactive amine released from mast cell and basophil granules.

Histocompatibility: The ability to accept grafts between individuals.

Histocompatibility testing: A method of matching the self-antigens (HLA) on the tissues of a transplant donor with those of the recipient; the closer the match, the better the chance that the transplant will take.

HIV (human immunodeficiency virus): The virus that causes AIDS.

HLA (human leukocyte antigen): The major histocompatibility genetic region in humans; protein markers of self.

Homologous: Of the same species.

Human leukocyte antigens (HLA): protein in markers of self used in histocompatibility testing. Some HLA types also correlate with certain autoimmune diseases.

Humoral immunity: Immune protection provided by soluble factors such as antibodies, which circulate in the body's fluids or "humors," primarily serum and lymph.

Humoral: Pertaining to the extracellular fluids, including the plasma and lymph.

Hybridoma: A hybrid cell created in vitro by fusing a B lymphocyte with a long-lived neoplastic plasma cell, or a T lymphocyte with a lymphoma cell. A B-cell hybridoma secretes a single specific antibody.

Hypogammaglobulinemia: Abnormally low levels of immunoglobulins.

Idiotypes: The unique and characteristic parts of an antibody's variable region, which can themselves serve as antigens.

IFN: See interferon.

Immune complex: A cluster of interlocking antigens and antibodies.

Immune response: The reaction of the immune system to foreign substances.

Immunoassay: A test using antibodies to identify and quantify substances. Often the antibody is linked to a marker such as a fluorescent molecule, a radioactive molecule, or an enzyme.

Immunocompetent: Capable of developing an immune response.

Immunoglobulins: A family of large protein molecules, also known as antibodies (e.g., IgA or IgG).

Immunosuppression: Reduction of the immune responses, for instance, by giving drugs to prevent transplant rejection.

Immunotoxin: A monoclonal antibody linked to a toxic drug or a radioactive substance.

In vivo: Referring to studies performed on tissues not removed from the living organism, or in the organism itself.

In vitro: Referring to studies performed on tissues removed from the living organism under artificial conditions in the laboratory.

Inflammatory response: Redness, warmth, swelling, pain, and loss of function produced in response to infection, as the result of increased blood flow and an influx of immune cells and secretions.

Intercellular: Between cells.

Interferon (IFN): A group of mediators that increase the resistance of cells to viral infection, by altering the activities of the cells' metabolic machinery; also has numerous other effects in modulating immune responses; group includes.

- **IFN-α:** Produced by leukocytes
- **IFN-γ:** Produced by T cells
- **IFN-ß:** Produced by fibroblasts

Interleukins (IL): A group of molecules involved in signaling between cells of the immune system

- **IL-1:** Released by numerous cells in the body, including macrophages; it has a wide variety of effects, including activation of T cells to express IL-2 receptors

- **IL-2:** Released by activated T cells and is required for T cell proliferation
- **IL-3:** Released by activated T cells and acts as a panspecific hemopoietin
- **IL-4:** Provisionally allocated to the B cell growth factor (BCGF) 1

Intracellular: Within a cell

Intrinsic asthma: Asthma without external cause.

Lymphokines tolerance: A state of specific immunological unresponsiveness.

Lymphokines: Powerful chemical substances secreted by lymphocytes. These soluble molecules help direct and regulate the immune responses.

Kupffer cells: Specialized macrophages in the liver.

LAK cells: Lymphocytes transformed in the laboratory into lymphokine-activated killer cells, which attack tumor cells.

Langerhans cells: Dendritic cells in the skin that pick up antigen and transport it to lymph nodes.

Leukocytes: All white blood cells; see lymphocytes.

Leukotrienes: Signaling compound chemically related to prostaglandins.

Line: A collection of cells produced by continuously growing a particular cell culture in vitro; such cell lines will usually contain a number of individual clones.

Lymph nodes: Small bean-shaped organs of the immune system, distributed widely throughout the body and linked by lymphatic vessels; lymph nodes are garrisons of B, T, and other immune cells.

Lymph: A transparent, slightly yellow fluid that carries lymphocytes, bathes the body tissues, and drains into the lymphatic vessels.

Lymphatic vessels: A body-wide network of channels, similar to the blood vessels, which transport lymph to the immune organs and into the bloodstream.

Lymphocytes: Small white blood cells produced in the lymphoid organs and paramount in the immune defenses.

Lymphoid organs: The organs of the immune system, where lymphocytes develop and congregate. They include the bone marrow, thymus, lymph nodes, spleen, and various other clusters of lymphoid tissue. The blood vessels and lymphatic vessels can also be considered lymphoid organs.

Macrophage: A large and versatile immune cell that acts as a microbe-devouring phagocyte, an antigen-presenting cell, and an important source of regulatory proteins—immune secretions.

Major histocompatibility complex (MHC): A group of genes that controls several aspects of the immune response. MHC genes code for self markers on all body cells.

Mast cell: A granule-containing cell found in tissue. The contents of mast cells, along with those of basophils, are responsible for the symptoms of allergy.

MHC restriction: A characteristic of many immune reactions, in which cells cooperate most effectively with other cells sharing an MHC haplotype.

MHC (major histocompatibility complex): A genetic region, found in all mammals, whose products are primarily responsible for the rapid rejection of grafts between individuals and which functions in signaling between lymphocytes and cells expressing antigen.

Microbes: Minute living organisms, including bacteria, viruses, fungi, and protozoa.

Microorganisms: Microscopic plants or animals.

Molecule: The smallest amount of a specific chemical substance that can exist alone. (To break a molecule down into its constituent atoms is to change its character. A molecule of water, for instance, reverts to oxygen and hydrogen.)

Monoclonal: Derived from a single clone, e.g., monoclonal antibodies that are produced by a single clone and are homogeneous.

Monoclonal antibodies: Antibodies produced by a single cell or its identical progeny, specific for a given antigen. As a tool for binding to specific protein molecules, monoclonal antibodies are invaluable in research, medicine, and industry.

Monocyte: A large phagocytic white blood cell which, when it enters tissue, develops into a macrophage.

Monokines: Powerful chemical substances secreted by monocytes and macrophages. These soluble molecules help direct and regulate the immune responses.

Murine: Pertaining to the genus that includes mice and rats.

NADPH: The reduced form of NADP (nicotinamide-adenine dinucleotide phosphate).

Natural killer (NK) cells: Large granule-filled lymphocytes that take on tumor cells and infected body cells. They are known as "natural" killers because they attack without first having to recognize specific antigens.

Neoplasm: A new and abnormal growth; used as a synonym for cancerous tissue.

Neutrophil: A large white blood cell that an abundant and important phagocyte.

Nucleic acids: Large, naturally occurring molecules composed of chemical building blocks known as nucleotides. There are two kinds of nucleic acids, DNA and RNA.

OKT3: A monoclonal antibody that targets mature T cells.

Opportunistic infection: An infection in an immunosuppressed person caused by an organism that does not usually trouble people with healthy immune systems.

Opsonize: To coat an organism with antibodies or a complement protein so as to make it palatable to phagocytes.

Organism: An individual living thing.

Paracrine: Produced by one cell/organ and acting on another.

Parasite: A plant or animal that lives, grows, and feeds on or within another living organism.

Passive immunity: Immunity resulting from the transfer of antibodies or antiserum produced by another individual.

Pathogen: An organism that causes disease, e.g., streptococcus, HIV.

Peptide: A compound of two or more amino acids in which the alpha carboxyl group of one is united with the alpha amino group of another, forming a peptide bond.

Peyer's patches: A collection of lymphoid tissues in the intestinal tract.

Phagocytes: Large white blood cells that contribute to immune defenses by ingesting foreign material, e.g., macrophages, neutrophils.

Phagocytosis: The process by which cells engulf material and enclose it within a vacuole (phagosome) in the cytoplasm.

Plasma cells: Large antibody-producing cells that develop from B cells.

Platelets: Granule-containing cellular fragments critical for blood clotting and sealing off wounds. Platelets also contribute to the immune response.

Pleiotropic: Refers to the ability of a gene to manifest itself in many ways.

Pluripotent: Able to act or to develop in any one of several different ways.

Polyclonal activators: Agents that stimulate the activation/proliferation of many cell types; nonspecific activators.

Polymorph: Short for polymorphonuclear leukocyte or granulocyte.

Proliferate: To reproduce.

Prostaglandins: A family of fatty acid derivatives producing a variety of biological effects, including inflammatory responses.

Proteins: Organic compounds made up of amino acids; proteins are one of the major constituents of plant and animal cells.

Protozoa: A group of one-celled animals, a few of which cause human disease (including malaria and sleeping sickness).

Pyrogenic: Causing fever.

Receptor: A cell surface molecule that binds specifically to particular proteins or peptides in the fluid phase.

Rh antigen: Rhesus antigen; a red blood cell surface antigen.

Rheumatoid-factor: An autoantibody found in the serum of most persons with rheumatoid arthritis.

RNA (ribonucleic acid): A nucleic acid that is found in the cytoplasm and also in the nucleus of some cells. One function of RNA is to direct the synthesis of proteins.

Scavenger cells: Any of a diverse group of cells that have the capacity to engulf and destroy foreign material, dead tissues, or other cells.

SCID mouse: A laboratory animal that, lacking an enzyme necessary to fashion an immune system of its own, can be turned into a model of the human immune system when injected with human cells or tissues.

Second messengers: Intracellular signaling mediators that, when activated, in turn alter the behavior of other target proteins within a cell, ultimately resulting in a cellular response such as activation.

Serum: The clear liquid that separates from the blood when it is allowed to clot. This fluid retains any antibodies that were present in the whole blood.

Severe combined immunodeficiency disease (SCID): A life-threatening condition in which infants are born lacking all major immune defenses.

Site-associated idiotopes: Idiotopes present in the antibody-combining site; this is usually defined functionally by inhibiting antigen binding with anti-idiotype or vice versa.

SLE (systemic lupus erythematosus): An autoimmune disease of humans.

Spleen: A lymphoid organ in the abdominal cavity that is an important center for immune system activities.

Stem cells: Cells from which all blood cells derive. The bone marrow is rich in stem cells.

Subunit vaccine: A vaccine that uses merely one component of an infectious agent, rather than the whole, to stimulate an immune response.

Superantigens: A class of antigens, including certain bacterial toxins, that unleash a massive and damaging immune response.

Suppressor T cells: A subset of T cells that turn off antibody production and other immune responses.

T lymphocytes (T cells): Lymphocytes that are processed in the thymus (thus T cell); they directly participate in immune responses and produce lymphokines.

Thymic epithelial cells: Thymic antigen presenting cells, expressing high levels of class II MHC antigens, thought to be important in the development of T cell immune recognition.

Thymus: A primary lymphoid organ, high in the chest, where T cells proliferate and mature.

TILs: Tumor-infiltrating lymphocytes. These Immune cells are extracted from the tumor tissue, treated in the laboratory, and reinjected into the cancer patient.

Tissue typing: See histocompatibility testing.

Tolerance: A state of nonresponsiveness to a particular antigen or group of antigens.

Tonsils and adenoids: Prominent oval masses of lymphoid tissues on either side of the throat.

Toxins: Agents produced by plants and bacteria, normally very damaging to mammalian cells, that can be delivered directly to target cells by linking them to monoclonal antibodies or lymphokines.

Transgenes: Genes from one organism that have been transferred to another organism; these genes are inserted into the host DNA.

Transgenic mice: Mice that have had specific genes, usually human, inserted into their genomes.

Triggering of mast cells: Stimulation of mast cell degranulation, effected by cross-linking of surface-bound IgE, direct triggering by C3a and C5a, or by drugs.

TSH: Thyroid-stimulating hormone.

Vaccine: A substance that contains antigenic components from an infectious organism; by stimulating an immune response (but not disease), it protects against subsequent infection by that organism.

Variable region: That part of an antibody's structure that differs from one antibody to another.

Virus: Submicroscopic microbe that consists of a protein coat and a nucleic acid core; viruses' inability to grow or reproduce outside of living cells makes them the cause of many infectious diseases.

Xenografts: Tissue grafts between species.

Index

Index

Index

M

594

600